THE ENCYCLOPEDIA OF DEPRESSION

Roberta Roesch
Introduction by
Ewald Horwath, M.D.

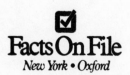

Facts On File
New York • Oxford

THE ENCYCLOPEDIA OF DEPRESSION

Facts On File, Inc.   Facts On File Limited
460 Park Avenue South   Collins Street
New York NY 10016   Oxford OX4 1XJ
USA   United Kingdom

Library of Congress Cataloging-in-Publication Data

Roesch, Roberta.
    The encyclopedia of depression/Roberta Roesch.
        p.   cm.
    Includes bibliographical references.
    Includes index.
    ISBN 0-8160-1936-3
    1. Depression, Mental—Encyclopedias.   2. Depression, Mental—
Information services—Directories.
        II. Title.
    [DNLM: 1. Depression—dictionaries.   WM 13 R718e]
    RC537.R63   1990
    616.85′27′003—dc20
    DNLM/DLC
    for Library of Congress   90-3576

A British CIP catalogue record for this book is available from the
British Library.

Facts On File books are available at special discounts when purchased in
bulk quantities for businesses, associations, institutions or sales
promotions. Please call our Special Sales Department in New York at
212/683-2244 (dial 800/322-8755 except in NY, AK or HI) or in Oxford at
865/728399.

Composition by TSI Graphics
Manufactured by R.R. Donnelley & Sons

Printed in the United States of America

10 9 8 7 6 5 4 3 2 1

This book is printed on acid-free paper.

CONTENTS

PREFACE

Today, at the end of the 20th century, the world is experiencing what many call the "New Age of Melancholy," as, according to the World Health Organization, at least 100 million people develop clinically recognizable depression each year.

In America depression is a major public health problem. Though statistics vary depending upon the source, the most recent available statistics from the National Institute of Mental Health (NIMH) are that 10 million Americans are affected by depression each year; 6.6% of all women suffer from depression during any six month's period; 3.5% of all men suffer from it during any six month's period; and 8.3% of all Americans suffer from an affective disorder at some point in their lives. Most people have friends, acquaintances or relatives who suffer—or have suffered—from some variant of it.

For some time it was thought that depression appeared more frequently in late-middle age and old age. But today's surveys indicate that a high proportion of younger persons are depressed. In fact, researchers believe that age 25 to age 65 may be the most susceptible age range. Researchers have also found that depression occurs during childhood and adolescence. Though the illness is less common among teenagers than adults, there is a definite and significant rise in its rates among adolescents, teenagers and young people. A smaller percentage of people over age 65 (as opposed to the younger age groups) is affected by it. But it is still both a common and serious affliction among the elderly.

Because depression is so widespread (and projected to increase in our changing social and physical environment) *The Encyclopedia of Depression* has been designed to give an overall view of both the disorder and the treatments and therapy that are available. Fortunately, as a result of ongoing research throughout the world, depression is being diagnosed much more effectively than in the past, and today there is more hope for depressives than at any other time of history—*if* people who suffer from depression seek available help.

As *The Encyclopedia of Depression* presents a broad view of all aspects of depression, it will cover bereavement, grief and mourning too, since the link between depression and grief has been solidly documented. To the best of the author's knowledge the coverage in this volume is the first A-to-Z encyclopedic reference to appear in the field of depression.

The Encyclopedia of Depression follows in format, approach and presentation of subject matter Facts On File's earlier reference books, including *The Encyclopedia of Alcoholism*, compiled by the late Robert O'Brien, Glen Evans and Dr. Morris Chafetz; *The Encyclopedia of Drug Abuse*, compiled by Mr. O'Brien and Dr. Sidney Cohen; and *The Encyclopedia of Suicide*, compiled by Glen Evans and Dr. Norman L. Farberow. Since the use of alcohol has been tied to depression in a variety of ways—and since drugs are prescribed and taken for the treatment of depression—entries for both are included in this volume. Suicide has several entries, too, because the alarming possibility that severely depressed persons will eventually attempt suicide is one of the greatest complications of depression. At the conclusion of the entries there are six appendixes of tabular material and key sources of information.

Since *The Encyclopedia of Depression* is intended for both the lay person and the professional, I have tried to keep the language concise and comprehensible without becoming simplistic. I hope that, as a result, this reference volume will have ongoing use for psychiatrists and the entire medical profession; psychologists and the full range of mental health and health care personnel; social scientists; religious leaders; educators; human service counselors; social workers and agencies; self-help and mutual-aid groups; the media; and the public at large.

Because of space limitations—and the immensity of the subject matter—I obviously have been unable to cover all of the information I would have liked to include. For this reason I have compiled an extensive bibliography for readers who need more data.

New information on depression becomes available on almost a daily basis, so, as the authors of the aforementioned encyclopedias have said before me, I consider *The Encyclopedia of Depression* also a "work in progress." Further editions will keep readers updated on the important and continuing issues that develop in the worldwide problem of depression and its treatment.

Roberta Roesch
Westwood, New Jersey

ACKNOWLEDGMENTS

Any project of this nature involves the work and contributions of many people and sources. Consequently, a listing of all the persons and organizations who contributed to this book, in either large or small ways, would require much more space than is allotted here. However, I am grateful to each and every source that shared information and provided help.

I am especially grateful for the research and writings of—or personal assistance from—Dr. Janice A. Egeland, Dr. Gerald L. Klerman, Dr. Ari Kiev, Dr. Helen DeRosis, Dr. Nancy D. Andreasen, Dr. Haroon Ahmed, Dr. N. Sartorius, Dr. Aaron T. Beck, Dr. Carl C. Bell, Dr. Irving Berlin, Dr. David D. Burns, Dr. Joseph R. Calabrese, Dr. Mark Zimmerman, Dr. Mardi Horowitz, Dr. Ira Lipton, Dr. Martin E.P. Seligman, Dr. Myrna Weissman, Dr. Mark S. Gold, Dr. Dolores Gallagher Thompson, Dr. Thomas Hutton, Dr. Richard Mayeux, Dr. Kay R. Jamieson, Dr. Ian H. Gotlib, Dr. D.F. Klein, Dr. David D. Ostrow, Dr. Robert Post, Dr. George Winokur, Dr. Sidney Zisook, Dr. Robert L. Spitzer, Dr. William Potter and Dr. Matthew Rudorfer.

The staffs of the following agencies and organizations provided much valuable research: National Institute of Mental Health (with special thanks to Joyce Lazar, director of the D/ART Program, Joan G. Abell of the Office of Scientific Information, and Dr. Ronald W. Manderscheid of the Division of Biometry and Applied Science); U.S. Department of Health and Human Services; U.S. Department of Health, Education and Welfare; U.S. Food and Drug Administration; U.S. Division of Vital Statistics; U.S. Centers for Disease Control; and the World Health Organization.

Mention should be made, too, of the valuable assistance received from Alzheimer's Disease and Related Disorders; American Association of Suicidology; American Medical Association; American Psychiatric Association; Barr-Harris Center for the Study of Separation and Loss During Childhood; Bereavement and Loss Center of New York; Center for Cognitive Therapy; Fair Oaks Hospital; Foundation for Depression and Manic Depression; Health Insurance Association of America; Institute for Scientific Information; Lithium Information Center; and National Depressive and Manic Depressive Association.

Other sources of information include the University of Pittsburgh's Western Psychiatric Institute and Clinic; Nathan S. Kline Institute for Psychiatric Research; National Alliance for Research on Schizophrenia and Depression; National Foundation for Depressive Illness; Social Psychiatry Research Institute; Texas Tech University Health Sciences Center; Wellness Associates; National Council of Community Health Centers; New Jersey Self-Help Clearing House; National Self-Help Clearing House; Depressives Anonymous; Bristol-Myers Company; Alcoholics Anonymous; Center of Alcohol Studies at Rutgers, the State University of New Jersey; Dr. Edward Bach Healing Society; Princeton Religion Research Center; British Information Service; Canadian Mental Health Association; Mental Health Commission of New Brunswick, Canada; Department of Health and Community Services, New Brunswick, Canada; and the embassies and agencies of foreign countries who responded to our requests for information.

Finally, I wish to express my appreciation to Charles F. Siegar and the reference staff of Messler Library, Fairleigh Dickinson University, and to thank personally Kate Kelly, my editor who had the idea for this project and who gave it constant support, and Nick Bakalar, my editor who saw it through to completion. In addition, I thank—as always—my husband Phil and our children, Bonnie, Meredith and Jeff for their neverending support and help.

—Roberta Roesch

INTRODUCTION

Depression as a feeling or mood has been described in both literary and medical texts throughout human history. However, the clinical syndrome of depression as a disease process distinct from normal, transient feelings of sadness or grief has been delineated carefully only relatively recently.

The focus on depression as a specific psychiatric disorder has contributed to the rapid expansion of knowledge about the nosology, epidemiology, neurobiology, genetics and treatment of affective disorders.

Diagnostic research has led to the development of several widely recognized systems of classification that define subtypes of mood disorder. The most successful and well known of these documents is the American Psychiatric Association's *Diagnostic and Statistical Manual of Mental Disorders*, Third Edition, Revised (DSM-III-R). DSM-III-R provides specific criteria for several categories of mood disorder, including bipolar disorder, major depression, dysthymic disorder and seasonal affective disorder. The widespread use of the diagnostic criteria has led to better agreement between clinicians and researchers, and has helped foster research on mood disorders.

Epidemiologic research has shown that depression is more common, begins at a younger age and causes more severe and prolonged disability than previously thought. Genetic epidemiology has demonstrated that subtypes of depression are distinct disorders with unique patterns of familial distribution.

Neurobiologic research has led to the discovery of neurotransmitters, or specific chemical substances, believed to be involved in the cause of certain types of depression. Some theories of the etiology of depression have emphasized abnormalities in neurotransmitter systems.

Research in molecular genetics has sought to identify specific genetic loci that may be responsible for transmitting a vulnerability to depression from one generation to the next.

Perhaps the most significant progress has been made in the treatment of depression. A variety of highly effective pharmacologic treatments now exist for depression and bipolar disorder. Cognitive therapy and interpersonal psychotherapy have been shown to improve the symptoms of depression and decrease the resulting social disability, respectively.

Active investigations continue, providing new findings and a sometimes bewildering array of new information in the field of depression research. As in all areas of research and clinical practice, the findings and observations are sometimes contradictory. This volume attempts to organize the knowledge about depression into a systematic compendium, which is approachable by those without training in the field of mental health. In so doing, the text attempts to preserve some of the complexity of the subject without overwhelming the lay reader with a multitude of conflicting research data. Hopefully, the resulting product is a useful guide to those who are interested in learning more about depression.

—Ewald Horwath, M.D.

A

absorption The process and rate by which a chemical compound such as a drug or nutrient passes through the body membranes into the blood stream. In drug absorption, the process is dependent on how the drug is administered: inhalation; oral or rectal administration; or intravenous, intramuscular or subcutaneous injections. Absorption is also influenced by the nature of the drug, the age of the person taking it, disease and environmental factors.

abuse potential of drugs The Food and Drug Administration defines "drug use" as the taking of a drug for its intended purpose, in the appropriate amount, frequency, strength and manner; "drug misuse" as taking a substance for the intended purpose, but not in the appropriate amount, frequency, strength and manner; and "drug abuse" as deliberately taking a substance for other than its intended purpose, and in a manner that can result in damage to the person's health or his ability to function.

Drug abuse is often an indication of underlying feelings of depression, helplessness and anxiety. But abusing drugs can also mean using them without appropriate and adequate supervision, in an illegal way that alters consciousness, gratifies physical needs and leads to losing control of behavior.

Acquired Immune Deficiency Syndrome (AIDS) No other medical event in recent history has produced as great a degree of public and personal fear as the epidemic of AIDS (a disease that attacks the body's immune system so that the immune system fails to function as a protection from other diseases). There is no known cure for AIDS and it is virtually always fatal.

Because of the hopelessness of those affected by AIDS Dr. David G. Ostrow (Department of Psychiatry, University of Michi-

gan School of Medicine, and Ann Arbor Veterans Administration Medical Center) has observed a continuum of AIDS-related psychiatric problems that include acute depression, anergic depression, chronic severe depression, chronic dysphoria, phobias, generalized anxiety disorders, full-blown immobilization and suicide.

AIDS patients often have symptoms consistent with those of depression. Among other things they experience anger, fear, difficulty in performing mental and physical tasks, loss of interest in previously pleasurable activities, sleep disturbances, lethargy and memory problems. These problems as well as spatial integration difficulties may respond to antidepressant or psychostimulant agents. But drug treatment has to be administered with care because of the possibility of anticholinergic side effects. Much attention must be paid to drug interactions.

"The experimental work on which many of these observations is based is an ongoing study of approximately 1,000 gay and bisexual men at high risk of AIDS," explained Ostrow. "These men comprise the Chicago cohort of a Multicenter AIDS Cohort Study (MACS)."

In addition to the Chicago cohort, similar cohorts started simultaneously in the Baltimore-Washington, D.C. area, Pittsburgh and Los Angeles. In Chicago 95% of the MACS cohort has also participated in a study of the psychosocial consequences of being at high risk for AIDS funded by the National Institute of Mental Health (NIMH).

"In our Chicago cohort we have seen a recent increase in fearful and angry responses to the question 'Is there anything else about AIDS and how it has affected you that you would like to tell us?' " Ostrow and his colleages have written. "These expressions of fear and anger at the reaction of general society to AIDS have shown a dramatic increase in parallel with increased media coverage of AIDS quarantine and mass HIV [human immunodeficiency virus] screening proposals.

"There is a growing recognition that HIV

can directly infect the central nervous system, producing a variety of serious neurological and psychiatric complications. Our subjects fear discrimination based on testing and are angry at the misuse of the test to deny them insurance, employment and other rights. No wonder that individuals can develop major depression as a result of the stress involved with the disease and programs to test them for exposure to the virus believed necessary to produce AIDS."

This observation leads Ostrow and other researchers to the conclusion that "fear of quarantine" is indeed a very real part of the psychiatric picture of AIDS in the United States. Whether or not such measures as quarantine are ultimately undertaken, the increasing discussion of quarantine proposals indicates the potential for negative social change and totalitarian responses to AIDS in our society.

"In addition to the fear of developing AIDS and a feeling of inefficacy in those behavioral changes already taken, persons in AIDS risk groups may have a number of other sources of chronic stress," Ostrow pointed out. "These include the social isolation and stigmatization that being in an AIDS risk group or having prodromal symptoms produces; the sense of helplessness one has in dealing with the disease for which there are at present no available interventions to prevent its development once infected; the significant loss of friends, lovers and others to the disease; the giving up of sexual or drug-use behaviors and the loss of pleasure and anxiety reduction that these behavioral changes may entail; the related loss of intimacy when major forms of close social interaction are deemed 'unsafe,' and the significant fear of quarantine and expectations of a 'holocaust scenario' reported by many of our subjects. Given the number and magnitude of sources of chronic stress that are present in persons at high risk of AIDS it is not surprising that we see an enormous range of psychiatric morbidity in our study population."

Because of the forgoing and similar studies there is every reason to believe that depression and psychiatric complications are common among those infected with AIDS and that individuals who experience AIDS-related symptoms will suffer the same kinds of extreme emotional distress that are known to characterize people who have been diagnosed with cancer or other life-threatening illnesses.

Ostrow, David G., "Models for Understanding the Psychiatric Consequences of AIDS" from *Psychological, Neuropsychiatric, and Substance Abuse Aspects of AIDS* (New York: Raven Press, 1988).

Ostrow, David G. et al., "Assessment and Management of the AIDS Patient with Neuropsychiatric Disturbances," *The Journal of Clinical Psychiatry*, 49 (May 1988).

active death wish A state of mind in which depressed persons actually consider suicide, investigate methods and make plans to follow through. With their "life isn't worth living" attitude they may actively think they'd be better off dead. Some psychiatrists believe that some depressed people (especially those who harbor suicide as an intellectual idea) are sometimes helped in their efforts to tolerate their depression by knowing they could always commit suicide. However, the more specific the plans are, the more apt the person is to attempt suicide.

Family, friends or acquaintances who are aware of this state of mind should seek professional help for the potential suicide. (See also SUICIDE PREVENTION CENTERS; SUICIDE WARNING SIGNS.)

acupuncture Because Chinese medicine incorporates both a physical and psychological function into an organic whole, authorities on acupuncture and Chinese medicine believe it is possible through study, perception and recognition for people to utilize this healing system to bring the body's energies into harmony. Thus its advocates see acupuncture as a healing system of traditional Chinese medicine that works by balancing the chi energies in the body through the use of discrete points on the body's surface. These points may be influenced by needles (acupuncture) or pressure (acupressure). Within the traditional system, these points are found on a network of chi energy channels called meridians. Each meridian corresponds to a major body organ as well as to its functions.

acute depression Depression is referred to by various terms and has several different subtypes that overlap and are not mutually exclusive. Consequently, the term of reference used to refer to or describe a type or subtype can depend on whether a person is talking to a clinician, researcher or other mental health specialist. Acute depression is a term that overlaps with CLINICAL, ENDOGENOUS or UNIPOLAR DEPRESSION. Acute itself is a term used to describe a condition that quickly develops into a crisis. Thus, acute depression seems to come about suddenly and rapidly as opposed to a depression that progresses slowly and continues for a long time.

Although the symptoms for some clinical depressions are long-lasting enough and sufficiently severe to require treatment, acute depression can be as brief as two weeks or last as long as a year, or longer. When it is of short duration, it can clear up spontaneously without treatment. The symptoms develop over a period of four weeks or less. Generally they include such things as pessimism, loss of interest, loss of pleasure, helplessness, hopelessness, self-condemnation and tearfulness. The physical symptoms can include change in appetite, sleep disturbance, agitation, retardation of movement and bodily complaints. (See also COMMON SIGNS AND SYMPTOMS.)

acute onset See ACUTE DEPRESSION.

additive effect A term used when two drugs are taken together and the result is equal to the sum of the two separate effects.

Adler, Alfred An Austrian psychiatrist (1870–1937) who founded the school of individual psychology and introduced the term "inferiority complex" into psychology. He defined the term as a complex of ideas centered on real or imaginary handicaps and colored by feelings of discouragement.

Early in his career Adler was an associate of Sigmund Freud until he rejected Freud's emphasis on sex and went on to maintain, instead, that all personality difficulties have their roots in a feeling of inferiority resulting from physical handicaps or from conflict with the environment. He contended these feelings of inferiority restrict a person's conscious desire for power and self-assertion. Thus, Adler saw these individuals' behavior disorders as overcompensation for deficiencies.

When people fail to compensate successfully, Adler believed, these individuals are likely candidates to develop a neurosis, withdraw from reality and limit their social participation. He also felt people's thinking patterns influence their moods. Consequently, he believed depressives tend to feel they are inadequate and willingly lean on others for support. (See also FREUDIAN THEORY OF DEPRESSION.)

adolescent depression See YOUNG PEOPLE'S DEPRESSION.

adverse drug reaction See DRUG THERAPY, SIDE EFFECTS.

aerobic regimen A form of treatment for depressive disorders originated by Dr. Robert S. Brown, a clinical psychiatrist at the University of Virginia. While treating depressed persons, he observed that he seldom treated individuals who were physically fit. To determine whether or not physical fitness might have an effect on depression he monitored the effects of aerobic exercise on approximately 10,000 people for more than 10 years.

In one study in his research at the University of Virginia he established a data base of approximately 5,000 students in a mental health course to confirm earlier findings that regular exercise is associated with significantly improved general activation and the relief of depression. Negative effects such as anger, hostility, fatigue and inertia were significantly decreased, and physical fitness emerged as an ideal state that tends to prevent depression and anxiety.

In another study, Brown used exercise therapy as an adjunct to psychotherapy in his outpatient psychiatric practice. The primary exercise recommended was brisk walking. Patients were encouraged to walk until they could cover a mile in 15 minutes, gradually increasing their walking to three miles a day in 45 minutes. Exercise partners were assigned to patients who were socially isolated and needed reinforcement. Trained student volunteers, screened for emotional stability, formed a cadre of exercise partners.

Jogging may also be an effective form of treatment for depression. Brown reports that in one study depressed people who jogged became more energetic and less hostile and that jogging has both an antidepressant and antianxiety effect. In *The Physician and Sportsmedicine,* he wrote:

On the basis of a study of about 700 subjects, including a number of persons with recognized clinical depression, we recommend that any rational, safe and effective treatment regimen for depression should include a prescription for vigorous exercise to bring about and maintain optimal affective functions. We found that depressed patients of widely differing ages who exercised became less depressed and less anxious when physical fitness was achieved.

Unfortunately research—including our own—into the ways that physical exercise relieves depression has yielded no definitive scientific information . . . Experience has shown that this phenomenon exists, but the mechanisms of mind/body reciprocity remain mysterious. However, it is apparent that they are multifarious and enormously complicated.

The apparent antidepressant effect of exercise may depend to some degree on the intensity, duration, and frequency of the physical activity. Subjects who played softball, like those who took no exercise at all, had unchanged depression levels, and tennis players showed only slight—although significant—reductions. Those who jogged five days a week for ten weeks had the greatest reduction in depression. When depressed subjects could select their exercises, the most depressed chose the most vigorous.

Brown discovered that his psychiatric outpatients who exercised on a regular basis showed significant improvement in depression, and also that exercise programs based on patients' physical conditions and life circumstances are a safe and effective way to treat depression. On this basis, an aerobic regimen has become a regular part of Brown's treatment for depressed patients.

Brown, R.S., Ramirez, D.E. and Taub, J.M., "The Prescription of Exercise for Depression," *The Physician and Sportsmedicine* (New York: McGraw-Hill, 1978).

Brown, R.S., "Jogging: Its Uses and Abuses," *Virginia Medical,* July 1979.

affective illnesses A term used for mood disorders and major depressive or manic episodes.

age factors For some time it was thought that depression appeared more frequently in late middle age and old age, but current surveys indicate that a high proportion of younger persons (under age 40) are depressed and that depression appears to occur as much, or more so, in the 20 to 40 age range as in older persons. Since depression now affects far more people under the age of 45 and fewer over age 65, researchers believe that the 25 to 44 may be the most susceptible age range.

Research also shows that depression occurs during adolescence and childhood (see ADOLESCENT DEPRESSION, CHILDHOOD DEPRESSION, YOUNG PEOPLE'S DEPRESSION.) Up until recent decades, depression in children and infants was vastly under-identified. But child psychiatrists have now discovered that children are common victims of depression. For example in *Why Isn't Johnny Crying?''* the authors say that from three to more than six million American children suffer from depression—much of it unrecognized and untreated.

Although depression is less common among teenagers than adults, there is a definite and significant rise in the rate of depression among adolescents, teenagers and young people. Dr. Gerald Klerman, professor of psychiatry at Cornell Medical College and associate chairman for research, Department of Psychiatry, Cornell University Medical Center, notes that the change in age distribution, with the rise in the rate of depression among young people, had its start in the 1970s when psychiatric facilities reported that more patients were being diagnosed as depressed and that they were younger than the standard textbook description of depressed patients as middle-aged. (This trend very obviously contributes to the dramatic increase in suicide attempts and in death by suicide among adolescents and young adults.)

Up until age 65 twice as many women as men are treated for depressive disorders, with the exception of bipolar disorder (manic-depression, see MANIC-DEPRESSIVE), which occurs equally in both sexes. Although fewer people over the age of 65 are affected by depression, it is still common among the ELDERLY. For this age range depression can occur because of loneliness; poor health and physical deterioration; waning strength; death of friends and loved ones; and an awareness of their own mortality.

McKnew, Donald H. et al., *Why Isn't Johnny Crying?* (New York: W.W. Norton, 1983).

Age of Depression While we approach the end of the 20th century we're experiencing what some psychiatrists have called the "new age of melancholy," as people grope for solutions to depression, grief, anxiety, loneliness, alienation and drug and alcohol abuse. With its significant increase in prevalence, depression has become a major public health problem; most people have a friend, acquaintance or relative who has suffered or is suffering from some variant of it. Statistics inevitably vary. But, according to the most recent available statistics from the National Institute of Mental Health (NIMH), 10 million Americans are affected by depression each year; 6.6% of all women suffer from depression during any six-month period; 3.5% of all men suffer from it during any six-month period; and 8.3% of all Americans suffer from an affective disorder at some point in their lives.

The annual cost of depression to the nation is more than $16 billion, of which over $10 billion is due to time lost from work. Above and beyond that, the cost in human suffering is immeasurable. Unfortunately, current evidence suggests that many people suffer needlessly, since available treatments could help 80% to 90% of those afflicted by serious depression. However, only one in three people with a depressive disorder seeks mental health treatment. (See also NEW AGE OF MELANCHOLY.)

aging See ELDERLY.

AIDS See ACQUIRED IMMUNE DEFICIENCY SYNDROME (AIDS).

alcohol and drug abuse Customary thinking regarding the relationship between depression and alcohol and drug abuse has generally been that the depression and anxiety found in drug abusers are always a result of the drug use. Now, however, some researchers believe it is possible that over a million Americans abuse alcohol or drugs primarily because they suffer from serious underlying depression or anxiety.

While the former thinking can be right in many cases, Dr. Edward V. Nunes, of the New York State Psychiatric Institute and Columbia-Presbyterian Medical Center, has found that there appear to be some people in whom the drug abuse is the result, rather than the cause, of psychiatric problems. In fact, Dr. Nunes estimates that 10% to 20% of alcoholics may fit the pattern, and that could mean more than a million patients throughout the United States. How many cocaine abusers may be involved is unclear.

The purpose of the group's study has been: (1) to define that subgroup of drug and alcohol abusers who fit the above pattern; (2) to give such patients treatment that will help their psychiatric problems; and (3) to observe whether drug abuse is helped at the same time. Nunes believes that problems with depression and severe anxiety experienced by a limited subset of alcoholics and drug abusers lead them to alcohol or other drugs such as cocaine for relief.

The self-medication may help for a short time. But neither alcohol nor cocaine is effective against the underlying problems of depression or anxiety. Furthermore, use of these drugs may result in addiction. Similarly, a depressed subgroup may exist among heroin addicts.

The researchers have found that IMIPRA-MINE, a standard antidepressant drug (which is also used for anxiety and panic attacks), helps some alcoholics and cocaine users. Thus the group's goal was to determine whether the medication helped reduce the patients' addictions to drugs or alcohol. The medication was not expected to help patients in whom the drug or alcohol abuse was the primary problem. Rather, the treatment theory was that it should help the subgroup of would-be cocaine or alcohol self-medicators.

For their research the group worked with volunteer patients who suffered severe problems of depression or anxiety first, and turned to drug or alcohol abuse later in efforts to cope with their disabling symptoms. The volunteers had to be chosen with great care because imipramine can have serious side effects if used at the same time as either alcohol or cocaine. In the study each patient was given an exhaustive psychiatric evaluation to find those whose original problem was either depression or anxiety and who took to cocaine or alcohol to cope with the situation.

In initial studies Dr. Nunes found that the treatment helped many people, because in more than half of the alcoholics treated, depression or anxiety was greatly diminished and so was the alcohol intake. But he emphasized that imipramine was neither a cure nor an effective treatment by itself. All of the patients received intensive counseling on their drug abuse habits, and Dr. Nunes stressed that even patients who benefit from the antidepressant drug need to go through the standard psychotherapeutic rehabilitation program, to take professional counseling and to participate in self-help groups, since all of them must deal with psychological issues and lifestyle changes.

Dr. Sidney Zisook of the University of California and his colleagues have also found that alcohol-related problems and symptoms of depression frequently coexist in the same individual.

Data he has gathered indicate that family history is a potential aid in clarifying the nature of the relationship between affective disorder and alcoholism. In a study on the relationship between the clinical course and a family history of affective disorder among 377 carefully diagnosed male primary alcoholics admitted to the Alcohol Treatment Program at the San Diego Veterans Administration Medical Center, Dr. Zisook and Dr. Marc A. Schuckit, director of the Alcohol Research Center at the Veterans Administration Medical Center, gathered their data from interviews with patients at intake and 12 months after discharge. The 37 primary alcoholic men (10%) who had a first-degree family member with affective disorder were themselves more likely to have had secondary depressions and to have experienced more alcohol-related problems at one-year follow-up than the 90% of primary alcoholic men without such family histories.

Zisook, Sidney and Schuckit, Marc, "Male Primary Alcoholics With and Without Family Histories of Affective Disorder," *Journal of Studies on Alcohol*, 48:4(1987).

Alcohol, Drug Abuse and Mental Health Administration (ADAMHA)
An umbrella agency that, in addition to its own administrative staff, includes the National Institute of Mental Health, the National Institute on Drug Abuse and the National Institute on Alcohol and Alcohol Abuse. ADAMHA is part of the Public Health Service of the U.S. Department of Health and Human Services.

Alcoholics Anonymous (AA)   The link
between alcohol and depression has been so firmly established that the Center of Alcohol Studies at Rutgers University, an international resource for scientific and scholarly literature on all aspects of alcohol and its use and misuse, has an extensive bibliography of several hundred published items on alcoholism and depression.

Alcoholics Anonymous (AA), is made up of over 53,000 local groups in 114 countries. It does not keep a list of members or statistics, but groups report how many people belong to each one. From these reports, total AA membership is estimated at over 1,000,000, with an estimated membership of approximately 800,000 in the United States.

The purpose of this fellowship of men and women who share experience, strength and hope with each other is to offer help to anyone who has a drinking problem and wants to do something about it. Since all the members are alcoholics themselves, they have a special understanding of each other. They know what the illness is like—and they have learned how to recover from it in AA.

Since AA members need healthy minds and healthy emotions to control their drinking and become sober, they begin to straighten out their confused thinking and unhappy feelings by following AA's "Twelve Steps" to recovery. Their goal is total abstinence one day at a time as they attend meetings regularly and maintain close contact with a sponsor, an experienced AA member in whom they can confide on a continuing, individual basis.

AA's "Twelve Steps" and "Twelve Traditions" are the heart of its program of recovery. Both are a guide to better ways of working and living, based on the philosophy that the group must survive in order for the individual to survive.

AA was started in 1935 in Akron, Ohio by a New York stockbroker, Bill W., and an Ohio surgeon, Dr. Bob, who had both been "hopeless" drunks. Prior to that time both Bill and Dr. Bob had been in contact with the Oxford Group, a mostly nonalcoholic fellowship that emphasized universal spiritual values in daily life. Under this spiritual influence Bill W. had sobered and had then maintained his recovery by working with other alcoholics, though none of these had actually recovered. Dr. Bob's Oxford Group, however, had not helped him enough to achieve sobriety. When Dr. Bob and Bill W. finally met, the effect on the doctor was immediate. Responding to Bill's convincing ideas, Dr. Bob soon sobered, never to drink again, and both men immediately set to work with alcoholics at Akron's City Hospital where one patient quickly achieved complete sobriety. These three men actually made up the nucleus of the first AA group. A book, *Alcoholics*

Anonymous (or the "Big Book" as it is known by members), was originally published in 1939. The 575-page hard-cover book is the "book of experience" from which the fellowship derived its name.

The book contains an analysis of the principles that led to the sobriety of the earliest members, together with a representative cross section of members' personal stories. It has appeared in 13 other languages. New, expanded editions were published in 1955 and 1976.

The General Service Office of AA has surveyed AA membership in the United States and Canada on a triennial basis since 1968 to determine characteristics of the membership and trends in those characteristics that are of interest to the membership, the professional community and the public. These surveys and analyses are intended only to provide overall information on AA fellowship and have been confined to macroscopic observations and properties. The seventh in this series was conducted in 1986 and preliminary results were reported in 1987.

The survey showed that the 18-year period spanned by the surveys has seen the registered membership grow at an average rate of about 9% a year, although in the three years since the 1983 survey the rate has been about 7% per year. This period witnessed some significant changes in composition. The percentage of women was 22% at the beginning of the period, but it rose to 34% in 1986 with signs that the growth of this percentage has either stopped or slowed greatly. The percentage of young people (under 31 years of age) was 7% at the beginning of the period, rose to 20% in 1986 and likewise showed signs of stabilizing at or near this point.

On the other hand the incidence of past drug addiction among AA members, which rose from 18% in 1977 (the first year it was measured) to 38% in 1986, does not yet show signs of stabilizing, nor does the percentage of the membership for whom professional help (defined as counseling or rehab treat-ment) was important in bringing them to AA. The latter has grown from 19% in 1977 to 36% in 1986.

Approximate measurements of the likelihood that members will remain sober and active in AA while in various stages of recovery are possible from the survey data and appear to show a significant move in 1986, as opposed to previous surveys for which such data seemed to be stable. While the percentage of members active in the fellowship who are sober more than a year has been between 59% and 63% for the first six surveys, with no discernible trend, in 1986 this figure went to 67%, a departure beyond likely normal statistical fluctuation.

AA is not without its critics. As Glen Evans and Norman L. Farberow, Ph.D., point out in *The Encyclopedia of Suicide:*

Many professionals believe the group concentrates on the symptoms and not the causes of an individual's drinking problem. Others feel the members do not learn to cope with their disease or gain self-reliance since the program encourages dependency and discourages outside interests that might diminish the central place of AA in the life of members. Still others criticize the very name—Alcoholics *Anonymous*—claiming it diminishes individual identity. They maintain this is just another way AA perpetuates itself—i.e., by downplaying the individual's names (members use only first names) and identities and leaving them with only the label "alcoholic," AA increases their dependence upon the organization.

But still and all—and despite the critics—most authorities in the field of alcoholism recognize the success that AA has had.

To find out about AA look for a listing in your area telephone book. If you do not find one, you can write to General Service Office, Box 459, Grand Central Station, New York, NY 10163.

Evans, Glen and Farberow, Norman L., *The Encyclopedia of Suicide* (New York: Facts On File, 1988).

alcoholism There are a variety of definitions for this term. ALCOHOLICS ANONYMOUS (AA) defines it as an illness and believes alcoholics cannot control their drinking beause they are ill in their bodies and minds (or emotions). If they do not stop drinking, their alcoholism almost always gets worse. The American Medical Association (AMA)—which in 1956 passed a resolution officially recognizing alcoholism as a disease—defines it as an illness characterized by significant physiological, psychological or social dysfunction that is directly associated with persistent and excessive use of alcohol. This AMA landmark resolution, plus a similar one by the American Bar Association (ABA), has since led to alcoholism-related laws at the federal, state and even local government levels. It has also impacted considerably on program, financing and insurance coverage, as well as the legal status of alcoholics.

Mark Keller, noted authority at the Rutgers Center of Alcohol Studies, defined alcoholism in the *Quarterly Journal of Studies on Alcoholism* (March 1960) as a chronic disease manifested by repeated implicative drinking so as to cause injury to the drinker's health or to his social or economic functioning. Robert O'Brien, Glen Evans and Dr. Morris Chafetz, in *The Encyclopedia of Alcoholism,* describe it as a chronic disorder associated with excessive consumption of alcohol over a lengthy period.

The disease concept has been around for a long time. According to O'Brien, Evans and Chafetz, the earliest known use of the term "alcoholism" was by a Swedish scientist, Magnus Huss of Stockholm. Huss published a treatise, *Chronische Alcohols Krankheit* (*Chronic Alcohol Disease*, Sweden, 1849; Germany, 1852), in which he identified a condition involving abuse of alcohol and labeled it "Alcoholismus Chronicus." References to it as a disease have also been found in the works of the Roman philosopher Seneca, the English medieval poet Geoffrey Chaucer and the 18th-century American Benjamin Rush.

Today most authorities—including the British Medical Association—recognize alcoholism as a disease. But its status as an illness is still disputed by some who believe that a condition that is self-inflicted cannot properly be termed a disease.

O'Brien wrote that certain religious groups, particularly fundamentalist Protestants, continue to oppose the disease concept. They view alcoholism as simple drunkenness and therefore a "sin." Some social scientists view alcoholism as a social dysfunction. They suggest that terming it a disease does no more than give it a medical-psychiatric label and that the medical approach is constricted and ineffective.

There are other arguments against the disease concept. One is that alcoholism is associated with no structural abnormality; therefore it cannot be a disease. Another is that irresponsible individuals will abuse both legal and medical benefits if they are labeled "sick," and that the disease concept excuses and dignifies drunkenness.

We have learned a great deal about how to identify and arrest alcoholism. But so far no one has discovered a way to prevent it, because nobody knows exactly why some drinkers turn into alcoholics. Doctors and scientists in the field have not agreed on the cause (or causes) of alcoholism. (See also ALCOHOL AND DRUG ABUSE.)

O'Brien, Robert, Evans, Glen and Chafetz, Morris, *The Encyclopedia of Alcoholism* (New York: Facts On File, 1988).

Evans, Glen and Farberow, Norman L., *The Encyclopedia of Suicide* (New York: Facts On File, 1988).

U.S. Department of Health and Human Services, *Sixth Special Report to the U.S. Congress on Alcohol and Health,* DHHS

Publication No. (ADM) 87-1519 (Washington, D.C.: Government Printing Office, 1987).

American Psychiatric Association, *Diagnostic and Statistical Manual of Mental Disorders,* (DSM-III-R), 3rd ed., rev. (Washington, D.C.: American Psychiatric Association, 1987).

alienation   Once a generic term for various forms of insanity or mental derangement. Later, mental alienation came to be a term largely restricted to forensic psychiatry, a usage with roots in the *alienatio mentis* of ancient Roman law. More recently, used to refer to a withdrawal or separation of a person or his affections from an object or position of former attachment or from the values of one's society and family. The person feels powerless, depersonalized, isolated and meaningless. Dr. Nathan S. Kline suggested in *From Sad to Glad* that: (1) the mental and emotional attitude of alienation may set in motion a chain of neurological consequences; and (2) habitual boredom may descend into a profound depression if postures of passive withdrawal are carried too far.

Kline, Nathan S., *From Sad To Glad* (New York: Putnam, 1974).

alprazolam (Xanax)   A member of the drug group known as the BENZODIAZEPINES; it has had positive results in treating patients suffering from anxiety and panic disorders, and in some cases of depression, particularly in mixed states of anxiety and depression. The drug causes sedation and lethargy—results that, in effect, are just the opposite of what would be needed in treating depression. Scientists hope that by learning why it is effective they can discover more about the basic nature of depression. The chemical reasons for its antidepressant effects are still unknown, but studies have shown that it has no effect on the nerve cell receptors that are the targets of some antidepressive drugs and that it does not hamper the RE-UPTAKE PROCESS.

Alzheimer's disease (AD)   Depression often accompanies Alzheimer's disease, especially in the earlier stages, when mood swings, anxiety, confusion, helplessness and the gradual loss of independence may cause patients to grow depressed or withdrawn as they become aware of their deficits.

Through the years the depression that is associated with Alzheimer's disease has traditionally been viewed as either a psychological reaction to the dementia or a coincidental phenomenon. However, research studies in the late 1980s suggest that neuroanatomic and neurochemical interrelationships may exist between Alzheimer's disease and depression. In "Depression in Alzheimer's Disease: An Overview of Adrenergic and Cholinergic Mechanisms," Dr. Edward H. Liston et al. (Department of Psychiatry and Biobehavioral Sciences at the UCLA School of Medicine) explain: "The loss of ascending noradrenergic and cholinergic cortical projections due to neuronal degeneration in the nucleus locus coeruleus and the nucleus basalis of Meynert may have implications for the development of depressive disorder in the primary degenerative dementia."

By definition, Alzheimer's disease is a progressive, neurologic, degenerative disorder that attacks the brain and results in impaired memory, thinking and behavior. Its history goes back to 1907 when Alois Alzheimer described the clinical and neuropathologic findings in a 51-year-old woman whose dementia had progressed over five years to a severe state. When Alzheimer examined her brain he found generalized atrophy and numerous microscopic neuritic plaques and neurofibrillary tangles. Subsequently EMIL KRAEPELIN applied the eponym Alzheimer's disease to honor Alzheimer, who was his student.

Currently Alzheimer's disease affects an estimated 2.5 million American adults, and is the most common cause of dementia. Victims may experience confusion, personality and behavior changes, impaired judgment, crying bouts, sadness, and difficulty in finding words, finishing thoughts or following directions. How quickly these changes will occur varies from person to person, but the disease eventually leaves its victims totally unable to care for themselves. The disease usually affects short-term memory first, followed by visual-spatial dysfunction, disorientation and impairment of other cognitive processes. Language, with the exception of word finding, is unaffected until late in the course.

According to Dr. Thomas Hutton, director of the Texas Tech Alzheimer's Disease Center at Texas Tech University, the average length of the illness varies, but is about 10 years. The first two years are typically subclinical with the afflicted person suffering from poor memory and growing confusion. Slowly and inexorably the forgetfulness progresses to more global confusion and eventually to dementia.

Since the cause of Alzheimer's is not known, the disease is undergoing intensive scientific investigation. According to the Alzheimer's Disease and Related Disorders Association, suspected causes include a genetic predisposition, a slow virus or other infectious agent, environmental toxins such as aluminum, and immunologic changes. Other factors also are under investigation.

One of the major challenges of Alzheimer's is diagnosing it accurately, since approximately 30% of the elderly who present symptoms associated with the disease may have other treatable disorders. Without a single clinical test to identify the disease, it is not always easy to distinguish it from other forms of dementia. Several other conditions must be excluded before a diagnosis. These include adverse drug reactions, metabolic changes, nutritional deficiencies, head injuries, brain tumors and strokes. Severe depression can often be mislabeled as Alzheimer's.

As things stand now, only after death can the brain be examined to show the above-mentioned neurofibrillary tangles and neuritic plaques that typify the illness. Reports by researchers suggest that the use of various pharmacologically-evoked hormonal responses may eventually aid in differential diagnosis of the disease.

Currently there is no effective treatment for Alzheimer's. Dr. Nunzio Pomara of the Geriatric Psychiatry Center at the NATHAN S. KLINE INSTITUTE for Psychiatric Research suspects that the central receptors for acetylcholine, the neurotransmitter whose deficits are implicated in Alzheimer's disease, may have a diminished capability to trigger appropriate biologic responses. He sees promise in administering THYROTRO-PIN-RELEASING HORMONE (TRH) concomitantly with cholinergic agents, such as choline, lecithin and physostigmine, for individuals who have Alzheimer's along with impaired responsivity in the cholinergic receptors.

Dr. Thomas Hutton has reported that a therapeutic trial of a tricyclic antidepressant medication may reduce the memory, cognitive and affective symptoms resulting from depression in Alzheimer's patients. Dosages of antidepressant medication in elderly, confused patients should be approximately 50% of those used in younger adults. Nortriptyline or amitriptyline have some sedating effects as well as antidepressant effects and may prove useful in the depressed sleepless patient. Regular exercise also reduces depression.

In summing up the relationship of depression and Alzheimer's disease in "Alzheimer's Disease and Psychiatric Nursing: Treating the Depression," Donna Yount Hughes (who has worked in a nursing home as a staff nurse in an end-stage Alzheimer's unit) wrote:

The feelings evoked by the progressing symptoms of Alzheimer's disease certainly test the patients' coping abilities. When coping skills wear thin, clinical depression can evolve, although this is not to imply that all patients with Alzheimer's disease are also clinically depressed. However, the symptoms the staff observed did correlate with those on a depression continuum. Unless medicated, Alzheimer's patients can experience chronically interrupted sleep patterns. Helplessness and apathy combined with a low energy level can leave patients unmotivated. They often give up levels of functioning long before their disease renders them incapable. Sexual energy and appetite are affected in much the same way as seen in depression. Anhedonia is marked, even in patients with only minor memory deficits. Giving up driving seems to be the turning point when patients admit they are ill. They are left sitting at home unable to work, but too well to tolerate the sudden change of lifestyle without adjustment difficulties. The person with Alzheimer's disease needs something to look forward to beside just getting worse.

Hughes, Donna Yount, "Alzheimer's Disease and Psychiatric Nursing: Treating the Depression," *Perspectives in Psychiatric Care*, 24:1(1987).

Liston, E., Jarvik, L. and Gerson, S., "Depression in Alzheimer's Disease: An Overview of Adrenergic and Cholinergic Mechanisms," *Comprehensive Psychiatry*, 28:5(September-October 1987).

Hutton, J. Thomas, "Alzheimer's Disease: Evolving Clinical Concepts and Management Strategies," *Comprehensive Therapy*, 13:9(September 1987).

American Association of Suicidology (AAS) A not-for-profit, tax-exempt organization whose goal is to understand and prevent suicide. Founded in 1968 by Edwin S. Shneidman, AAS promotes research, public awareness programs, training for professionals and volunteers, and other programs necessary for the understanding and prevention of suicide. It also serves as a national clearinghouse for information on suicide.

Its membership is made up of mental health professionals, researchers, suicide

prevention and crisis intervention centers, school districts, crisis center volunteers, survivors of suicide and a variety of laypersons who have an interest in suicide prevention. The primary objective of AAS is to help suicide prevention, and crisis intervention centers throughout the United States and Canada provide quality services. The AAS has developed standards for the certification of these centers. For information and a list of centers contact: American Association of Suicidology Central Office, Julie Perlman, Executive Officer, 2459 S. Ash St., Denver, CO 80222. Phone: 303-692-0985.

American Council for Drug Education (CDE) Established in 1977 as the American Council on Marijuana and other Psychoactive Drugs (ACM), the name was changed in 1983. As CDE educates the public about the health hazards associated with the use of psychoactive drugs and drug abuse, it covers the broad scope of drug abuse, including persons suffering from serious underlying depression. To do this, the council promotes scientific findings, organizes conferences and seminars, provides media resources and publishes educational materials.

American Indians See NATIVE AMERICANS.

American Medical Association (AMA) An association of physicians and surgeons that keeps the medical profession abreast of progress in clinical medicine, pertinent research and landmark developments. Its primary function is to promote the art and science of medicine, improve public health and provide advisory, interpretative and referral information on medicine and health care.

The association publishes a newsletter and the *Journal of the American Medical Association* (JAMA), in which many articles on depression appear. It is a source of statistics, brochures, pamphlets and library searches. A publications list is available. For information: 535 N. Dearborn St., Chicago, IL 60610.

American Psychiatric Association (APA) A professional medical organization whose members are United States and Canadian psychiatrists. Its purpose is to: (1) improve treatment, rehabilitation and care of the mentally ill; (2) promote research; (3) advance standards of all psychiatric services and facilities; and (4) educate medical professionals, scientists and the general public.

Among other services the APA provides advisory, analytical, bibliographical, historical, how-to, interpretative, referral and technical information on psychiatric care, psychiatric insurance and mental illness. It holds an annual meeting each May and publishes advance and post-convention news releases and articles on the proceedings. More than 400 individual papers presented at the meetings are available each year. These papers cover a wide range of topics. Throughout the year periodic news releases are furnished concerning new studies published in the APA journals. For information: 1400 K Street, NW, Washington, DC 20005. Phone: 202-797-4900.

American Psychological Association Within its specific field of expertise, the purpose, functions and services of this professional society correspond to those of the American Psychiatric Association. It is a source of information and referrals on depression and other concerns to professionals and the general public. For information: 1200 17th Street, NW, Washington, DC 20036. Phone: 202-833-7600.

amines Chemicals produced by the central nervous system that are involved in the functioning of the brain. Known technically as BIOGENIC AMINES (or neurotransmitters),

amines are chemical transmitters that nerves use to send messages to each other. They are located in the LIMBIC SYSTEM, a brain region that appears to be involved in mood regulation, and include NOREPINEPHRINE, DOPAMINE and SEROTONIN.

For some time researchers studying the chemistry of mood disorders have believed that depression can result from decreased levels of amines. To date, their studies of the amine theory substantiate that. In one study, reported by psychiatrist Dr. David D. Burns in his book *Feeling Good—The New Mood Therapy*, a group of depressed patients received a drug that causes a buildup in brain-amine concentrations. After several weeks of treatment, the patients were clinically improved. Then they were given a second drug that depletes the brain amines. The patients all relapsed into depression within a couple of days. When the second drug was withdrawn, so that the brain-amine levels were allowed to rise, the patients again recovered. (See also BRAIN CHEMISTRY and CENTRAL NERVOUS SYSTEM).

Burns, David D., *Feeling Good—The New Mood Therapy* (New York: New American Library, 1980).

amphetamines Also known as "uppers" or "speed," these drugs are STIMULANTS, and individuals suffering from mild or temporary depression have found small doses of them effective in its treatment. They are *not* ANTIDEPRESSANTS, though they are sometimes prescribed along with the latter. They are referred to as uppers or speed only when used illegally in excessive doses. They do have legitimate medical functions, but their use is limited because of the tendency for tolerance to develop. Under proper supervision they are a valuable adjunct to the more important antidepressants.

The National Institute of Mental Health (NIMH) advises that amphetamines should not be taken alone for depression. Long-term use or excessive doses are worthless and possibly harmful if persons suffering from depression abuse them. Depressed persons seeking the feelings of self-worth and energy this drug can produce often use and abuse illicit amphetamines.

A breakdown of amphetamines follows:
Amphetamines
amphetamine sulfate (Benzedrine)
dextroamphetamine sulfate (Dexedrine)
methamphetamine hydrochloride (Desoxyn)
Amphetamine relatives
benzphetamine hydrochloride (Didrex)
clortermine hydrochloride (Voranil)
diethylpropion hydrochloride (Tenuate; Tepanil)
mazindol (Sanorex)
methylphenidate hydrochloride (Ritalin)
phendimetrazine tartrate (Barcarate; Bontril; Melfiat; Plegine; Prelu-2; Trimtabs; Wehless-35)
phenmetrazine hydrochloride (Preludin)

anergic   Characterized by abnormal inactivity and marked by lack of energy.

anger   Anger, or at least a distinct ambivalence, toward the self has been considered to be one feature of the psychology of depression, particularly in the psychoanalytic tradition. This view was suggested by the low self-regard and frequent self-reproaches of many depressed persons. This led, at times, to the rather simplistic view that depression was nothing but anger turned inward, and that depressed persons merely needed to acknowledge that rage and express it more openly to others. As the emphasis on this aspect waned, another aspect of this explanatory tradition was given more and more attention—namely, Freud's "loss of self-regarding feelings," which came to be referred to as a "loss of self-esteem."

On quite another dimension, it should be noted that there is often an admixture of anger among the symptoms of depression.

(See also FREUDIAN THEORY OF DEPRESSION.)

anhedonia   The technical name for a diminished ability to experience satisfaction and pleasure. It is a state of mind and mood experienced by victims of depression who fail to initiate any meaningful activity or task because they feel the reward of accomplishing a task would be far less than the investment of effort required to do it. In a negative way, they discount any sense of fulfillment from anything they might undertake.

Ann Arbor Study   See LENGTH OF GRIEVING PROCESS.

anorexia nervosa   An eating disorder in which people (usually girls and young women) debilitate themselves by refusing to eat over a long period of time. Generally the disorder is prompted by an intense fear of becoming obese. Psychologically, victims of this disorder, like most addictive persons, have a deep sense of inadequacy, low self-esteem, self-hatred and similar symptoms of depression.

Risk factors for the development of anorexia nervosa are unclear. But having a family member with anorexia or BULIMIA and a possible family history of affective disorder or substance abuse seems to be a risk.

The DIAGNOSTIC AND STATISTICAL MANUAL OF MENTAL DISORDERS (DSM-111-R) gives the following criteria for anorexia: (1) refusal to maintain body weight at a minimal normal weight for age and height, e.g., weight loss leading to maintenance of body weight 15% below that expected, or failure to make expected weight gain during period of growth, leading to body weight 15% below that expected; (2) intense fear of gaining weight or becoming fat, even though underweight; (3) disturbance in the way in which one's body weight, size or shape is experienced, e.g., the person claims to "feel fat'' even when emaciated, believes that one area of the body is "too fat," even when obviously underweight; (4) in females, absence of at least three consecutive menstrual cycles when otherwise expected to occur.

Yates, William R. and Sieleni, Bruce, "Anorexia and Bulimia," *Primary Care*, 14:4 (December 1987).

anticipatory grief See GRIEF.

anticonvulsants Medications used to control or ward off convulsions. Two examples are CARBAMAZEPINE and CLONAZEPAM.

antidepressant medication precautions Patients often are tempted to stop medication too soon, but it is important to keep taking it until the treating physician says to stop, even if patients start to feel better. When stopping a drug, some medications must be stopped gradually to give the body time to adjust. In cases of manic-depressive (see BIPOLAR DEPRESSION) illness and chronic major depression, medication may have to become part of everyday life to avoid disabling symptoms.

The following are antidepressant medication precautions that patients must keep in mind:

1. Although the side effects of mixing an antidepressant with another medication depend on the specific drugs involved, serious and dangerous side effects can sometimes result from combining two drugs, unless they are administered with extreme caution. Therefore, depressives must refrain from mixing medications of any kind—prescribed, over-the-counter or borrowed—without consulting a doctor.
2. Dentists or other medical specialists who prescribe drugs should be told when a patient is taking antidepressants.

3. Alcohol must be avoided because wine, beer and hard liquor may interact dangerously with antidepressants.
4. Dangerous interactions can occur between tricyclic drugs and MAO inhibitors, so depressives need at least a 10-day drug-free period before switching from one to another.
5. Tricyclic drugs and MAO inhibitors also tend to cause blood pressure changes, so patients who are on hypertensive medication need to be aware that dosages sometimes have to be adjusted to compensate for changes. Some of the newer antihypertensives themselves can cause a problem when combined with other drugs, though if the combinations are done judiciously they can usually be worked around.
6. Certain heart patients—for instance, people who have a significant amount of electrical disturbance in the way impulses are conducted from one chamber of the heart to the next—must be sure that antidepressants are administered with extreme care.
7. Lithium may cause toxicity when taken in combination with diuretics or non-steroidal anti-inflammatory drugs.

antidepressants Antidepressant medication is regarded by many professionals as the best treatment for the most serious forms of depression. Rarely used for nonmedical purposes, the drugs are not tranquilizers, they don't produce "highs" and they're not habit-forming. They seem to increase SEROTONIN and NOREPINEPHRINE in the SYNAPSES of depressed patients.

The development of antidepressants came about almost by accident in the early 1950s when physicians noticed that tuberculosis patients treated with IPRONIAZID sometimes became extremely cheerful. The conclusion that this euphoria might be a side effect of the drug led to the development of the MONO-

AMINE OXIDASE INHIBITORS, usually called MAO inhibitors. They were followed by the tricyclic antidepressants, which became the mainstay of depression treatment, while lithium became the preferred treatment for bipolar, or MANIC-DEPRESSIVE, illnesses. MAO inhibitors and tricyclic antidepressants are generally used to treat unipolar illness (see UNIPOLAR DEPRESSION) in which the patient may be severely depressed but does not become manic.

The antidepressant drugs include:

Tricyclic
amitriptyline hydrochloride (Elavil; Endep; SK-Amitriptyline; Amitid)
amoxapine (Asendin)
desipramine hydrochloride (Norpramine; Pertofrane)
doxepin hydrochloride (Adapin; Sinequan)
imipramine hydrochloride (Imavate; Janimine; SK-Pramine; Tofranil)
nortriptyline hydrochloride (Aventyl; Pamelor)
protriptyline hydrochloride (Vivactil)

MAO Inhibitors
isocarboxazid (Marplan)
phenelzine sulfate (Nardil)
tranylcypromine sulfate (Parnate)

Lithium salts
lithium carbonate (Eskalith; Lithane; Lithonate)

In the so-called newer generation of antidepressants trazodone (Desyrel) and maprotiline (Ludiomil) are being used. Fluoxetine (Prozac), a serotonin re-uptake blocker that was first used in Europe, is helping some people who did not respond to standard drugs. Other newer-generation drugs are under investigation.

Within the past few years, several antidepressants, such as Merital (NOMIFENSINE) and Wellbutrin (BUPROPION HYDROCHLORIDE), have been introduced, marketed briefly, then later recalled for further investigation because of serious side effects. Reportedly, Merital caused some serious hyper-

sensitivity reactions, notably hemolytic anemia, an anemia due to destruction of red blood cells. Wellbutrin was pulled because a side effect for some people was seizures, but it is now back on the market.

Experience has shown that patients who do not respond to one antidepressant medication often have a better than average chance of responding to another. Consequently doctors sometimes need to try a variety of antidepressants before finding the most effective medication or combination of medications. Sometimes the dosage must be increased to be effective. So, as is the case with any type of medication prescribed for more than a few days, antidepressants have to be carefully monitored to see whether patients are getting the correct dosage.

Some experts believe that antidepressants are often prescribed at insufficient dosages and that, as a result, many depressed patients are classified as cases in which antidepressants do not work. Moreover, since some depressives turn to medication following a period of psychotherapy that did not relieve their depression an inadequate dosage of drugs that also fails to provide relief may increase their feeling of hopelessness.

The response time for all antidepressants is variable. Some people will respond in the first week. On the other hand, there are people who will take four to six weeks to respond. Some researchers will dispute the fact that some patients will respond in the first week. Other research confirms that there are cases where this happens. Unfortunately, for a significant minority of patients the antidepressant medication does not work. In addition to the disadvantage of the slow onset of antidepressant action, some people experience unpleasant or dangerous side effects: of sedation, troublesome anticholinergic effects, occasional dangerous and even lethal cardiovascular effects, and other reactions. Consequently, even though the current pharmacological approach to major depressive illness still relies mainly on the tricyclic antidepressants, which show efficacy in an estimated 60% to 70% of patients, there remains a need for more effective, safer compounds. As Dr. Sidney Zisook of the University of California at San Diego, who has conducted extensive research on antidepressants, puts it: "Given the prevalence and morbidity of depression as well as the limitations of the currently available therapies, there is ample room for the development of newer antidepressants with even greater biological specificity, effectiveness and safety." (See also DRUG THERAPY; TRICYCLIC COMPOUNDS.)

Zisook, Sidney et al., "Efficacy and Safety of Fezolamine in Depressed Patients," *Neuropsychobiology*, 17(1987), 133-138.

anxiety Depressive disorders and anxiety are closely related, so even though some degree of anxiety is a normal, even necessary part of life, abnormal, overwhelming, hard-to-control anxiety can be an indication of the affective disorders of severe depression, mania or bipolar depression. In clinical samples a generalized anxiety disorder sometimes seems to follow a major depressive episode.

Anxiety is characterized by a feeling of apprehension, uncertainty and fear, without apparent stimulus. The DIAGNOSTIC AND STATISTICAL MANUAL OF MENTAL DISORDERS (DMS-III-R) indicates that the essential feature of a generalized anxiety disorder is unrealistic or excessive concern and worry about two or more life circumstances for six months or longer, during which the person has been bothered by these concerns more days than not. Typical examples of such apprehensive expectations are worry about possible misfortune to one's child who is in no danger and worry about finances for no good reason.

As people anticipate the worst and feel keyed up and on edge, anxiety disorders are marked by both psychologic and physiologic symptoms. Typical symptoms are jumpiness, irritability, restlessness, tension, headache, sweating, increased pulse, heart pounding or racing, panic bouts, phobias and sleeping problems.

One form of anxiety now receiving considerable attention in research circles is posttraumatic stress disorder (PTSD), though according to DSM-III-R this classification is still controversial since the predominant symptom is the reexperiencing of a trauma, not anxiety. However, anxiety symptoms are extremely common. In PTSD a person experiences an event that is outside the range of usual human experience and that would be markedly distressing to almost anyone (for example, military combat, airplane crashes, flood disasters). This traumatic event can be reexperienced in a variety of ways.

Generally, a person has recurrent and intrusive recollections of the event or recurrent distressing dreams during which the event is relived. According to Dr. John M. Rainey and other researchers at the VA Medical Center in Allen Park, Michigan major depression is a frequently encountered concurrent diagnosis in patients with PTSD. To investigate the relationship of PTSD to other psychiatric disorders the Michigan researchers administered the structural clinical interview for DSM-III-R (SCID) to 21 Vietnam veterans with a clinical diagnosis of PTSD. Twelve of the 21 (55%) met the criteria for major depression.

When anxiety interferes with a person's ability to perform normally, treatment to alleviate the symptoms and return the person to normal activities should be considered. This treatment can include both psychotherapy and drug therapy. Usually a combination of psychotherapy or behavior therapy and drug therapy is the most effective form of treatment. (See also PANIC ATTACKS, PHOBIA.)

Rainey, J.M., Aleem A. et al., "A Laboratory Procedure for the Induction of Flashbacks," *American Journal of Psychiatry* (in press).

American Psychiatric Association, *Diagnostic and Statistical Manual of Mental Disorders,* 3rd ed., rev. (Washington, D.C.: American Psychiatric Association, 1987).

Lear, Martha Weinman, "Redefining Anxiety," *New York Times Magazine,* August 31, 1988.

anxiolytics   Anti-anxiety drugs that have become the prevalent form of treatment for many anxiety disorders. Also known as "minor tranquilizers; anxiolytics are useful primarily for generalized anxiety disorder and as very temporary therapy in simple phobias. Minor tranquilizers are also used widely to treat situational anxiety, particularly the type that often accompanies serious illnesses. In patients with anxiety and depression (or those with panic attacks) a combination of anxiolytics and antidepressants may be used. The most common anxiolytics in use today are the BENZODIAZEPINES.

areas of research and study   Much research, targeted to a wide range of goals, is being conducted on depression. There is a great deal of important work going on in the neurobiology and genetics of depression. Some subjects under study are:

1. Alternatives to lithium to help manic-depressive patients who are non-responsive to lithium therapy.

Important work in this field is being done by Dr. Robert M. Post, chief, Biological Psychiatry Branch, National Institute of Mental Health, and his colleagues who have been studying the use of CARBAMAZEPINE on patients who were inadequately responsive to lithium carbonate. The researchers feel that, while lithium carbonate is clearly the drug of choice, we might increasingly consider carbamazepine as one of the first-line alternative or adjunctive treatments.

2. Antidepressants that will reduce the lag before drugs take effect.

This is an urgent research goal. For a person who is feeling bad, the lag can be a serious drawback, but for one who is suicidal it can be fatal.

Usually patients treated with antidepressants have to take their drug for two to three weeks before they get real relief from their agonizing sadness and sense of hopelessness. Some experts have speculated that key groups of nerve cells in the brain have to reset the balance of the receptors that govern the effects on the cells of neurotransmitters.

3. The isolation of the precise roles of different neurochemicals in different kinds of depression and the tailoring of a drug for each subtype.

By testing blood, spinal fluid and urine, scientists have already uncovered different chemical ratios underlying some of the various sorts of depression, and if they can isolate precise roles there will be new and more effective treatments for depression.

4. New drugs that can be used as SEROTONIN re-uptake blockers.

So far Prozac (see FLUOXETINE) and Anafranil (clomipramine), pure serotonin re-uptake blockers, are the first such drugs that have become available. Since there is speculation that many people may have a depression that is related to a deficit in the serotonin transmission, other serotonin re-uptake blockers are under investigation.

Post, Robert M. et al., "Correlates of Antimanic Response to Carbamazepine," *Psychiatry Research,* 21(1986), 71–73.

art, literature, music and depression
See CREATIVITY.

Association for Advancement of Behavior Therapy (AABT)   A professional, interdisciplinary organization concerned with enhancing the human condition through the scientific investigation and application of the principles of human behavior. Founded in 1966, AABT refers to itself as the most significant voice of behavior therapy in North America. The association is active in facilitating the interaction of clinicians, clinical researchers and basic researchers, and serves as a centralized resource for all matters relating to the field. Each year at its annual convention it presents many offerings in the area of depression.

Whether referred to as behavior therapy, behavior modification, applied behavior analysis or conditioning therapy, this field is constantly evolving, resulting in a continuing need for the evaluation and consolidation of new information at all levels. It is to this end that AABT, while primarily an interest group, is also active in: (a) encouraging the development of the conceptual and scientific basis of behavior therapy as an empirical approach to applied problems; and (b) facilitating the appropriate utilization and growth of behavior therapy as a professional activity. Address: 15 W. 36th St., New York, NY 10018. Phone: 212-279-7970.

asthma and depression Researchers have found that depression and hopelessness could be factors in asthma deaths among adults. Similarly, a study of asthmatic children by Dr. Robert C. Strunk, a pediatric allergist at Washington University in St. Louis, and Dr. Bruce Miller, a psychiatrist at the National Jewish Center for Immunology and Respiratory Medicine in Denver, has indicated that a combination of depression and asthma could also be potentially lethal in children.

Their study implies that while all children with serious asthma are prone to bouts of depression, children who feel helpless about their personal lives because of loss through divorce, abandonment, death or the experience of living in conflict-ridden families may be at greater risk for fatal asthma attacks. In studying 24 cases from various parts of the country the researchers found that 12 children had died from asthma attacks, while 12 others had survived asthma attacks that near-

ly killed them. Differences between the groups were revealing. Seven children who died came from families experiencing problems with marital discord, alcoholism, drugs or lack of emotional support or medical treatment. Only two children who survived had experienced such strife.

The researchers say depression is not the primary cause of asthma death. But their research indicates that it can be an important contributing factor. In their studies, reported in *Circumstances Surrounding the Deaths of Children Due to Asthma,* emotional disturbance was rated if the child had been referred for psychiatric treatment within the six-month period before the attacks or if the child appeared to have been experiencing problematic functioning. Depression was rated on the basis of reported clinical symptoms or if the child had been treated for depression within six months of the episode.

"The emotional state of hopelessness/despair was scored positive if the child was reported to have expressed feelings of hopelessness, a wish to die, or direct or indirect references to suicide or [patient's own] death within one month before the index episode," they wrote. "This emotional state is a frequent finding in patients with depression or other forms of emotional disturbance, although hopelessness/despair alone is not sufficient to make a diagnosis of depression."

In indicating that a combination of depression and asthma could be potentially lethal in children, Dr. Miller emphasized that he does not want to alarm parents of asthmatic children. At the same time he stressed, however, that if a parent notices an asthmatic child has become despondent or hopeless that parent should be alert to the possibility of an asthma attack and get help and watch the child closely. It is unlikely that the child will die, but the parent should be aware that there are risk factors that predispose the child to an asthma attack.

Miller, Bruce D. and Strunk, Robert C., "Circumstances Surrounding the Deaths of Children Due to Asthma," *American Journal of Diseases of Children*, November 1989.

Strunk, Robert C. et al., "Physiologic and Psychological Characteristics Associated With Deaths Due to Asthma in Childhood," *Journal of the American Medical Association*, September 6, 1985.

at-risk individuals or groups As with other diseases, these are people with characteristics that increase the probability of developing depressive or grief-related illnesses.

Australia At the mood disorders clinic at the Prince Henry Hospital in Sydney, Dr. Philip Boyce, a psychiatrist, is doing extensive studies on SEASONAL AFFECTIVE DISORDER (SAD). He started his study of SAD people in 1985 and he is successfully treating many cases in Australia through phototherapy (see LIGHT THERAPY).

Boyce first became interested in SAD in the mid '70s through work being done by Dr. Bob Seamark, a scientist at the University of Adelaide who was investigating MELATONIN, a hormone secreted by the PINEAL GLAND, which has been tied to SAD. To further his studies on melatonin and SAD Boyce asked an Australian publication in 1985 to run an article describing the effects of weather on health. In the article he invited people who had regular seasonal mood changes to take part in a research survey. As a result of the article he received 300 replies, primarily from women from the most densely populated states.

To qualify for the survey people had to have suffered three episodes of depression in the same season of the year over the past five years. Boyce eventually selected 22 people and recruited other psychiatrists and students at the university to take part in an experiment to find out how light affected the levels of melatonin in their blood. The samples were sent to Seamark who analyzed the melatonin levels. Because the group was small, there

were not enough results to establish normal and abnormal levels. But the curves plotted showed that everyone followed the same pattern—the more light there was, the more the level of melatonin went down.

The Australian studies on SAD and light treatment are ongoing, and many of the scientists involved in them consider seasonal affective disorder one of the country's major health issues.

Bell, Glennys, "A New Light on the Blues," *The Bulletin*, July 25, 1989.

B

---

baby blues See POSTPARTUM DEPRESSION.

baby boomers Young adults, between the ages of 25 and 44 who were born in the 1950s or later and dubbed the "baby boomers," face three to 10 times the risk of major depression that their grandparents faced. In fact, depression is an epidemic among young adults. It is also striking earlier, and the average age at onset has dropped in the last 30 years from the early thirties to the early twenties.

This data, cited by Dr. Martin E.P. Seligman, a University of Pennsylvania psychology professor, and researchers from the National Institute of Mental Health, comes in part from federally-funded research projects that were conducted over the last 10 years to examine the epidemiology of various mental disorders. In the first of the studies in this project, the EPIDEMIOLOGIC CATCHMENT AREA (ECA), 9,500 adults nationwide were involved. The researchers found that people aged 20 to 25 had a 5% to 6% chance of having had at least one major depression. Those 25 to 44 had an 8% to 9% chance. But people born around 1925 had only a 4% chance and those born before World War I had a 1% chance.

Seligman, M.E.P., "Why Is There So Much Depression Today?" *The G. Stanley Hall Lecture Series*, in Washington, D.C., 1988.

barbiturates Derivatives of barbituric acid are used to induce sleep and to provide daylong sedation in the treatment of tension and anxiety. Since they act as central nervous system depressants they slow down or decrease the activity of the nerves that control emotions, breathing, heart action and various other body functions.

The first barbiturate was synthesized in 1864 from barbituric acid by two German scientists. In 1882 it was manufactured and used in medicine as barbital. In 1903, it was released under the trade name Veronal. Then in 1912 a phenobarbital was introduced and released as Luminal.

Since that time many barbituric acid derivatives have been synthesized and manufactured as tablets, capsules, suppositories and liquids for injection. Short-acting barbiturates are commonly known as sleeping pills. Their effects last only five or six hours and they produce little or no hangover when not abused. However, when they are abused, a person can become addicted and a sleeping problem can grow even worse. They are legitimately available only by prescription. But the government estimates that 20% of legally manufactured barbiturates are deflected to the black market and sold illicitly. (See also BENZODIAZEPINES, DRUG THERAPY.)

Barr-Harris Center for the Study of Separation and Loss During Childhood An arm of the Chicago Institute for Psychoanalysis and a nonprofit program specializing in childhood mourning that was established in 1976 to offer help to recently bereaved children and parents. Currently it also includes services to children and parents of divorced families.

Its principle purpose is to provide preventive services to appropriate families and to investigate the effect of loss and separation upon children over the course of their development. With this as its goal it is committed to the wide dissemination of knowledge on the effect of losses and separations in childhood and to the education of both professionals and laypersons on the ways and means of preventing lasting damage to children from such traumatic events. It is interested in furthering scientific knowledge in this area and is continuously studying: the initial and later effects of loss and separation upon children and their parents; the amount of time and degree of mourning required for favorable adaptation; and the means by which adaptation can be influenced through intervention.

In a pilot study of school functioning, the center compared control children with children who suffered a death or divorce in the family. Preliminary data showed that the children of death or divorce had more difficulty in school. The bereaved children were more on the depressive side, while the divorce children had more behavioral problems.

Most bereaved families come to the center clinic within the first six months following the death. However, when a parent is facing imminent death, families also contact the center for assistance in discussing the handling of the death with their children. For information contact: Barr-Harris Center, Institute for Psychoanalysis, 180 North Michigan Ave., Chicago, IL 60601. Phone: 312-726-6300.

BEAM scanning (brain electrical activity mapping) A process that provides color pictures of brain electrical activity in minutes. It was developed by Dr. Frank Duffy, associate professor of neurology at Harvard Medical School, and his colleagues. The process combines computers, image-processing techniques and a statistical program to compare observed electrical activity with what is normal for a given part of the brain.

Beck, Aaron A professor of psychiatry (1921–) at the University of Pennsylvania School of Medicine and one of the world's foremost authorities on mood disorders. He is founder of the Cognitive Therapy of Depression and director of the Center for Cognitive Therapy at the University of Pennsylvania (see COGNITIVE THERAPY).

Soon after Beck began his career as a practitioner of traditional psychoanalytic psychiatry, he began to investigate and research the theories and therapies of depression. His investigations suggested to him that depressed individuals see themselves as losers—inadequate persons doomed to frustration, humiliation and failure. In describing them he has referred to them as people with a four-D image: Defeated, Defective, Deserted, and Deprived.

From his research and investigations Beck developed his premise that depression involved not only behavioral, biological and motivational factors but also idiosyncratic cognitive contents and processes.

In his preface to Dr. David D. Burns' book *Feeling Good*, Beck wrote:

> My conclusion was that depression must involve a disturbance in thinking: the depressed person thinks in idiosyncratic and negative ways about himself, his environment, and his future. The pessimistic mental set affects his mood, his motivation, and his relationships with others, and leads to the full spectrum of psychological and physical symptoms typical of depression. We now have a large body of research data and clinical experience which suggests that people can learn to control painful mood swings and self-defeating behavior through the application of a few relatively simple principles and techniques.

The promising results of Beck's work have triggered strong interest in cognitive theory among psychiatrists, psychologists, and other mental health professionals, and the findings have been viewed by many as a major development in the scientific study of psychotherapy and personal change. (See also BECK DEPRESSION INVENTORY.)

Beck, Aaron T., *Depression: Causes and Treatment* (Philadelphia: University of Pennsylvania Press, 1967).

Beck, Aaron T. et al., *Cognitive Therapy of Depression* (New York: Guilford Press, 1979).

Beck Depression Inventory (BDI) A mood-measuring device and multiple-choice questionnaire developed by DR. AARON T. BECK to detect the presence of depression and rate its severity. It was first introduced in 1961, and in 1971 a revised BDI was developed. In its more than 25 year history, it has become one of the most widely used instruments not only for assessing the intensity of depression in psychiatrically diagnosed patients, but also for detecting depression in non-diagnosed populations. According to the files of the Center for Cognitive Therapy, it has been employed in over 1,000 different research studies.

To develop the BDI Beck made systematic observations and records of the characteristic attitudes and symptoms of depressed patients. Then he selected a group of the attitudes and symptoms that appeared to be specific for depressed patients and were consistent with the descriptions of depression contained in the psychiatric literature.

On the basis of this procedure he constructed an inventory composed of 21 categories of symptoms and attitudes. These 21 symptom-attitude categories are:

1. Mood
2. Pessimism
3. Sense of Failure
4. Lack of Satisfaction
5. Guilty Feeling
6. Sense of Punishment
7. Self-Hate
8. Self-Accusations
9. Self-Punitive Wishes
10. Crying Spells
11. Irritability
12. Social Withdrawal

13. Indecisiveness
14. Body Image
15. Work Inhibition
16. Sleep Disturbance
17. Fatigability
18. Loss of Appetite
19. Weight Loss
20. Somatic Preoccupation
21. Loss of Libido

In the BDI, each of the above categories describes a specific behavioral manifestation of depression and consists of a graded series of four or five self-evaluative statements. Typical statements are "I am blue or sad all the time and I can't snap out of it," "I feel that the future is hopeless and that things cannot improve," "I do not feel like a failure," "I feel bored most of the time" and "I don't feel disappointed in myself."

The statements are ranked to reflect the range of severity of the symptom from neutral to maximal severity, and numerical values from 0 to 3 are assigned each statement to indicate the degree of severity.

Although the BDI was initially designed to be administered by trained interviewers, it is often self-administered. When self-administered, it generally takes five to 10 minutes to complete and is scored by summing the ratings given to each of the 21 items. (See also COGNITIVE THERAPY.)

Beck, Aaron T., *Depression: Causes and Treatment* (Philadelphia: University of Pennsylvania Press, 1967).

Beck, Aaron T. et al., *Cognitive Therapy of Depression* (New York: Guilford Press, 1979).

Beck, Aaron T. et al., "An Inventory for Measuring Depression," *Archives of General Psychiatry*, 4(1961).

Beck, Aaron T. et al., "Psychometric Properties of the Beck Depression Inventory: Twenty-Five Years of Evaluation," *Clinical Psychology Review*, 8(1988).

Beethoven, Ludwig Van A German composer (1770–1827) who is regarded by many as the greatest of all composers. However, his life was plagued by problems and conflicts, and as he suffered from anxiety, depression and grief from disappointment in love many critics believe he poured his emotional upheavals into his voluminous compositions. By the time he reached midlife he had also become so deaf that all communication with him had to be in writing.

In *Outlook,* a newsletter of the Department of Psychiatry of the New York Hospital-Cornell Medical Center, Dr. William A. Frosch, vice chairman and professor of psychiatry at Cornell University Medical College and medical director of the Payne Whitney Clinic, writes of Beethoven: "In 1801, when he was 30 years old, Beethoven published his first six quartets. The final movement of the sixth quartet was called *La Malinconia,* the Italian word for melancholia. This movement is Beethoven's representation of manic depressive illness." Dr. Frosch believes that Beethoven drew this portrait from personal experience and goes on to explain that, although Beethoven was not necessarily manic depressive, he had mood swings superimposed upon a prevailing mild depression. "Beethoven became more and more eccentric after he became deaf and probably had a psychotic episode during the battle for custody of his nephew," he wrote. "Beethoven's knowledge of cyclic insanity, however, like his knowledge of the vagaries of nature, was part of the imagery that shaped his creativity. Beethoven had the ability to illustrate what he knew about or had observed in others, including manic-depressive illness."

Frosch, William A., "Moods, Madness, and Music," *Outlook,* Fall 1988.

Behavioral disorders Depressives may "act out" (a phrase clinicians use to describe the use of *behavior* rather than *words* to express emotional conflicts). Some "act out" through aggressive, hostile, defiant behavior. Others show their behavioral disorders through passive, withdrawn, gloomy, noncommunicative behavior. Depending on the situation, some may switch behavior disorders and go from one extreme to the other. (See also COMMON SIGNS AND SYMPTOMS.)

behavior therapy   A process that applies learning techniques and the principles of conditioning to train chronically depressed persons to perform with more incentive and greater optimism. In order to help dissipate depression behavior therapy encourages the modification of maladaptive personality attitudes, traits and behavior. It shows patients how to relax and avert fears, panic and anger explosions within their depression. Behavior therapy is also useful for patients with mild to moderate degrees of reactive and NEUROTIC DEPRESSIONS and as a combined or follow-up procedure for people who have adjusted poorly to life situations before, during or after a depressive illness.

A number of methods are used to teach patients to be more effective in obtaining rewards and satisfaction through their own actions. For example, the therapist may help the patient set up a schedule for monitoring pleasant and unpleasant events and then encourage the patient to increase those occurrences that give pleasure and decrease those that do not. In other instances, a patient may be taught relaxation or social skills. By ignoring depressive behaviors and rewarding coping activities, the therapist assists the patient to interact more positively with others, to fulfill more personal needs and to gain desirable ends. Initially, patients' efforts are therapist-directed and rewarded, but eventually patients learn that they are capable of initiating actions that result in desired rewards and goals. This new sense of control reduces feelings of helplessness and hopelessness and breaks the cycle that may lead to depression. (See also COGNITIVE THERAPY, INTERPERSONAL PSYCHOTHERAPY.)

Department of Health and Human Services, *Depressive Disorders: Causes and Treatment* (Rockville, Maryland: DHHS, 1983).

Bell Jar, The   See PLATH, SYLVIA.

benzodiazepines   Minor anti-anxiety tranquilizers whose chemical source is benzodiazepine. As central nervous system depressants they act on the brain's limbic system (the center of emotional response) and relieve tension and anxiety due to emotional stress.

As popular substitutes for barbiturates, they're readily absorbed into the gastrointestinal tract, quickoy (though unevenly) distributed in the body, metabolized in the liver and slowly excreted in the urine. The main benzodiazepine derivatives are oxazepam (Serax); lorazepam (Ativan); temazepam (Restoril); alprazolam (Xanax); triazolam (Halcion); chlordiazepoxide (Librium); diazepam (Valium); clorazepate (Tranxene, Azene); flurazepam (Dalmane); clonazepam (Clonopin); prazepam (Verstram, Centrax); and halazepam (Paxipam).

Xanax is unique in that it seems to be the only benzodiazepine that does have an antidepressant effect to a significant degree. (See also DRUG THERAPY.

bereavement   A condition caused by the loss or death of a loved person—or pet, relationship or important material attachment. Uusually a bereaved person's state is diagnosed—from the medical and psychological points of view—as a normal response to the circumstances of his or her situation. When overt signs and symptoms reach pathological proportions bereavement may be considered an illness and treatment may be in order. However, many bereaved people neither need nor seek out psychotherapy or support groups.

In writing about the bereavement that follows the death of a loved one in *On Death and Dying*, Dr. Elisabeth Kubler-Ross divides the normal psychological passages into five stages: (1) denial, (2) rage and anger, (3) bargaining, (4) depression, (5) acceptance.

In *Living With an Empty Chair* Dr. Roberta Temes separates grief into three stages. Writes Temes:

In the first stage of grief, which can last several weeks or months, the bereaved goes about daily life in a mechanical fashion . . . He feels as if he is involved in a bad dream which will soon be over. People are temporarily anesthetized. The second stage, disorganization, which can last many months, is the most difficult stage. The shock has worn off. People aren't around like before. The bereaved experiences symptoms of depression . . . Feelings of craziness, anger, guilt, self-pity and resentment are possible . . . The third stage, reorganization, which can last several weeks or months, brings with it the acceptance of the death as real. The bereaved once again is whole. He cares about himself and his future. He recognizes that there might be occasional setbacks or bad days. But these are temporary and eventually do pass. The mourning process has been completed.

(See also GRIEF; GRIEF, CAUSES AND EFFECTS OF: GRIEF THERAPY/TREATMENT: LOSS: LENGTH OF GRIEVING PROCESS: MOURNING: STAGES OF GRIEF.)

Kubler-Ross, Elizabeth, *On Death and Dying* (New York: Macmillan, 1969).

Temes, Roberta, *Living With an Empty Chair* (Amherst, Massachusetts: Mandala Press, 1977).

bereavement counseling courses Bereavement courses and counseling: (1) give direct help to families and individuals who have suffered a loss; and (2) provide ways that enable persons to deal with the hurt of the loss. In counseling sessions the bereaved are encouraged to express their grief through crying and showing their anger and pain without feeling they have to maintain a facade. In the process they are helped to see themselves and the things that have happened to them more clearly and comfortably, so they can deal with what they have lost and, subsequently, move on.

For persons who cannot return to a functioning state in a reasonable time or who are reluctant to reveal themselves before strangers in SELF-HELP/SUPPORT ORGANIZA-TIONS bereavement counseling courses (or private counseling) are often recommended.

A number of bereavement counseling courses and specialized professional or semi-professional services, such as those available at the BARR-HARRIS CENTER FOR THE STUDY OF SEPARATION AND LOSS DURING CHILDHOOD and the BEREAVEMENT AND LOSS CENTER, can be found in areas throughout the country. A number of cities have centers and some colleges and hospitals offer courses. There are also local professional organizations of social workers, psychologists, psychiatrists and nurses that can be called for recommendations for a bereavement course.

Fees are moderate and in some cases there is a sliding payment scale. For some counseling services medical insurance reimbursement is available.

Bereavement and Loss Center A private, non-sectarian organization in manhattan that provides professional counseling services for individuals who have suffered loss of various kinds—or who may be anticipating a loss. Individuals or families may be mourning the loss of a spouse, child, parent, relative or friend; a couple may have experienced miscarriage, stillbirth, neonatal death or infertility problems. Treatment may be short- or long-term.

Counselors are psychiatric social workers and psychiatrists who have special expertise and experience in problems of bereavement and loss. There is also an advisory staff of social workers, psychiatrists, other medical specialists, psychologists, attorneys and financial experts. Fees are moderate. For information contact: Anne W. Rosberger, Executive Director, Bereavement and Loss Center of New York, 170 E. 83rd St., New York, NY 10028. Phone: 212-879-5655.

binge-purge syndrome See BULIMIA.

biochemical factors Some 30 years ago physicians first observed that certain medications had strong mood-altering properties. Depression was observed in patients taking reserpine, a drug to control blood pressure. In contrast, iproniazid, used to treat tuberculosis, was associated with euphoria in some patients.

The implications of these observations—that mood disorders could be a function of a biochemical disturbance and could be stabilized by drugs—prompted clinical and laboratory studies that have revolutionized the treatment of mental disorders and, through ANTIDEPRESSANTS, helped alleviate the suffering of individuals with depressive disorders.

In addition to the efficacy of the antidepressant drugs, further evidence of biochemical disturbance in depressive disorders has been found in animal brain tissue studies. A group of chemical compounds, the BIOGENIC AMINES, has been shown to regulate mood. Two of the amines, SEROTONIN and NOREPINEPHRINE, appear to be of particular importance and are concentrated in areas of the brain that also control such drives as hunger, sex and thirst. (See also BRAIN, BRAIN CHEMISTRY.)

biofeedback A treatment technique in which people are trained to improve their health by using signals from their own bodies. Psychologists use it to help tense and anxious clients learn to relax. It is also used in the treatment of migraine headaches, tension headaches and many other types of pain, which can cause an overwhelming sense of depression, stress, hopelessness and anxiety, which in turn exacerbates the pain.

The word biofeedback was coined in the late 1960s to describe laboratory procedures then being used to train experimental research subjects to alter brain activity, blood pressure, heart rate and other bodily functions that normally are not controlled voluntarily. At the time many scientists looked forward to the day when biofeedback would give us a major degree of control over our bodies. Today research has demonstrated

that biofeedback can help in the treatment of many painful conditions and has shown that we have more control over so-called involuntary bodily functions than we once thought possible. But it has also shown that nature limits the extent of such control and psychiatrists, psychologists and other health care professionals, who rely on other techniques in addition to biofeedback, regard it as a tool in which relaxation is a key component in treatment of many disorders, particularly those brought on or made worse by stress. For patients, the biofeedback process acts as a kind of sixth sense, which allows them to "see" or "hear" activity inside their bodies.

Many clinicians believe that some of their patients and clients have forgotten how to relax, so feedback of physical responses, such as skin temperature and muscle tension, provides helpful information, as biofeedback aims at changing habitual reaction to stress that can cause pain and illness. As patients and professionals work together as a team, patients must examine their day-to-day lives to learn if they may be contributing to their own distress. They must commit themselves to practicing biofeedback or relaxation exercises every day. For information: Biofeedback Society of America, 10200 W. 44th Ave., #304, Wheat Ridge, CO 80033. Telephone: 303-422-8436.

biogenic amines As a chemical produced by the CENTRAL NERVOUS SYSTEM and involved in the functioning of the brain, their biochemical role is to assist in the transmission of the electrochemical impulses from one nerve cell to another. NOREPINEPHRINE, DOPAMINE and SEROTONIN are biogenic amines. (See also AMINES.)

bipolar depression In bipolar depression, also called MANIC-DEPRESSIVE disorder, a patient experiences mood swings of uncontrollable mania, alternating with episodes of severe depression.

During the manic or "high" state people may feel well and strong, go without sleep for long periods and plunge into vast, often foolish, undertakings in their personal or business affairs. They have abundant energy and grandiose notions, feel agitated and excited, and believe they are capable of any undertaking. Along with their constant talking, they exhibit an extremely elevated, ecstatic mood, inappropriate degrees of self-confidence, nonstop hyperactivity, increased sexual activity, a decreased need for sleep, heightened irritability and aggressiveness, and self-destructive, impulsive behavior, such as reckless spending binges.

When they're in a depressive phase, they have bouts of inertia and may suffer from any of the symptoms associated with major depressive disorder, as they feel "down," dispirited and sad. manic-depression usually develops into a chronic pattern of uncontrollable highs and lows. Frequently an episode of one type is followed immediately by a brief episode of the other type.

According to Dr. Lewis Judd, director of the National Institute of Mental Health, only one-third of the estimated two million Americans suffering from manic-depressive illness are receiving treatment that could help them lead normal lives. Judd said the low percentage of manic-depressives undergoing treatment is particularly disturbing because about 75% to 80% of such patients respond well to the mood-stabilizing drug lithium. Untreated, said Judd, manic-depressives live in misery, with a suffering that ravages their lives. Part of the problem of getting people into treatment is that patients and their families often do not recognize the symptoms of the disorder. (See also TREATMENT OF DEPRESSION, DRUG THERAPY, PSYCHOTHERAPY.)

United Press International. "Seek Help, Victims of Depression Are Urged." *The* [Hackensack, N.J.] *Record,* Nov. 29, 1988.

black Americans In the past it was an accepted belief that rates of affective disorders in black Americans were lower than in whites, and for many years black manic-depressive patients were frequently misdiagnosed as being chronic undifferentiated schizophrenics. As such, they were treated with major tranquilizers when lithium would have been the drug of choice.

More recent research, however, has found similar rates for blacks and whites. but even with this newer research, clinicians indicate that the frequent misdiagnosis of blacks with major affective disorders continues to be prevalent. "There is no doubt in my mind that the incidence of depression in the African–American community has been seriously under-reported," commented Dr. John T. Chissell, a family practitioner in Baltimore for 32 years, and chief consultant to the Positive Perceptions Group. "This under-reporting has been due to misdiagnosis because of failure to recognize the physical symptoms of depression, miscommunication between white clinicians and African–Americans, failure of the depressed individual to seek treatment, lack of availability of appropriate treatment in chronically underserved African–American communities, and the reluctance of providers or consumers of health care to consider and discuss the psychophysiological consequences of the doctrine of white supremacy on both whites and non-whites."

In "The Misdiagnosis of Black Patients with Manic Depressive Illness," Dr. Carl C. Bell, executive director of the Community Mental Health Council in Chicago, and Dr. Harshad Mehta wrote: "In addition to the management dynamics of patient care, there are obviously other factors leading to the misdiagnosis of black manic depressive patients. It is a common belief that manic depressive illness is clustered in higher socioeconomic patients. This belief tends to support the notion that black patients (frequently at the bottom of the socioeconomic totem pole) do not get affective illnesses."

The authors believe that these myths significantly contribute to the misdiagnosis of patients exhibiting euphoria, pressured speech, poor interpersonal relatedness, and hyperactivity. Bell and Mehta also wrote that the myths are rooted in a pervasive, covert form of racism, which has been institutionalized in psychiatry to the point that low prevalence and incidence of manic depressive illness in blacks is assumed. While the schizophreniform nature of manic depressive illness might understandably lead to a misdiagnosis of paranoid schizophrenia or catatonic schizophrenia, the repeated diagnosis of schizophrenia, chronic undifferentiated type, in a patient with manic symptoms is almost inconceivable. There is the distinct danger of "schizophrenia, chronic undifferentiated type" being used as "a catchall diagnosis, simply because blacks are of a lower socioeconomic class and of a minority ethnic background."

In a survey of the outpatient psychiatric clinic at Jackson Park Hospital in Chicago, Bell and Mehta found that black patients have similar prevalence rates of manic-depressive illness when compared to white patient populations. In addition, they noted that the demographic characteristics of this subgroup of manic-depressive patients were very similar to those found in white manic-depressive patients. Yet, when the past histories of these black manic-depressive patients were reviewed, there were large numbers of patients who had received a diagnosis of schizophrenia and, thus, were not considered for treatment with lithium.

In other research on depression and black Americans Dr. Billy E. Jones of the Department of Psychiatry, Lincoln Medical and Mental Health Center in the Bronx, New York, and his colleagues stated in "Major Affective Disorders in Blacks: A Preliminary Report" that ongoing studies on major affective disorders in blacks demonstrate that: (1) the delusions of the disorder in black Americans may be of paranoid quality as well as of a grandiose nature, and that the hallucinations may or may not be mood-congruent; (2) formal thought disorder, such as flight of

ideas, incoherence, loosening of association and illogical thinking may be present; (3) the diagnostic picture may be further complicated by alcohol and/or drug abuse; and (4) hostile and/or aggressive behavior may be manifested.

All in all—as things stand now— researchers collectively agree that there is an ongoing and pressing need for further epidemiologic, clinical and diagnostic studies of depression in black Americans.

Bell, Carl C. and Mehta, Harshad, "The Misdiagnosis of Black Patients with Manic Depressive Illness," *Journal of the National Medical Association*, 2:72(1980).

———,"Misdiagnosis of Black Patients with Manic Depressive Illness: Second in a Series," *Journal of the National Medical Association*, 2:73(1981).

Jones, Bill E. et al., "Major Affective Disorders in Blacks: A Preliminary Report," *Integrative Psychiatry*, 6(1988).

black bile In light of the fact that modern research gives much credence to decreased levels of brain chemicals (AMINES) as a cause of depression, it is of interest that the physicians of antiquity also thought in terms of a physiological imbalance as an explanation for melancholia. Hippocrates (?460-?377 B.C.) thought an excess of "black bile" in the body was the cause. (The word "melanchola" is Greek for black bile.) The black bile theory was an ancestor of modern chemical explanations. Today scientists are searching for more answers and a greater understanding of the chemical imbalances that cause episodes of depression.

blahs, the See BLUE DAYS.

blood tests Depressed persons taking lithium must be monitored regularly by blood testing in order to maintain a proper blood level. In testing the latter, the physician determines how much lithium a patient needs by taking a sample of blood from time to time to determine the amount of lithium present in the blood. This is called a lithium blood level. Measuring these levels helps the physician not only to select and maintain the most effective dose but also to keep the levels low enough to avoid a toxic dose. If one stops taking medicine for only a day, the lithium blood level will be lower than it should be for effective therapy. Because the blood level of lithium rises rapidly for a few hours after swallowing a lithium pill and then slowly levels off, having a blood test right after taking the drug can mislead the physician into thinking that the dosage is too high. To gauge the steady-state blood level accurately it is important to have blood drawn 12 hours after the last dose of lithium. Most patients take their nighttime dose of lithium and then come to the doctor's office the next morning to have a blood test before taking their first pill of the day.

A blood test that has potentially important therapeutic implications is one that appears to detect a difference between manic-depressive patients and those whose episodes are strictly depressive. Dr. Matthew Rudorfer, chief of the Clinical Research Unit, and Dr. William Potter, chief of the section on clinical pharmacology at the National Institute of Mental Health (NIMH), have worked with a group of patients diagnosed as either unipolar (depressive) or bipolar (manic-depressive). They have found that simply moving from a lying-down position to a standing one can produce measurable changes in blood levels of NOR-EPINEPHRINE, a NEUROTRANSMITTER that's one of the so-called stress chemicals.

"Many theories of depression have focused on norepinephrine," explained Dr. Rudorfer.

On the one hand, the original catecholamine hypothesis which was first published in 1965 posited a lack of sufficient norepinephrine presumably at certain critical locations in the brain to be associated with depression. On the other hand, other studies that have looked at that hypothesis

experimentally have concluded that norepinephrine as measured in the blood stream was actually elevated in many cases of depression. Our hypothesis was that it is probably not a simple matter of norepinephrine being up or down in depression but rather that there is some dysregulation of the norepinephrine system.

The purpose of the researchers' testing procedure was twofold: (1) to determine whether the resting level of norepinephrine in the blood is altered in depression, and (2) to address the question of possible dysregulation by monitoring the response of the norepinephrine system to a naturalistic stress procedure. Their procedure, as indicated above, was a well-controlled method of measuring norepinephrine in the blood, with the subject first in a lying-down position after a period of rest, and second, in a standing position for five minutes. This simple procedure enabled them to address both of the preceding questions.

"Despite the fact some studies have claimed that norepinephrine is elevated in depression we are finding a more complex answer," stated Dr. Rudorfer. "We find the test identifies a difference betwen bipolar and unipolar patients—namely bipolar depressed patients seem to have a lower resting norepinephrine level than do the healthy volunteers in the control group. On the other hand, most of our unipolar depressed patients are the same as controls, with a subset of unipolars having elevated norepinephrine."

The other aspect of the testing procedure concerned the dysregulation of norepinephrine. The researchers found bipolar and unipolar patients to be similar in their exaggerated response to the testing—that is, where healthy individuals will typically double their norepinephrine levels upon standing many depressed patients will show as much as a tripling of norepinephrine.

The initial studies on this ongoing blood test suggest that for most patients norepinephrine levels return to normal upon successful treatment. This has been seen most clearly when patients have been treated with electroconvulsive therapy. But the researchers stress that further research is needed and that all of their results so far have to be regarded as preliminary. They hope their studies will lead to the development of a clinically-useful test. The test is not presently available in most laboratories.

blue days The normal low periods and occasional down-in-the-dumps moods that everyone experiences. These emotional letdowns, transient feelings of unhappiness, and periods of sadness associated with unhappy events and failures are part of the ups and downs of everyday living. As Dr. Frederick K. Goodwin, director of scientific and intramural research at the National Institute of Mental Health (NIMH), stated in *The Washington Post:* "Almost everybody knows what it is like to wake up in the middle of the night and not be able to go back to sleep because of an obsessive worry or preoccupation; most everybody knows what it feels like to lose your capacity for pleasure; most everybody knows what it feels like to have slowed thinking, to be unable to concentrate because of some depressing thought."

These feelings fall into the class of normal emotional reactions, and people experiencing them are able to function despite the way they feel inside. The vast majority of people have this periodic feeling from which they emerge. But people with CLINICAL DEPRESSION have this feeling week after week. The symptoms last longer. There may be more of them simultaneously, and normal functioning may be impaired.

brain As the center of the CENTRAL NERVOUS SYSTEM the brain, which inlcudes all the higher nervous centers that receive stimuli from the sense organs, interprets and correlates these data, and is the source of motor impulses. The cerebrum, the biggest portion of the brain, controls all mental activity.

As one of the largest organs in the human body, the brain occupies the entire cavity enclosed by the skull and weighs roughly three pounds. It consists of approximately 12 billion cells and is composed of gray and white matter. The lower end of the brain stem is a continuation of the spinal chord. The brain is made up of neurons and supporting and nutritive structures, and through its complex chemistry and nerve cell network it controls almost all of the functions of the body.

Of the body's hundred or so known HORMONES, at least half are in the brain, many of which have been identified only in the past 10 years. Like NEUROTRANSMITTERS, neurohormones have wide-ranging effects through both the brain and the rest of the body. Transmission from one neuron to another is a chemical process, and there are numerous neurotransmitters (BIOGENIC AMINES) that carry the signals. These transmitters include DOPAMINE, NOREPINEPHRINE and SEROTONIN. Stimulation of a neuron results in an electrical transmission through the long cell axons that extend from the nerve cell.

In *From Sad to Glad* Dr. Nathan S. Kline likens the cell operation of the brain to a short-wave radio station, broadcasting and receiving coded messages. Tiny sacs of serotinin, norepinephrine and dopamine are attached to the nerve-cell axons and are released by electric disturbance as a signal pulses through. The action frees molecules that flash across the intervening SYNAPSE and sensitize the receiving apparatus of the adjacent cells. That, in effect, provides the "on" switch. The "off" switch is provided by a set of antagonistic compounds. Some of these compounds destroy the biogenic amines, and some merely block the amine action. Many depressions are attributed to amine deficits that damp down the circuits by locking switches in the "off" position. An amine surplus may produce the opposite manic effects. We can correct some of these malfunctions through drugs that adjust the biogenic amine levels up or down as the case may require.

Wina Sturgeon—author of *Depression: How to Recognize It, How to Treat It, and How to Grow From It* and a former victim of depression herself—explains the workings of the brain this way:

Brain cells transmit their data in the form of a minute burst of electricity. These electrical bursts are the method by which the brain processes information. Electricity in the brain acts pretty much like electricity anywhere else. It needs a conduit to get where it's supposed to go. When you want to guide an electrical charge, you use a wire to carry it. Electricity from the brain cells is directed to its destination by a "wire" made of a balanced chain of chemicals, the biogenic amines. When a brain cell is stimulated to fire by some external stimuli or by the thought processes, the charge travels to the cerebral cortex along this chemical chain. The composition of this conduit is so delicate that scientists have no accurate way of measuring the chemical amounts involved. But if that balance is upset even in the slightest, it will change the results of the electrical impulses by the time they get to the cerebral cortex.

Sturgeon goes on to explain that when this occurs the complete unit of thought or action may be distorted, since the cerebral cortex's power of judgment or discrimination, may be impaired. Consequently, if the cerebral cortex puts together a mixed-up signal, the organism acts upon it without question. Feelings of depression come as a direct result of the distortion of the thought process.

Dr. David D. Burns, a psychiatrist and author of *Feeling Good: The New Mood Therapy*, also compares the workings of the brain to electricity. Writes Burns: "The brain is essentially an electrical system. The nerves, or wires, communicate their electrical signals to each other by way of chemical messengers. If the nerves become depleted of these chemical messengers the wiring in the brain develops faulty connections. The result will be mental and emotional static, much like the music that comes out of a radio with a loose wire in the tuner. The emotional static would correspond to depression. Conversely, manic states are thought to be due to an excessive level of activity of these chemical messengers, leading to hyperactive nerve function." (See also BIOCHEMICAL FACTORS; BRAIN CHEMISTRY.)

Kline, Nathan S., *From Sad to Glad* (New York: Putnam, 1974).

Sturgeon, Wina, *Depression: How to Recognize It, How to Treat It, and How to Grow From It* (Englewood Cliffs, N.J.: Prentice-Hall, 1979).

Burns, David D., *Feeling Good: The New Mood Therapy* (New York: New American Library, 1980).

brain chemistry Although it is evident that some types of depression are accompanied by abnormalities in BRAIN function and that individuals with major depressive disorders often have too little or too much of certain neurochemicals that depression-relieving drugs seem to relieve, unanswered questions concerning the role of brain chemistry in depression still remain. We know through neurotransmitter research that imbalance in a neurotransmitter triggers an imbalance of a chemical in the HYPOTHALAMUS, leading to an imbalance of a hormone in the pituitary. This causes the adrenal glands to pump out too much CORTISOL, a hormone with wide-ranging physiological effects. Researchers at the National Institute of Mental Health (NIMH) believe that ongoing neurohormonal research could lead to a breakthrough drug that inhibits cortisol, preventing the syndrome of stress and depression that could otherwise ensue.

The tricyclic antidepressants appear to enhance the potency of the brain's mood messengers, although they do not cause an actual increase in the levels of these substances. We also know that the MAO inhibitors lead to an actual elevation of the levels of amine messengers in the emotional regions of the brain and that, as the brain becomes loaded with extra amounts of chemical transmitters, the presumed chemical amine deficiency is corrected. When it comes to lithium, the effects are less clearly understood, but some researchers theorize that lithium stabilizes the chemical-messenger levels, so that cyclic oscillations in amine concentrations are less apt to occur. L-TRYPTOPHAN, which is still being researched extensively, is used by the brain in the synthesis of one of the chemical messengers. (See also BIOCHEMICAL FACTORS.)

brain imaging Up until the late 1970s the brain was largely inaccessible to researchers interested in the origins of mental illness. Scientists such as Dr. Herbert Pardes, vice president for health sciences, dean of the Faculty of Medicine, and professor and chairman of the Department of Psychiatry at Columbia College of Physicians and Surgeons, asked "How could we get under the hood and study the engine?" Now that question is being answered through brain imaging (neuroimaging, a powerful technique that provides unprecedented looks at the living, working brain and allows researchers and neuroscientists to study computer images of the brain's structure and certain brain functions, both in health and in disease.

Previously, investigators had to base their hypotheses on an indirect study of the brain's activities or, in some situations, use an ELECTROENCEPHALOGRAM (EEG), a technique that records the brain's electrical activity with electrodes pasted on the scalp. This technology is the oldest and simplest brain imaging instrument.

Today, however, such imaging techniques as CT scan (COMPUTERIZED AXIAL TO-

MOGRAPHY), MRI (MAGNETIC RESONANCE IMAGING), PET SCAN (POSITRON EMITTING TOMOGRAPHY), SPECT (SINGLE PHOTO EMISSION COMPUTERIZED TOMOGRAPHY) and BEAM (BRAIN ELECTRICAL ACTIVITY MAPPING) allow researchers to visualize structures and activity deep within the brain and study the brain's structure, metabolism, blood flow, neurochemistry and electrical activity. It is the hope of researchers that in the future the growing availability of brain imaging will facilitate early diagnoses of disorders so physicians can start treating patients in the initial stages of an illness.

Romney, Elizabeth, "Breaking Through," *NARSAD Research Newsletter* (Spring 1989).

broken heart syndrome Centuries ago Shakespeare wrote in *Macbeth*: "Give sorrow words; the grief that does not speak, whispers to the o'erfraught heart and bids it break." Today studies indicate that the health of the sorrow-stricken can be weakened by intense emotional anxiety and that illness and even death can become a great likelihood in unresolved grief. (See also GRIEF, CAUSES AND EFFECTS OF.)

bulimia A major psychiatric eating disorder that is often associated with depression. It is believed to be a disorder with emotional, not physical roots. Risk factors for its development are unclear, but having a family member with ANOREXIA or bulimia and a possible family history of affective disorder or substance abuse appears to be a risk factor. Persons affected by it are usually depressed. For example, one survey on eating disorders reported by Glen Evans and Dr. Norman L. Farberow in *The Encyclopedia of Suicide* showed 60% of the women studied reported feeling depressed most of the time.

According to another study conducted by Dr. William Yates, a University of Iowa College of Medicine assistant professor of psychiatry, and other UI researchers, nearly two-thirds of the 30 patients with bulimia nervosa they studied had other problems in addition to the eating disorder. The most common problems that accompanied bulimia were depression, substance abuse or some form of personality disorder.

Bulimia is defined by the DIAGNOSTIC AND STATISTICAL MANUAL OF MENTAL DISORDERS (DSM-III-R) as follows: (1) recurrent episodes of binge eating (rapid consumption of a large amount of food in a discrete period of time); (2) a feeling of lack of control over eating behavior during the eating binges; (3) regularly engaging in either self-induced vomiting, use of laxatives or diuretics, strict dieting or fasting, or vigorous exercise in order to prevent weight gain; (4) a minimum average of two binge-eating episodes a week for at least three months; (5) persistent over-concern with body shape and weight.

Generally the victims are of college age or in their teens. Occassionally, however, they are younger. Ninety-five percent to 98% are female, usually single, white, ambitious, educated and middle- or upper-class.

According to Evans and Farberow, bulimics also subject themselves to other serious side effects that range from ulcers to hernias, dehydration, stomach rupture and disturbance of the blood's chemical balance (which could result in heart attacks). The obsession with food is similar to an addiction to alcohol and generally ends in dominating the young person's life.

A combination of pharmacotherapy and psychotherapy probably affords the best chance of improvement for many eating-disorder patients. In discussing pharmacotherapy in "Anorexia and Bulimia" Dr. Yates reports that pharmacotherapeutic approaches to treatment of eating disorders appear to be more helpful for bulimia than for anorexia. Both tricyclic antidepressants and monoamine oxidase inhibitors have shown some effectiveness and a decrease in binging and vomiting behaviors. The mechanism of action in antidepressants for eating disorders is unknown, although most patients who im-

prove with medication report a decrease in carbohydrate craving, resulting in fewer binging episodes. Up to 30% to 40% of bulimics may experience complete remission of binging with tricyclic antidepressants. The use of antidepressants in bulimic patients requires caution, however. Prudent management includes monitoring of electrolytes and obtaining baseline electrocardiograms during tricyclic administration.

Evans, G. and Farberow, N., *The Encyclopedia of Suicide* (New York: Facts On File, 1988).

Yates, William R. and Sieleni, Bruce, "Anorexia and Bulimia," *Primary Care*, 4:14 (December 1987).

bupropion hydrochloride (Wellbutrin)
An antidepressant that is chemically unrelated to tricyclic, tetracyclic or other known antidepressant agents.

The neurochemical mechanism of the antidepressant effect of bupropion is not known. It does not inhibit monoamine oxidase. Compared to the classic tricyclic antidepressants, it is a weaker blocker of the neuronal uptake of SEROTONIN and NOREPINEPHRINE. It also inhibits the neuronal reuptake of DOPAMINE to some extent.

At this writing, physicians considering Wellbutrin for treating depression must be well aware of the fact that the drug may cause generalized seizures with an approximate incidence of 0.4%. This incidence of seizures may exceed that of other marketed antidepressants by as much as fourfold. This relative risk is only an approximate estimate because no direct comparative studies have been conducted. The 1990 *Physicians Desk Reference* states that the effectiveness of Wellbutrin in long-term use, that is, for more than six weeks, has not been systematically evaluated in controlled trials. Therefore, the physician who elects to use Wellbutrin for extended periods should periodically reevaluate the long-term usefulness of the drug for the individual patient.

The drug is contraindicated in persons with

a seizure disorder. It is also contraindicated in people with a current or prior diagnosis of BULIMIA or ANOREXIA NERVOSA because of a higher incidence of seizures noted in such persons treated by the drug. In addition, taking Wellbutrin and a MAO inhibitor at the same time is contraindicated. At least 14 days should elapse between discontinuing a MAO inhibitor and beginning Wellbutrin. Adverse reactions commonly encountered with Wellbutrin can include agitation, insomnia, dry mouth, headache/migraine, nausea/vomiting, constipation and tremor.

Burton, Robert An English churchman and academician who spent more than 20 years compiling *The Anatomy of Melancholy*. In this work, more than 500,000 words in length, he wrote of the omnipresence of depression, quoting the ancient Greeks and Romans that depression in their world was so common scarcely one in a thousand persons was free of it.

Burton himself was a victim of depression who took refuge in work in an effort to avoid his melancholy. In one part of his volume he wrote: "We call him melancholy that is dull, sour, lumpish, ill-disposed, solitary, any way moved, or displeased. And from these melancholy dispositions no man living is free . . . None so well composed but more or less some time or other he feels the smart of it."

In another part he wrote:
I'll change my state with any wretch,
Thou canst from gaol or dunghill fetch;
My pain's past cure, another hell,
I may not in this torment dwell.
Now desperate I hate my life,
Lend me a halter or a knife,
All my griefs to this are jolly,
Naught so damn'd as melancholy.
Burton also listed foods and veverages his readers should abstain from because they presumably could cause melancholy. His warnings included beef, fowl, venison, milk products, fish, most fruit and vegetables, spices, grains, strong drinks and beer.

BuSpar See BUSPIRONE HCI.

Buspirone HCI (BuSpar) A tranquilizer that, when first approved for use by the Food and Drug Administration in 1986, appeared to be a major advance over Valium and other tranquilizers. Later it got mixed reviews from psychiatrists who prescribed it.

In clinical trials BuSpar (whose generic name is buspirone) was considered to be as effective for treating anxiety as the BENZODIAZEPINES, and clinicians considered it a positive advance because it did not have some of the side effects of other tranquilizers. For instance, it caused far less drowsiness than other tranquilizers and did not produce physical dependency in patients after prolonged use. It was also considered safer to take in conjunction with alcohol because it did not exacerbate the effects of alcohol as the benzodiazepines did. Another plus was the fact that it appeared less likely to be overused because it did not give the patients a euphoric high. However, it can cause such side effects as dizziness, nausea, headache and lightheadedness.

After its first 20 months on the market some psychiatrists began having sharply differing opinions about it. Some continued to consider it a major advance because it does not have sedative effects or withdrawal symptoms. Others feel it has not lived up to its expectations, and that for many people it is not potent or as effective as the benzodiazepines.

Two psychiatrists who have conducted controlled clinical studies of BuSpar believe its chief value may be as a forerunner of a whole class of new anti-anxiety drugs. In an article in *The New York Times* (May 26, 1988) Dr. Karl Rickels, professor of psychiatry at the University of Pennsylvania medical school, said he finds BuSpar "not significantly worse than but certainly not better than" the benzodiazepines. "It's an important option to have but it's not replacing the benzodiazepines yet.

Dr. David Sheehan, professor of psychiatry at the University of South Florida in Tampa, called BuSpar "a laudable step in the right direction because it appears dramatically safer than the other tranquilizers." Although BuSpar's effectiveness has been questioned, Dr. Sheehan said, "We should not abandon the whole class of drugs, but should monkey with the molecule a bit to find a more potently active variant."

C

Cade, John An Australian physician (1912–1980) who introduced lithium into psychiatry in the late 1940s. Prior to this time, while researching disturbed behavior in MANIC-DEPRESSIVES, Cade injected guinea pigs with various substances (first with urine from manics, depressives, schizophrenics and normal subjects, and later with uric acid) to investiage the reaction of the guinea pigs and learn more about the manic-depressive state.

In order to control the potency of the uric acid Dr. Cade administered it in a solution of lithium salts. When he found this solution caused the injections to be less toxic he began injecting lithium alone. As he observed the sedated guinea pigs (that would normally kick and squeal when placed on their backs) lying there passively, he discovered that lithium had tranquilizing effects.

Dr. Cade then gave lithium to 10 manic patients, six schizophrenics and three chronic psychotic depressives. With the schizophrenics and depressives, he noted minimal results. But he saw a dramatic change and calming effect in the manics. He then documented his results with other patients with manic symptoms and announced in 1949 that lithium was an effective treatment for manic excitement.

Unfortunately, Cade's discovery coincided with reports in America of several deaths from the unrestricted use of lithium chloride as a salt substitute for cardiac patients. Four patients died and several developed toxic reactions. It was not known at that time that lithium can accumulate to dangerous levels in the body or that lithium has to be used with special caution in patients with cardiac disorders. As a result of these experiences lithium was virtually neglected in the United States until the early 1960s. Then, renewed interest in the compound led to extensive clinical trials and testing to determine how it could be used safely and effectively to treat psychiatric disorders. The Food and Drug Administration approved it for psychiatric use in 1969.

caffeine A behavioral stimulant of the CENTRAL NERVOUS SYSTEM that is found in tea, coffee, some soft drinks, cocoa, certain headache pills, diet pills and patent stimulants. Excessive ingestion of coffee may cause anxiety and insomnia. When taken in beverage form caffeine begins to reach the body tissues within five minutes. Peak blood levels are reached in about 30 minutes. It appears to increase stress and motivate intellectual performance in some individual;s while impairing it in others.

Canada According to Dr. Brian F. Shaw, psychologist-in-chief of the Toronto General Hospital, Canada is one of the leading countries in research on affective disorders. Much of Dr. Shaw's research focuses on the psychosocial aspects of depression and he has done extensive work on the use of COGNITIVE THERAPY with major depressive disorders. His research, which examines the stability of cognitive patterns in major depression, represents an effort to determine which cognitive aspects exist and are stable in clinical depression. The overall pattern of the results suggests that the cognitive assessment measures used in a major study supported by a grant from the Ontario Mental Health Foundation were specific to major depressive disorder, possess strong internal reliabilities and correlate well with both themselves and measures of the severity of depression. However, Shaw points out that the fact that the study identified stable components of cognition in persons who were previously depressed does not argue for a causal role of cognition in depression. It is possible that behavioral and biochemical aspects of persons who were depressed remain stable as well. There is further work to be done, and Shaw hopes the work he has done thus far will serve as an impetus for prospective research on cognition.

Dr. Shaw's colleague, Dr. Randy Katz at Toronto General Hospital, is researching the genetics of depression and MANIC-DEPRESSIVE disorder. Much Canadian research in this field is focused on two areas: first, the mode of inheritance of manic-depressive illness, with the use of molecular biological techniques to detect and localize major genes; and second, the ways in which familial predisposition and environmental inuslts combine to produce depressive disorder.

Dr. Katz's studies have shown: (1) that depressive disorders are more common in the relatives of depressed probands than in the population at large; and (2) that there is compelling evidence that the familial aggregation of bipolar disorder and severe unipolar depression is at least partly due to genetic factors. However, the evidence concerning nonendogenous depression is less clear and family environment probably plays a stronger role.

At the University of Western Ontario, Dr. Ian H. Gotlib has done interesting work, along with his colleagues, on memory deficits in victims of depression. In the past other investigators have reported depression-associated deficits in memory functioning, but have not differentiated between depressed and non-depressed subjects with respect to their memory function. By comparison Dr. Gotlib's work has been designed to address methodological limitations of previous investigations in this area and to examine potential depression-associated deficits in sensory and short-term memory processing in a single sample of subjects. In a study he conducted 20 depressed and 20 nondepressed subjects participated in two tasks, designed specifically to asses the two memory processes most likely to be impaired in depressed individuals. The first task examined the possibility that depressed persons will exhibit impairment in a memory process labeled variously as the "visual information store," "iconic memory" and "sensory memory." The second task was selected to assess retrieval and short-term memory functioning. The results of this study suggest that whereas sensory memory is intact in depressed individuals, short-term memory processing is impaired as the depressed subjects experienced difficulty with the retention of material, likely owing to impaired rehearsal ability (with maintenance rehearsal being the term for those activities aimed at achieving permanent storage in memory). In summing up this study, Dr. Gotlib stated that further work is necessary to more fully explore the proposed rehearsal hypothesis.

Another area of research receiving attention in Canada is the neurobiology of time. In pointing out that this subject has major implications in our understanding of the pathophysiology of depression, Dr. Meir Steiner, professor of psychiatry and biomedical sciences at McMaster Psychiatric Unit at St. Joseph's Hospital in Hamilton, Ontario wrote in *The neurochemistry of Mood:*

Circadian rhythms are built into all living organisms. In mammals, the suprachiasmatic nucleus is probably the brain's timekeeper, and the relationship of this center to visual pathways and to the entire retinal-hypothalamic-pineal axis, is especially significant in health and in disease. It is now known that the circadian clock is controlled by genes and proteins and is influenced by neurotransmitters, neuromodulators, and neuropeptides. External factors such as light also influence biological clocks in a profound way. Thus, it is hoped that increased knowledge about the nature of the clock will lead to better understanding of dysregulated or disrupted rhythms which cause depression and will also lead to the development of new chronotherapeutic interventions. It has already been suggested that lithium may control mania by resetting the circadian clock.

Neuroendocrine investigation of depressive illness is another active field of investigation. Still other areas of prime importance in Candaian research include depressive disorders in children and adolescents; the social behavior of depressed children; the clinical status and emotional adjustment of children of depressed mothers; depression and marital functioning and interaction; depression in pregnancy and the postpartum; and depression in old age.

In the WHO COLLABORATIVE STUDY ON STANDARDIZED ASSESSMENT OF DEPRESSIVE DISORDERS, Metropolitan Montreal was one of the five areas used: (1) to develop and test simple instruments for clinical description of depressive states; (2) to examine with these instruments a series of "average" depressive patients in different cultures; and (3) to set up a network of field research centers. Metropolitan Montreal is characterized by a rapidly increasing urban population. Two psychiatric facilities took part in the identification and selection of patients for the study: the Doublas Hospital and the Department of Psychiatry of the Montreal General Hospital. A major characteristic of this research setting was the distinction between population groups on the basis of mother tongue. While the proportion of bilingual individuals is increasing, it is still usual for French-speaking and English-speaking residents to seek medical care in different services and facilities. Therefore, any series of patients selected for study at a predominantly French-speaking or predominantly English-speaking facility is bound to be unrepresentative of the area population. Since the two facilities participating in the present study

were predominantly English-speaking, it could be assumed that the patients were not representative of all those receiving psychiatric care in Metropolitan Montreal. However, the researchers believe that on the whole the patients could be considered as demographically fairly "typical" of the English-speaking segment of the patient population. (See also Appendix 1, "WHO Collaborative Study on Standardized Assessment of Depressive Disorders," tables)

Colby, C.A. and Gotlib, I.H., "Memory Deficits in Depression," *Cognitive Therapy and Research*, 12:6(1988).

Dobson, K.S. and Shaw, B.F., "Cognitive Assessment with Major Depressive Disorders," *Cognitive Therapy and Research*, 10:1(1988).

McGuffin P. and Katz, R., "The Genetics of Depression and Manic-Depressive Disorder," *British Journal of Psychiatry* (in press, 1989).

Steiner, M., "The Neurochemistry of Mood," *Psychiatric Journal of the University of Ottawa*, 14:2(1989).

Sartorius, N. et al., *Depressive Disorders in Different Cultures* (Geneva: World Health Organization, 1983).

cancer A malignant tumor of potentially unlimited growth that expands locally by invasion and systemically by metastasis. Some professionals state that in the early weeks, months or even years of tumor development, mental symptoms may be the only clues. They advise that anyone who experiences depression without a history, an abrupt personality change or a weight loss of more than 20 pounds should be evaluated for cancer.

In linking cancer and depression some of the professionals have theorized for years that depressed people are at a higher risk. Some have believed that some cancers might actually be caused by grief and other stresses simply because any strong emotional stress brings about chemical changes in the body. For instance, researchers have pointed out that an over-allotment of corticosteroids diminishes our natural immunity to illness, especially illnesses caused by viruses, and many forms of cancer are thought to be viral in origin.

Now all of this thinking is undergoing a change, according to researchers from the national Institute on Aging's Gerontology Research Center in Baltimore. In a study of more than 6,000 men and women the researchers found the results contradicted some early findings that depressed people are at a higher risk for getting cancer.

The study, which was conducted from the early 1970s to the mid-1980s, followed up on data from the national Health and Nutrition Examination Survey. For the study the researchers used personality measures to gauge depressive symptoms in more than 6,000 healthy men and women between the ages of 25 and 75 and then tracked down subsequent cancer deaths or hospitalizations for cancer.

The results showed similar rates of cancer and cancer deaths among those who had depressive symptoms and those who did not. From 9% to 10% of both groups developed cancer. About 4% of both groups died of cancer.

In an editorial accompanying the report of this study in the *Journal of the American Medical Association* in September 1989, Bernard H. Fox of the Boston University School of Medicine said: "Most of the earlier studies suffered from faulty design, small samples, failure to adjust for confounders, and a number of biases."

Added to this a researcher, who earlier found a link between depression and cancer in a 20-year study of 2,000 middle-aged men who were initially healthy, said this latest study and other recent evidence concinced him that depression did not increase the risk of cancer.

Evans, Glen and Farberow, Norman L., *The Encyclopedia of Suicide* (New York: Facts On File, 1988).

Kong, Dolores, "No Higher Cancer Risk for Depressed," *The* [Hackensack, N.J.]

Record (special from *The Boston Globe*), September 1, 1989.

carbamazepine (Tegretol) An anticonvulsant used to treat depression. According to Dr. Robert M. Post, chief, Biological Psychiatry Branch, National Institute of Mental Health (NIMH), who has worked with the drug, some 60% of manic-depressives who cannot tolerate lithium appear to do well on carbamazepine, sold as Tegretol. Patients who have many cycles during a year appear to do less well on lithium and better on carbamazepine.

According to Post, it looks as though three different indicators of poor response to lithium actually predict better response to carbamazepine. In an article in *Currents in Affective Illness*, Post discussed studies conducted on carbamazepine in mania and depression.

In a study of 17 acute manics cited in the article the researchers saw good effects of the drug in 12 of the 17.

When the researchers looked at the 12 good responders, compared to the seven manic patients who were partial responders or nonresponders to the drug, it turned out that the best responders were: (1) more severely manic to start out with; (2) also more dysphoric (they had higher depression ratings during mania); and (3) more rapid cycling in the year prior to NIMH admission, with an average of seven episodes in the year prior to admission, compared with less than three over the same period for the nonresponders. These three aspects, which tend to go with poor lithium response—severity, dysphoria and rapid cycling—seemed associated with a better response to carbamazepine.

Post, Robert M., "Carbamazepine (Tegretol) and Affective Disorders," *Currents in Affective Illness*, 5:2(1986).

Post, Robert M. et al., "antidepressant Effects of Carbamazepine," *American Journal of Psychiatry*, 143:1(January 1986).

Catapres See CLONIDINE.

catatonia Literally, a state of lowered tension. The term was used by KARL KAHLBAUM in 1874 to name a clinical condition, which was later absorbed by EMIL KRAEPELIN into his subtypes of dementia praecox and which later still became the 20th century diagnostic category of catatonic schizophrenia. Characterized by an apparent lack of responsiveness to the point of near stupor and either muscular rigidity or the "waxy flexibility" of the musculature in which, if placed in one position, the person will stay that way until moved to another. It is now recognized that catatonia is a clinical syndrome seen in association with affective disorders, organic mental syndromes, schizophrenia and some neurological diseases. Since the advent of modern antipsychotic medications, it has been diagnosed much less frequently, due to either the masking of symptoms or the aborting of a catatonic state by the medications.

causes of depression In adults the broad causes for depression have many ramifications and need not be related to any particular life experience. In fact, a combination of factors can be involved in the onset of a depressive disorder, so the causes are often interrelated.

At New York Hospital-Cornell Medical Center Dr. Gerald R. Klerman, associate chairman for research and professor of psychiatry, has researched the hypothesis that there may be a gene/environmental connection to the rates of depression and its age distribution in the United States.

According to Dr. Klerman, while most discussions of possible environmental influences focus on psychosocial factors, the possibility that depression might be caused by BIOLOGICAL FACTORS, such as viral agents, or by some environmental substance or nutritional change should also be considered. "The environmental risk factors could be biological including changes in nutrition, the possible role of viruses, or the effects of an unknown depressogenic chemical agent in

the water or air," suggests Klerman. "Other environmental risk factors could be nonbiological."

As far as genetics are concerned, research over the past decade strongly suggests a genetic link to depressive disorders and indicates that depression can run in families. Bad life experiences (such as a serious loss, chronic illness, difficult relationships, midlife crises, financial problems, career setbacks, marital problems, frustrations, disappointments or any unwelcome change in life patterns) can also trigger a depressive episode.

People who have low self-esteem, who consistently view themselves and the world with pessimism, and who are readily overwhelmed by stress, are also prone to depression. Other personality traits that increase the chances of becoming depressed are overdependence, introversion, and excessive need for approval, feelings of uselessness and the inability to live up to expectations.

Partly because of experience with drugs that are effective against depression, it has become clear that severe depression can result from abnormalities in BRAIN CHEMISTRY and a shortage of certain natural chemicals in parts of the brain (see BRAIN).

Depression is often associated with alcoholism. It may be a reason for drinking if depressed individuals consume alcohol for its euphoric effect and the feeling of confidence it can induce. On the other hand, it can be caused by drinking because prolonged drinking almost always leads to depression and a deterioration of mood as soon as the "high" wears off.

In some cases a main cause of depression can be withdrawal from alcohol use, and in these post-withdrawal states individuals sometimes attempt suicide. A withdrawal from drugs, such as cocaine, may also cause a syndrome like depression.

Center for Cognitive Therapy See BECK, DR. AARON; COGNITIVE THERAPY.

central nervous system Consists of the BRAIN and spinal cord and is associated with an extensive network of peripheral nerves. Together they control the action of the entire body. Sometimes the central nervous system is compared to a communications system in which the brain is the main switchboard, the spinal cord the main trunkline and the peripheral nerves the various plug lines that carry nerve impulses to and from the central system.

Along with the endocrine glands, the central nervous system coordinates much of the biochemical activity we need to live. Hormones, the chemicals produced by the endocrine glands, play their role by circulating in the cardiovascular system. Prominent among the chemicals used in brain function are the biogenic amines, which serve as neurotransmitters at crucial juncture points in the nervous system. These biogenic amines have an important role in allowing our brain to function so we can think and reason. When too much or too little of these amines are available, the resultant imbalances lead to symptoms in the areas of thought, behavior and emotion. Depression is one of the disturbances that can result from such imbalance. (See also BIOCHEMICAL FACTORS; BRAIN CHEMISTRY.)

ceremonies See FUNERALS.

change-of-life depression See MENOPAUSE.

child abuse Parents inclined toward child abuse often waver between being overly attentive and demonstrative or threatening and abusive. This is confusing and depressing to children since the children don't know where they stand or what to expect from one day to another.

As most youngsters want to please their parents and feel loved and wanted, they can easily grow lonely and isolated when they sense they have lost their parents' love. Along with fostering depression and low self-esteem this experience causes them to feel frightened, neglected and anxious. Some wonder if they are responsible for the way their parents act and, when this happens, they can even blame themselves for the problems that cause their parents' abusive actions. When all of these feelings are put together it is understandable that abused children are at risk for depression.

childhood bereavement See BARR-HARRIS CENTER FOR THE STUDY OF SEPARATION AND LOSS DURING CHILDHOOD: BEREAVEMENT: GRIEF: LOSS.

childhood depression Normal behaviors vary so much from one childhood stage to another that it sometimes is difficult to know whether a child is suffering from depression or just going through the normal ups and downs of growing up. Also, temporary interludes of depression are just as common among children as adults. But until now depression in children and infants has been vastly under-identified and untreated, especially when depressive symptoms are mixed with other types of behavior, such as hyperactivity, delinquency, school problems or psychosomatic complaints.

Today, however, specialists agree that children experience depression, and that if a child's behavior changes and his moods seem to shift, a closer examination of his thinking and functioning may well reveal underlying depression. Child psychiatrists also report an increasing number of cases, sometimes in children too young to talk. In fact, in *Why Isn't Johnny Crying?* the authors say that from three to more than six million American children suffer from depression.

Most childhood depression is not caused by a single precipitating incident or factor, but is usually associated with a child's general circumstances in life, genetic vulnerability, a biochemical disorder and ongoing environmental stresses. The loss of love or attention from someone on whom a child is dependent for care and nurturance may precipitate a depressive episode, whether the loss is caused by the death or the prolonged absence of the beloved person.

In some cases, the caretaker may remain physically present but withdrawn emotionally from the child and such depreciation and rejection of the child by a caretaker can also be important factors in many cases of childhood depression.

Children identified as especially at-risk for depression include those of manic-depressive parents or of parents hospitalized for a chronic physical illness. Hospitalized children, particularly those with a chronic illness, are also at risk. Still another precipitating factor is the effect an adult's bad moods or negative emotions can have on children. When a child is exposed to negative emotions (such as anger or heated arguments) the child can experience confusing and conflicting emotions, even though the adult's bad mood or negative emotion is directed toward someone else rather than the child.

There are definite common symptoms and signs by which a parent can recognize depression in a child. It may be indicated if symptoms similar to those seen in depressed adults continue for several weeks. In cases of severe depression children, like adults, may experience feelings of hopelessness and despair and harbor suicidal thoughts. Other symptoms are weeping; bed-wetting; lack of interest in and enthusiasm for participating in any activity; withdrawal from (or fighting with) playmates and friends; excessive dependency on a loved adult; restlessness; difficulties with school and homework; mood shifts; behavioral problems with periods of irritability, rage, aggression and destructive impulses; and inertia and listlessness—for example, sitting dazed in front of a TV for hours, with no interest in or recall of what he or she is watching.

As with most problems in childhood development early identification of depression is essential since untreated childhood depression may lead to problems in adolescence and adult life. Loving support and understanding is always recommended when a child exhibits occasional bouts of sadness and unhappiness, but at those times parents should also examine the child's present lifestyle and try to determine how stresses, separations and the kinds of background feelings the child is exposed to might be changed. A parent should consult a specialist if a preschool child acts weepy, sad, restless or irritable for as long as a month at a stretch. When a child is in school the parent should compare notes with teachers if they notice slipping grades, a lack of interest in outside activities, a lowering of energy and periods of sudden, violent behavior.

Parental counseling and family therapy are commonly used methods for helping the younger depressed child. Children over eight years of age usually participate in family therapy. In some situations, individual treatment may be appropriate for older children. Medications, such as ANTIDEPRESSANTS or LITHIUM, can be an important treatment, too, especially for the more serious and recurrent forms of depression. (See also CAUSES OF DEPRESSION: COMMON SIGNS AND SYMPTOMS.)

McKnew, Donald H. et al., *Why Isn't Johnny Crying?* (New York: W.W. Norton, 1983).

Sturgeon, Wina, *Depression: How to Recognize It, How to Treat It, and How to Grow From It* (Englewood Cliffs, N.J.: Prentice-Hall, 1979).

chlordiazepoxide (Librium) A widely prescribed sedative-tranquilizer that contains a BENZODIAZEPINE derivative. It is prescribed to reduce simple and severe forms of tension, anxiety and fear. If it is used beyond the recommended dosage (or used with alcohol or other CENTRAL NERVOUS SYSTEM depressants) physical and psychological dependency and additive effects can develop. Overdoses can also result in diminished reflexes, drowsiness, confusion and even coma.

chromosome 11 See OLD ORDER AMISH STUDY.

chronic depression Like ACUTE DEPRESSION, chronic depression is a term that overlaps with some of the other various types and subtypes of the disorder. It is used to describe a condition that is characterized as arising gradually, with slowly progressing symptoms, as opposed to acute, a condition that quickly develops into a crisis. It can continue for an indefinite period of time, sometimes lingering for as long as two or more years, with ultimate remission.

chronic fatigue Depression is often associated with fatigue, a condition the *Harvard Medical School Health Letter* describes as a state of feeling too tired to begin or finish normal activities. Fatigue becomes chronic when it outlasts more than the few days or weeks that can be attributed to sleep loss, overwork or a case of the flu. It is a common symptom of chronic illness, but it may also exist as a condition by itself. Relatively little research has been done on chronic fatigue, but, as reported in the *Health Letter,* researchers at the Brooke Army Medical Center in San Antonio, Texas asked patients coming into the medical clinic on certain days to answer a questionnaire about symptoms that were a major problem in their lives. Over a thousand people completed the questionnaire, and a quarter of them identified chronic fatigue as one of the major problems. The symptom was more prevalent in women (28%) than in men (19%). For statistical analysis they were matched to 26 people without fatigue, and results from the two

groups were compared. In one of the comparisons, depression or some form of anxiety disorder was found in 80% of the subjects, as opposed to 12% of the matched controls without fatigue.

The investigators found a rather high rate of psychological distress in the patients. However, they could not uncover unsuspected medical conditions, and the few minor abnormalities brought to light did not point the way to therapy that would reverse the fatigue. After a year only about 28% of the people with fatigue spontaneously improved. But major diseases had not developed more often in the fatigue patients than in the controls, indicating that chronic fatigue, despite its persistence, was not necessarily a danger signal of things to come.

The Harvard Medical School Health Letter also described a research project conducted at the University of Connecticut Health Center that focused on 100 patients (65 were women and 35 were men) who had been experiencing fatigue for an average of 13 years. All went through medical examinations, laboratory testing and psychiatric interviews at the center's fatigue clinic. No abnormality could be found in nearly one-third. Five had a specific medical disorder capable of causing chronic fatigue. Two had a seizure disorder. Each of the others had sleep apnea, asthmatic bronchitis or polymyalgia rheumatica. A subsequent report indicated that four of the patients met the criteria for CHRONIC FATIGUE SYNDROME. In the remaining two-thirds the main diagnostic finding was depression.

Much remains to be learned about chronic fatigue. But research such as the foregoing seems to indicate that when persistent fatigue is the *only* symptom people have, a medical explanation is unlikely to be found. However, the symptom should receive a medical evaluation since constant fatigue that develops over weeks and months can be the forerunner of other ailments. Research also indicates that depression, anxiety and psychiatric and psychological disorders very commonly accompany chronic fatigue in some individuals.

Anon., "Chronic Fatigue—What Does It Mean?" *Harvard Medical School Health Letter,* 14:5(March 1989).

chronic fatigue syndrome (CFS) This is not quite the same as CHRONIC FATIGUE since in this syndrome fatigue is usually accompanied by other symptoms that may indicate a persistent viral illness. However, CFS is considered to have a direct connection to depression, because the majority of CFS patients describe themselves as depressed or anxious, though many point out that their depression and anxiety developed after the onset of CFS.

The U.S. Centers for Disease Control describes CFS as an illness characterized by debilitating fatigue and a group of related symptoms, including headache, sore throat, fever, weakness, lymph node pain, muscle and joint pains, memory loss and difficulty in concentrating. It is not a progressive disease, and for most people symptoms plateau early in the course of the illness and recur with varying degrees of severity for at least six months. At this writing CFS is a provisional diagnosis to be considered by a physician only after all other potential causes of illness have been reasonably excluded.

It is not known how many people have CFS because the illness cannot be diagnosed with certainty. In an effort to obtain better estimates of its frequency the Centers for Disease Control has initiated a CFS surveillance and follow-up system in four sites across the United States. Results of the findings will not become available until sometime in the 1990s, but it is expected that when they are available they will provide the first reliable estimates of the frequency of CFS in the general population. The illness can affect people from all walks of life and of any age—ranging from children to adults in their 50s and 60s. However, most patients who

have sought medical care are Caucasian women in their 30s.

For more than a century, there have been reports in the scientific literature of syndromes of chronic fatigue associated with a variety of other symptoms, but the etiology of these syndromes has remained unknown in spite of intensive search. Because of this history it seems unlikely that the illness now called CFS is a genuinely new illness.

Today there is a great deal of controversy regarding the role of psychological factors and psychiatric diseases in causing CFS. Many of the physical symptoms—headache, muscle aches, difficulty in concentrating and sleep disorders—are also characteristic of primary mood disorders. However, other symptoms—sore throat, fever, lymph node enlargement and joint pains—suggest an underlying physical illness. Some patients state that CFS began at points in their lives when they were under great psychological stress, suggesting that this may play a role in the illness.

No proven effective treatment for CFS exists at this time. There are some reported successes in small numbers of patients, with a wide range of treatments that include antiviral and immunomodulating drugs, vitamins, holistic remedies, diet modification and activity reduction. In persons who have significant depressive symptoms, low doses of ANTIDEPRESSANT drugs have the potential for producing significant improvement in these symptoms. Most experts recommend a regimen of balanced diet, adequate rest, physical conditioning and self-pacing physically, emotionally and intellectually.

Department of health and Human Services, *Chronic Fatigue Syndrome* (Atlanta: Public Health Service, Centers for Disease Control, February 1989).

Churchill, Winston A British statesman, soldier and author (1874–1965) known for his stirring oratory and energy and considered by some to be the outstanding public figure of the 20th century. In 1953 (the same year he was honored with a knighthood) he received the Nobel Prize in literature for both his writing and oratory.

A strain of depression ran through Churchill's family, and despite his honors and achievements, he, too, experienced periods of depression, an afflication he called "his black dog always waiting to bare its teeth at him." In a 1944 conversation with his friend and physician, Lord Charles Moran, Churchill is reported as saying "When I was young for two or three years the light faded out of the picture. I did my work, I sat in the House of Commons, but black depression settled on me."

While concealing his depression beneath a gruff exterior Churchill also experienced some of the phobias that can at times be characteristic of the illness. For example, he was afraid of leaning over a balcony. He didn't like to stand near the edge of a platform when an express train was passing through. And he disliked standing by the side of a ship and looking down into the water.

circadian rhythms The Latin-derived word "circadian" means "about a day." Thus circadian rhythms are internally driven rhythms of about 24 hours. Their existence has been recognized in plants since the 18th century, but the exploration of these mechanisms has greatly expanded during the past few decades. Because they are important adaptation devices that allow an organism to synchronize internal, or endogenous, biological and behavioral processes with each other and with cyclic changes in the external environment, researchers suggest that circadian rhythms may be associated with unipolar and bipolar disorders. They hypothesize that affective psychoses (including unipolar and bipolar illnesses) may be linked to the biological rhythms, which are out of phase with each other, or to failures in their synchronization with the external day-night cycle.

Dr. Frederick Goodwin of the National Institute of Mental health (NIMH) and his colleagues have supported the hypothesis that the cyclic nature of the affective disorders in humans may be tied to this condition in which biological rhythms or cycles, regulated by multiple "pacemakers" (or oscillators) in the different systems of our body, fail to be successfully entrained to external time or coordinated to each other. In normal people, this entrainment may be brought about by a circadian "master-pacemaker" or biological clock, whose function is to synchronize these mutually related rhythms to external time. The implications of this "circadian pacer" (or "desynchronization") hypothesis are not only that episodes of depression and manic-depression reflect desynchronized rhythms without an effective circadian pacer, but also that such episodes will regularly recur as, without an effective circadian pacer, these rhythms go in and out of phase with each other and the external, 24-hour day.

A battery-powered wristband device that monitors and records the activity of the wearer continuously over several days makes possible the continuous recording of the motor activity and rest cycles of MANIC-DEPRESSIVE patients.

In one of their studies Dr. Goodwin and his colleagues accumulated records of 10 manic-depressives for periods of one to two years through both phases of the illness. During mania the length and intensity of activity was much higher than during depression. The recordings revealed that during a manic episode the patient's daily activity occurred progressively earlier. Other studies of depressed patients have found abnormal increases in evening activity. These findings provisionally suggest, in mania, a phase advance or shortening of the daily activity cycle, and in depression, a phase delay. Within the 24-hour, steady cycle of the environment, a mania activity cycle would peak earlier and earlier over time, a depression cycle later and later. (See also BIPOLAR DEPRESSION: UNIPOLAR DEPRESSION.)

Corfman, Eunice, *Depression, Manic-Depressive Illness, and Biological Rhythms*

(Rockville, Maryland: Alcohol, Drug Abuse and Mental Health Administration, 1982; DHHS #82-889).

clinical depression The term "clinical" is a general term applied to a depression that lasts for more than a couple of weeks and with symptoms severe and lasting enough to require treatment. In addition to feelings, it can change behavior, physical health and appearance, academic and job performance and the ability to handle everyday decisions and pressures. It is manifested by more dramatic behavioral changes than NORMAL DEPRESSION, and it is a term that overlaps with major, unipolar or endogenous depression.

Some mental health experts suggest that the key feature of clinical depression is change in behavior and other aspects mentioned above; as it goes beyond the normal state, people do not function as usual. In *Depressive Disorders: Treatments Bring New Hope*, a 1986 publication of the National Institute of Mental Health (NIMH), Marilyn Sargent of the Office of Scientific Information of NIMH cites the example of the former man-about-town who loses interest in women and the once-social woman who becomes reclusive. Without treatment, the loss of interest in sex or food, the changes in sleep patterns or mood, or other symptoms experienced by clinically depressed people, may continue for months, even years.

Although some people have only a single episode of clinical depression in a lifetime, it is more commonly a recurrent disorder. The recurrent forms can require maintenance on medication to prevent new episodes from occurring. When a clinical depression becomes especially severe, delusions are not uncommon. (See also BIPOLAR DEPRESSION: MANIC-DEPRESSIVE: UNIPOLAR DEPRESSION.)

clonazepam An anticonvulsant marketed under the name Klonopin.

clonidine (Catapres) Clonidine is in common use as an antihypertensive medication that decreases the activity of central noradrenergic neurons. It has antimanic properties and alone or in combination with lithium may have advantages over neuroleptics in the acute stages of mania. Its main side effects include drowsiness, sedation and, in some cases, depression. These side effects do not limit the continuation of treatment, however, and it has not been consistently reported that the drug causes depression. Its efficacy and pitfalls continue to be investigated.
Giannini, A.J. et al., "Clonidine in Mania," *Drug Development Research*, 3(1983), 101-103.

clozapine (Clozaril) An atypical antipsychotic drug. Under investigation it proved to be an effective drug with few side effects. However, hope for it was dashed temporarily and its introduction to the U.S. market was delayed when it was noted that the drug produced damage to white-blood-cell (WBC) production. Later it was found that, if WBC counts are determined weekly and clozapine is stopped within seven days of developing a low WBC count, the WBC count will return to normal in approximately two weeks.

In 1982 the FDA rejected a proposal for the drug's approval and challenged the researchers working on it to design a study showing the drug was superior in efficacy to other antipsychotic drugs and that its benefit could outweigh its risk. Since then a multicenter trial conducted in the United States has demonstrated its clinical efficacy in patients who failed to respond to conventional neuroleptics. One of its greatest advantages is that there have been no cases of TARDIVE DYSKINESKIA (the abnormal facial movements that some neuroleptic drugs produce). In late 1989 the FDA approved it for marketing.
Zonderman, Jon, "Schizophrenia: The Postneuroleptic Era," *NARSAD Research Newsletter*, 2(Summer 1989).

Clozaril See CLOZAPINE.)

coca Any of several South American shrubs with leaves resembling those of the tea plant. The dried leaves contain alkaloids, including cocaine.

cocaine An alkaloid found in the leaves of the coca bush that the Peruvian Indians use as an anesthetic, mood drug, and stimulant and energizer for periods of sustained labor. It has also been associated with mystical rites that the Western world in the 1500s saw as dark magic and demon worship. Because of this the benefits from the drug were considered more an illusion of the devil than a medicinal remedy.

During the 1800s, however, Europeans began to view cocaine as a powerful though dangerous drug that could be used for either good or evil, and by the mid-1880s, when pure cocaine began to be sold in the United States, it was perfectly legal to purchase it and use it to sniff, smoke, inject, rub, eat or drink. People were advised it was safe, non-addictive and had no bad aftereffects. By the end of the 1800s it was a medical fad that was regarded as a tonic and cure-all for many ills, including depression.

In the early Sherlock Holmes stories, Sir Arthur Conan Doyle's fictional detective was addicted to using cocaine to help his depression. But in the later stories Holmes was cured of the habit after people learned of its dangers. Sigmund Freud was also a cocaine user and advocate at one point in his life. In *From Sad to Glad* Dr. Nathan Kline wrote of Freud: "For about three years he regularly dosed himself with cocaine to ward off depression and combat fatigue. He found the results magical and enthusiastically recommended the drug to a medical friend who suffered from a condition of chronic pain. The friend became an addict, and Freud was horrified at his inadvertent part in the affair. Thereafter he opposed not only cocaine but also any other drug that affected mental processes."

Though the early 1900s saw a decline in the use of cocaine, partially due to the federal law enacted against it, its widespread use was renewed in the last part of the 20th century. It is commonly used as a social drug, and in some situations it continues to be used to overcome depression.

When physical dependence occurs, the withdrawal symptoms that replace the feelings of euphoria and increased alertness can be serious depression (often in a more severe form), extreme fatigue and prolonged periods of restless sleep. Generally more cocaine will be needed to combat the depression. This can lead to a perpetuation of the habit.

cognitive behavior therapy (CBT) See COGNITIVE THERAPY.

cognitive therapy Cognitive therapy is based on the premises that: (1) people's emotions and behaviors are determined by how they view the world and interpret their experiences; and (2) depressed persons tend to think negatively about themselves, the world and the future.

The cognitive therapy of depression was developed by Dr. AARON T. BECK. It is a specific type of the broad class of therapies called "cognitive-behavioral" (also referred to as cognitive behavior therapy (CBT). Through the years it has attracted wide attention as an effective, short-term therapy modality for clinical depression. Its supporters believe that through it people can help themselves understand and eliminate the symptoms of depression and experience personal growth so they can minimize future episodes and cope with depression more effectively in the future. In some situations cognitive therapy and drug treatment are combined.

Cognitive therapy is based on three principles. First, all of our moods are created by our thoughts. Second, when we are feeling depressed our thoughts are dominated by a pervasive negativity. We perceive not only ourselves but also the entire world in dark, gloomy terms. We come to believe things really are as bad as we imagine them to be. Third, the negative thoughts that cause our emotional turmoil nearly always contain gross distortions. This twisted thinking is a major cause of our suffering.

In *Feeling Good–The New Mood Therapy*, Dr. David D. Burns who worked with Dr. Beck, states that 10 cognitive distortions form the basis of depression. The distortions he cites are: (1) seeing things totally in black-and-white categories; (2) regarding one negative event as a neverending pattern of defeat; (3) clouding your sense of reality by dwelling on a single negative detail; (4) feeling that positive experiences do not count; (5) jumping to conclusions and believing things will turn out badly; (6) exaggerating or minimizing the importance of things; (7) assuming your pessimistic feelings reflect the way life is; (8) directing "should" and "should not" statements and expectations to yourself and other people; (9) attaching negative labels, such as "I'm a loser/He's a loser" to yourself and others; (10) experiencing guilt because you see yourself as the cause of a negative event for which you were not primarily responsible.

In treating depressed persons cognitive therapists use a variety of strategies to help patients correct maladaptive beliefs and negative thought patterns so that, through more realistic and logical thinking, behavioral and mood changes are enhanced and people become less depressed and less vulnerable to future depression.

In one treatment strategy reported in the January 1990 issue of the *American Journal of Psychiatry*, Dr. John H. Greist, of the Department of Psychiatry at the University of Wisconsin, and his colleagues used computer-administered cognitive-behavioral therapy. For this strategy a study conducted by Greist compared the progress of 12 depressed people who received therapy from a computer, 12 who consulted a therapist and 12 who received no treatment during the experiment. For the computer therapy a program designed by Paulette M. Selmi, Ph.D., asked such questions as how long a person had felt depressed and which activities in a list made

the person feel better. It also asked about particular symptoms.

According to Greist, the computer therapy used in the study works best for people with only mild to moderate depression, and humans are needed to screen patients for this therapy and to step in if the computer fails to give adequate treatment. But in the experiment depressed patients who were treated by computer improved as much as those who consulted a human therapist.

Further research on computerized therapy is needed, and some members of the psychiatric community are somewhat skeptical about it. Dr. Selby Jacobs, professor of psychiatry at Yale School of Medicine and assistant chief of psychiatry at Yale-New Haven Hospital, has said that while computers might help psychotherapists, it is unlikely that it will ever replace them.

The University of Wisconsin researchers themselves emphasize that, though computer treatments may have a role to play in providing a part of effective, efficient and economical treatment, computer therapy must be used in the context of careful professional assessment and comprehensive management of patients. Further development of direct patient-computer treatment programs, subject to rigorous evaluations, is warranted.

Beck, Aaron T., *Depression: Causes and Treatment* (Philadelphia: University of Pennsylvania Press, 1967).

Beck, Aaron T. et al., *Cognitive Therapy of Depression* (New York: Guilford Press, 1979).

Burns, David D., *Feeling Good–The New Mood Therapy* (New York: New American Library, 1980).

Dobson, Keith S., "A Meta-Analysis of the Efficacy of Cognitive Therapy for Depression," *Journal of Consulting and Clinical Psychology* (in press, 1989).

Selmi, P., Klein, M., Greist, J. et al., "Computer-Administered Cognitive-Behavioral Therapy for Depression," *American Journal of Psychiatry*, January 1990.

Associated Press, "Computer Helps Cure

Depression," *New Haven Register*, January 30, 1990.

cohort effect While studying age groups affected by depressive disorders scientists have been struck by the early onset of the disease and the rise in SUICIDE among people born since 1940. In a February 12, 1986 *Washington Post* article, Sandy Rovner wrote that this phenomenon is officially known as "the cohort effect"—found in a specific group, or cohort, of people—determined in this case by year of birth.

Rovner reports that Dr. Elliot S. Gershon, of the clinical neurogenetics branch of the National Institute of Mental Health (NIMH), has found that not only depressive illness in general has increased, among those born since 1940, but also manic-depression, the most severe form. This is a development he considers "ominous."

Although research indicates that genetics can play a role in depression Dr. Gershon believes that this rapid change in rate (of both clinical depression and manic-depression) cannot be due to genetics. "Genes don't change that fast," he said. "But it can be familial. Indeed there is still a lot more illness in relatives of patients than in relatives of controls." Dr. Gershon concludes that the increase is "either a genetic/environmental interaction, or a cultural event which is peculiar to families already vulnerable to mood disorders."

In discussing the cultural or environmental factor that might account for the rise in youthful depression, Dr. Gerald L. Klerman of New York's Cornell University Medical College was quoted in *Newsweek* as saying: "Coming to maturity in the period from 1960 to 1975 seems to have had a profound adverse impact on the likelihood of depressive illness." The article goes on to point out that the period was marked by unprecedented social upheaval, suggesting that it may have sown the seeds of mass emotional disturbance—along with suicides, alcoholism and drug addiction. Klerman speculates that the turmoil signaled a NEW AGE OF MELANCHOLY spurred by the disruption of family ties and the loss of faith. However, he and other researchers do not rule out the possibility of biological causes, such as a new virus or changes in nutrition, since biology now looms ever larger in the study of depression.
Leerhsen, Charles et al., "Depression," *Newsweek*, May 4, 1987.

common signs and symptoms Not everyone who is depressed or manic experiences every symptom. Some people have a few while others suffer from many. Also, the severity of symptoms varies with individuals.

The main signs and symptoms are feelings of: apathy, indifference, anxiety, sadness, emptiness, hopelessness, hostility, helplessness, irritability, unworthiness, guilt, fatigue, restlessness, boredom, apprehension, pessimism, inadequacy, inertia, self-depreciation.

Other indications are constant negative thinking; downhearted periods that won't go away; lack of interest in or pleasure from job, family life, hobbies or anything else; loss of self-esteem; sleep problems such as insomnia, a need to sleep too much, night sweats and waking up at early hours; headaches and unexplained physical pains that don't respond to treatment; constipation; decreased appetite and weight loss (or a compulsion to overeat and weight gain); drug or alcohol abuse; frequent or unexplainable crying spells; changes in sexual habits and behavior; decreased powers of memory and concentration; inability to give or accept affection; thoughts of death or suicide (or suicide attempts.)

People who are manic-depressive show such symptoms as inappropriate elation; grandiose notions; increased talking, moving and sexual activity; disconnected and racing thoughts; extreme energy; poor judgment and disturbed ability to make decisions; and unsuitable social behavior.

Experts at the National Institute of Mental Health (NIMH) recommend that professional help be sought if some or all of the above-listed symptoms cause impairment in ordinary functions and grow too strong and last too long. Some specialists advise that if people suffer four or more of the signs and symptoms of depression for more than two weeks they may well be depressed and in need of treatment.

community mental health services A community mental health service is an organization, staffed by professional mental health specialists, that provides counseling and support for people suffering from depression and other emotional problems. Depending on the service or center the programs offered include diagnosis and treatment, emergency care, outpatient clinic care, social services, and referrals to hospital programs. Fees vary and often are on a sliding-scale basis. Services also vary at each center, and not all of the services listed above are available at each mental health center.

Not every community has a mental health service or center. But most geographical areas throughout the country have at least one organization that provides help—or referrals to help—for depression and other emotional problems.

Many universities and hospitals have mental health services, centers and clinics, and some community services and programs are available through governmental or nonprofit organizations. Typical mental health organizations to contact for help for depressives are adult mental health clinics, community counseling services, family services, youth services, and health and welfare councils.

To find the nearest service in your area check the ''Mental Health Services'' and ''Social Service Organizations'' listings in the yellow pages of your phone book. In addition, the front pages of county and city telephone directories provide a list (with phone numbers) of available community services.

Telephone directories also provide listings of city, township, county, state and United States Government numbers for information and referrals in the blue pages of Government listings or (in some cases) in the white pages under the name of the county, city, town or village—or under state and U.S. Government listings. Many public libraries maintain a file of local community service agencies. In Appendix 6 at the end of this volume you will find addresses to which you can write for directories of community mental health centers. You will also find a list of state-by-state mental health centers and regional referrals for the treatment of depression.

compassionate friends A self-help nonprofit organization offering friendship and understanding to bereaved parents. The purposes are to promote and aid parents in the positive resolution of the grief experienced upon the death of their child and to foster the physical and emotional health of bereaved parents and siblings.

A bereaved parent who contacts the national office will be responded to individually and, whenever possible, will be referred to the name, address and phone number of the closest local chapter. There are 600 chapters throughout the United States and each chapter develops its own resources, newsletters, libraries and community of caring people. Some chapters have established professional advisory committees consisting of local doctors, nurses, clergy, social workers, psychologists, funeral directors and others who are available as supportive resources for the chapter leaders and who may present educational programs to the groups. Membership in the chapters is open to all family members, and meetings that center around small, informal discussion groups provide an opportunity to become friendly with persons who are willing to talk about the death, openly share feelings and help one another put the pieces back together.

The Compassionate Friends was founded in 1969 in Coventry, England by Rev. Simon Stephens, an assistant to the chaplain in the Coventry and Warwickshire Hospital. Many children died each year in the hospital, and after the coincident deaths of two young boys, the boys' parents met by chance and a meaningful friendship developed. In their mutual grieving, they discovered that by listening to each other, by crying together if they chose and by understanding how each felt, their grief was lessened. They, together with other bereaved parents, asked Rev. Stephens to work with them in establishing an organization for bereaved parents. The Compassionate Friends was the result, and the first U.S. chapter was organized in Miami, Florida in 1972. The organization has no religious affiliation and depends upon voluntary contributions to cover operational costs on both the local and national levels. For information contact: Compassionate Friends National Headquarters at P.O. Box 3696, Oak Brook, Illinois 60522. Phone: 312-990-0010.

computerized axial tomography (CT scan)   A computerized series of narrow-focused X rays (sometimes referred to as CAT scan) that provide a means of visualizing the brain and picturing different planes of the head. This form of brain imaging can show internal tissues, and the computer builds an image of a thin slice of the body as if the body were sliced in cross section. The source of the X rays rotates rapidly around the body and a detector measures how much radiation passes through the patient.

Brody, Jane, "Personal Health," *The New York Times*, April 20, 1989.

computer treatment of depression   See COGNITIVE THERAPY.

convulsions   Involuntary spasmodic contractions of muscles that can arise during CENTRAL NERVOUS SYSTEM depressant withdrawal, or following a stimulant overdose.

Corey, Richard   A fictitious victim of depression and the subject of one of Edwin Arlington Robinson's famous poems exploring the paradoxes of human character and the frustration and pain of the human experience. In "Richard Corey" everyone in Corey's community believed Corey and the life he lived was the epitome of satisfaction and perfection until the depths of Corey's hidden depression caused him to take his life. The poem provides a perfect example of a victim of MASKED DEPRESSION.

cortex   The outer layer of gray matter of the cerebrum and cerebellum.

cortisol   A crystalline hormone of the adrenal cortex. Changes in the production of cortisol have been observed in depressed persons. Cortisol production generally follows a pattern of peaking in the early morning, leveling off during the day and reaching its lowest point in the early evening. Cortisol levels also increase when the body is exposed to stressful situations, such as extreme cold, or when an individual is feeling angry or frightened. In depressed individuals, the hormone peaks much earlier in the day than is normal and remains high all day. The high levels of cortisol may explain the sleep disturbances experienced during depressive episodes.

creativity   Depression seems to be an occupational hazard for many artists, writers, musicians and other creative people. In fact, according to Dr. Frederick Goodwin, scientific director of the National Institute for Mental Health, 38% of the Pulitzer prize-winning poets have met the criteria for manic depression.

In both the past and present, many creative artists have put their depressions to use, working through them to glimpse some larger truth about the human experience. Sylvia Plath's life and work appear to indicate that she drew on her own inner bleakness and death wishes to enhance her creative power. George F. Handel wrote his *Messiah* in less than a month during one of his manic states. Vincent Van Gogh produced many of his best works when he alternated between psychotic depression and episodes of euphoria. Ernest Hemingway, while writing his acclaimed novels, was hospitalized for depression. And Charles Schultz, the creator of the popular *Peanuts* comic strip who has suffered from depression, told the *San Francisco Chronicle*, "I suppose I've always felt that way—apprehensive, anxious, that sort of thing. I have compared it sometimes to the feeling that you have when you get up on the morning of a funeral." But drawing Linus, Snoopy and the other *Peanuts* characters has been palliative, stated Schultz.

The list of creative people who have experienced bleak depression and despair is a literal "Who's Who" of creativity: William Styron, Virginia Woolf, Ann Sexton, John Berryman, Robert Schumann, Feodor Mikhailovich Dostoevski, Edgar Allen Poe, Nathaniel Hawthorne, F. Scott Fitzgerald, Samuel Johnson, Issac Newton, Robert Lowell, William James, John Keats, Leo Tolstoy, Friedrich Nietzsche and Ludwig van Beethoven all suffered from depression.

In discussing depression and creativity, Dr. Kay Redfield Jamison, associate professor in the Department of Psychiatry at the Johns Hopkins University School of Medicine, who did a study ("Mood Disorders and Patterns of Creativity in British Writers and Artists"), pointed out that extremes in mood, thought and behavior—including psychosis—have been linked with artistic creativity for as long as man has observed and written about those who write, paint, sculpt or compose.

In her study of eminent British writers and artists Jamison found that virtually all subjects (89%) reported having experienced intense, highly productive and creative episodes that were characterized by increases in enthusiasm, energy, self-confidence, speed of mental association, fluency of thoughts, elevated mood and a strong sense of well-being. A comparison with DSM-III-R criteria for HYPOMANIA revealed that the subjects' mood and cognitive symptoms showed the greatest degree of overlap between intensely creative and hypomanic episodes, indicating that cognitive changes occurring during hypomanic states are critical to creativity. When the subjects were asked specifically about the importance of very intense feelings and moods in the development and execution of their work, 90% stated that such moods and feelings were either integral, necessary or very important. Jamison said that for writers and artists who draw so deeply on their lives and emotions for their work the wide range, intensity, fluctuation and variability of emotional experience brought about by mood disorders can work to advantage as well as disadvantage. The study indicated that the milder forms of hypomania may represent the more productive phases of affective illness.

In Jamison's study the artists and writers were asked whether or not they had received treatment and, if so, the nature of that treatment for a mood disorder. A very high percentage of the total sample, 38%, had been treated for an affective illness; three-fourths of those treated had been given antidepressants or lithium or had been hospitalized. Poets were most likely to have required medication for their depression (33%) and were the only ones to have required medical intervention (hospitalization, electroconvulsive therapy, lithium) for mania. Fully one-half of the poets had been treated with drugs, psychotherapy and/or hospitalization for mood disorders. The playwrights had the highest total rate of treatment for affective illness (63%), but a relatively large percentage of those treated (60%) had been treated with psychotherapy alone. With the exception of the poets, the subjects reported being treated for depression, not mania or hypomania.

In another study on creativity Dr. Nancy Andreasen of the University of Iowa College of Medicine and her colleagues found an exceptionally high rate of affective illness, especially bipolar, in their sample of writers from the University of Iowa Writers' Workshop.

The Iowa Writers' Workshop is the oldest and most widely recognized creative writing program in the United States. Students and faculty have included such writers as Philip Roth, Kurt Vonnegut, John Irving, Robert Lowell, Flannery O'Connor and John Cheever. Since well-known writers are brought in for a semester or two each year as visiting faculty members, they represent a reasonably valid cross section of contemporary American writers. In Andreasen's study (in which confidentiality about the subjects' identity was a condition for participation), a group of 15 successful creative writers was found to differ significantly from a group of 15 noncreative controls when both were examined for psychiatric symptoms and family history, using a structured interview and specifically defined diagnostic criteria. Seventy-three percent of the writers suffered from some form of psychiatric disorder as compared with 20% of the controls. The most common illness was affective disorder, which occurred in 67% of the writers and 13% of the controls. The two groups also differed significantly in family history. The primary relatives of writers had a 21.4% prevalence for any type of psychiatric illness, as compared with 4.4% among the relatives of controls.

The data from researchers such as Jamison, Andreasen and others support Aristotle's dictum that those who have been eminent in the arts have all had tendencies toward melancholia. The data also appeared to indicate that there is an association between genius and psychiatric disorder. In addition, the data suggest that there may indeed be a familial, perhaps genetic, pattern tending toward the development of both creativity and illness. Subsequent studies have substantiated that there is a close association between mental illness and creativity and that the type of mental illness is predominantly affective disorder, particularly bipolar illness.

In speaking of the effects of drugs on creativity Dr. Jamison stated that the short- and long-term effects of lithium, carbamazepine

and antidepressants on productivity and creativity remain unclear. Ongoing studies of lithium's effect currently conflict in their findings. For example, one study reported by L.I. Jud et al. in *Archives of General Psychiatry* found no effects of short-term lithium treatment on creativity in normal subjects; another using bipolar patients as their own controls, reported by E.D. Shaw et al. in *The American Journal of Psychiatry*, found substantial detrimental effects of lithium.

In summing up depression and creativity Andreasen wrote: "The question of the relationship between creativity and neuropsychiatric disorders has been discussed and debated for centuries. The roads to creativity are many, and they include both experiencing pain and tension and overcoming them."

Andreasen, Nancy, "Ariel's Flight: The Death of Sylvia Plath," *Journal of the American Medical Association*, 228:5 (April 29, 1974).

———, "Creativity and Mental Illness: Prevalence Rates in Writers and Their First-Degree Relatives," *American Journal of Psychiatry*, 144:10(October 1987).

Andreasen, N. and Canter, A., "The Creative Writer: Psychiatric Symptoms and Family History," *Comprehensive Psychiatry*, 15:2(March/April 1974).

Andreasen, N. and Glick, I., "Bipolar Affective Disorder and Creativity: Implications and Clinical Management," *Comprehensive Psychiatry*, 29:3(May/June 1988).

Jamison, Kay Redfield, "Mood Disorders and Patterns of Creativity in British Writers and Artists," *Psychiatry*, 52(May 1980).

Judd, L.I. et al., "The Effect of Lithium Carbonate on the Cognitive Functions of Normal Subjects," *Archives of General Psychiatry*, 34(1977), 355-57.

Shaw, E.D. et al., "Effects of Lithium Carbonate on Association Productivity and Idiosyncrasy in Bipolar Outpatients," *American Journal of Psychiatry*, 143(1986), 1166–69.

Richards, R.L. et al., "Creativity in Manic-

Depressives, Cyclothymes, and Their Normal First-Degree Relatives: A Preliminary Report," *Journal of Abnormal Psychology*, 97(1988), 281–88.

cross-cultural research According to Dr. Norman Sartorius, director of the Division of Mental Health of the World Health Organization in Geneva, Switzerland cross-cultural research into depression creates a bridge between the study of cultural change and the investigation of depression. Currently, this cross-cultural investigation is attracting the attention of scientists, clinicians and public authorities.

As cultures intertwine, certain diseases and disorders disappear or become so similar to others that there is no point in seeing them as separate. Others seem to assume universal importance and grow in numbers and the awareness of them. "Depression is the foremost of these, and a major health problem," says Sartorius. "There are estimates that there are at least one hundred million people in the world who suffer from depressive disorders amenable to treatment."

However, results obtained in cross-cultural research have so far uncovered more questions than they have answered. Prevalence and incidence figures vary from culture to culture, and the differences are often enormous. Sartorius points out that studies of the incidence and prevalence of depression in African countries, for example, reported on the whole that depression was rare until those countries reached political independence. When this was achieved, it might have become possible for a native to be given a diagnosis of depression earlier reserved for the colonizers. In studies done after 1957, when many of these countries did become independent, rates of depression became similar to those in some other parts of the world.

Chinese in Indonesia have more depression than the Indonesians. In Argentina, the Indians of the Alto-Plano have more depression than those from villages. Western immigrants into Israel have more depression than those migrating from the Orient.

There are differences in the clinical picture of depression in different cultural settings, too. "These differences have been most frequently reported in the instance of somatization," pointed out Sartorius.

Somatization has been reported as more prominent in people from lower social classes, in patients in certain developing countries and in a variety of cultural groups and subgroups. Many of the differences on the dimension of somatization and on others in the symptomatology of depressive disorders proved on closer investigation to be the result of nosocomial factors. The studies which WHO has undertaken on samples of patients in Iran, Japan, Canada, Switzerland, India and others also seem to confirm this, showing that there are differences in the clinical pictures among the groups studied but that on the whole the similarities are more in evidence than the differences.

According to Sartorius, there is high probability that the incidence and prevalence of depression will grow in the years to come, since life expectancy is increasing in most countries. Thus the number and percentage of people running a higher risk of developing depression will also increase. Since there are now vast advances in the methodology of cross-cultural investigation and groups of scientists willing and able to carry out research, properly conducted cross-cultural research can yield results that can help to solve the challenge that depression across the world presents.

Sartorius, Norman, "Cross-Cultural Research on Depression," *Psychopathology*, 19(Suppl. 2), 1986.

counseling Counseling can be helpful in some situations, and both individual and group counseling are available at many county and community mental health centers and at private counseling services, staffed by psychiatrists, psychologists and therapists. Check the yellow pages of telephone directories for local listings of the names, addresses and phone numbers of the centers and services.

In addition, hot lines and self-help organizations provide support systems and permit persons suffering from depression to share their experiences with people who have similar experiences. These services can help give encouragement and healing through their meetings and contacts. See Appendix 6 for individual listings of self-help/support organizations. (See also PSYCHOTHERAPY; TREATMENT OF DEPRESSION.)

CT scan   See COMPUTERIZED AXIAL TOMOGRAPHY.

cyclothymia   A chronic mood disorder of at least two years' duration characterized by numerous periods of depression alternating with periods of mildly elevated mood. It is not of sufficient severity and duration to meet the criteria for a major depression or a manic episode, but it is sometimes called a "cousin" of manic-depression. Depressive and hypomanic periods may be separated by periods of normal mood lasting for as long as several months at a time. Persons with a cyclothymic disorder do not experience such psychotic features as delusions, incoherence or loosening of associations.

D

Darwin, Charles   An English scientist and naturalist (1809–1882) who, after preparing for a career in medicine and the ministry, became interested in botany. This led to his study of thousands of fossils, his theory of evolution and the subsequent publication in 1859 of his famous *Origin of Species*.

Despite his success and fame, Darwin, an exceptionally modest man, was often so beset by low moods that he would all but collapse in the midst of his work. Even before he went on his five-year-cruise to collect infor-

mation he experienced such gloom and misery that he suffered from excruciating chest pains and heart palpitations. Later, when he returned from the voyage, he had to lay his work aside for a year and a half because he became so depressed that he could not even read. His health declined after the voyage, and some historians and medical professionals believe this was because he contracted the trypanosome of Chagas' disease in South America during the voyage. However, Dr. Ralph Colp Jr., author of *To Be an Invalid: The Illness of Charles Darwin*, questions this and from his extensive research suggests that rather than Chagas' disease the main cause of Darwin's ill health was stress, especially stress arising out of the great difficulties of proving his theory of evolution.

Colp, Ralph, Jr., *To Be an Invalid: The Illness of Charles Darwin*, (Chicago: University of Chicago Press, 1977).

delusions   Delusions experienced by depressives often represent exaggerations of helplessness, hopelessness or guilt, such as beliving that one is responsible for all the evil in the world. Depressives may also experience paranoid delusions, delusions of reference and other delusions known as "mood incongruent delusions."

dementia   The loss of intellectual functions (thinking, remembering, reasoning) severely enough to interfere with an individual's daily life. Dementia is not a disease in itself but rather a group of symptoms, which may characterize and accompany certain diseases or conditions. Persons with dementia show changes in personality, mood and behavior. How much assistance and specialized care each patient needs will depend on the symptoms and the degree of impairment. When dementia and depression are present together, intellectual deterioration may be exaggerated.

The causes and rate of progression of dementia vary. Some of the more well known diseases that produce dementia are ALZ-

HEIMER'S DISEASE (AD), PARKINSON'S DISEASE (PD) and Huntington's Disease (HD).

dementia praecox See SCHIZOPHRENIA.

deprenyl See SELEGILINE.

depressants Drugs that work by depressing and slowing down the action of the CENTRAL NERVOUS SYSTEM, thus diminishing or halting vital body functions. Too much will stop the respiratory system and can cause death. Depressants also affect the reticular activating system, including sleep, and other areas of the cerebral cortex.

Alcohol and tranquilizers are the most commonly used depressant drugs, but the group also includes opiates and barbiturates. Their action is irregular because they do not depress all parts of the central nervous system at once. They work primarily on the brain, depressing psychomotor activity and relieving tension and anxiety. When the sedative level in the blood begins to fall, psychomotor activity increases, producing agitation. The term "depressant" may be misleading because such drugs actually elevate a person's mood initially. The term has no direct relationship to depression except that consistent use of central nervous system depressants can result in psychological depression.

depressed parents and children For some time researchers have observed that children of depressed parents were at a heightened risk of experiencing depression, anxiety disorder, substance abuse and other psychiatric problems. Such findings have led many researchers to suspect a genetic influence on depression, while others point out that families also share cultures, diet, stress and social interactions.

In discussing a study that focused on 220 children, aged 6 to 23, Dr. Myrna Weissman, a professor of epidemiology and psy-

chiatry at Columbia University College of Physicians and Surgeons, stated (in a 1987 Associated Press report) that study researchers tested 125 children of 56 depressed parents and 95 children of 35 parents who never had been psychiatrically ill.

When tested, depressed children of a depressed parent showed an average age of onset of about 13 years. That compared to 17 years for depressed children whose parents did not suffer depression. The time of onset was about the same for boys and girls. In addition, researchers found some cases of prepubertal depression, which started before age 12 in children of depressed parents, but no such cases in children of normal parents. In a later study Dr. Weissman found about a threefold increase in risk in the rates of depression in children of depressed parents.

Dr. Marian Radke-Yarrow, chief of the Laboratory of Developmental Psychology at the National Institute of Mental Health (NIMH), has also done a great deal of research on depressed parents and their children. Some of her research will be published in a forthcoming Cambridge University Press book, *Risks and Protective Factors in the Development of Psychopathology*. In one study, which examined depressed mothers and children, she identified the following factors as the main differences between life for a child in a family where a parent is seriously depressed and in a family where there are no such problems. Although Dr. Radke-Yarrow used mothers in her study, it is believed that the results of her research are also applicable to fathers who are depressives.

• Depressed mothers are more likely to back off when they meet resistance from children while trying to control them.
• Depressed mothers were less able to compromise in disagreements with their children, and they often confused their children's normal attempts at independence with breaking rules.

- While making and eating lunch, depressed mothers spoke to their children far less than did other mothers. The children of the depressed mothers also spoke infrequently.
- When the depressed mothers spoke they made more negative comments than did other mothers.

Associated Press, "Stronger Cases Made for Link Between Genetics, Depression," *The* [Hackensack, N.J.] *Record,* October 8, 1987.

Goleman, Daniel, "Depressed Parents Put Children at a Greater Risk of Depression," *The New York Times,* March 30, 1989.

Depression Awareness, Recognition and Treatment Project (D/ART) A major national program to educate the public, primary care physicians and mental health specialists about depressive disorders—their symptoms and treatments. It is sponsored by the National Institute of Mental Health in collaboration with private organizations and citizens. Its primary goal is to alleviate suffering due to depressive disorders by: (1) helping the public recognize the disorders' symptoms and learn where to get help; and (2) informing primary care physicians and mental health specialists about the latest treatments for depression. It is based on more than 40 years of research on the diagnosis and treatment of depressive disorders.

Extensive organizational and campaign planning for D/ART has involved experts from both the public and private sectors and set in motion the development of: (1) written and audiovisual materials for the public; (2) training programs for mental health specialists; (3) clinical training grants for universities and medical schools to develop short-term educational programs for mental health specialists and primary care physicians; and (4) media kits and training programs for community volunteers.

For further information about the program contact: DEPRESSION, 5600 Fishers Lane, Room 15C-05, Rockville, MD 20857. Phone: 301–443–4140.

depression, definition of Sometimes called "the common cold of mental disorders," depression is a widespread, complex and many-faceted disorder that is difficult to describe with a one-definition-fits-all explanation.

The *Psychiatric Dictionary* (fourth edition) states: In psychiatry, depression refers to a clinical syndrome, consisting of lowering of mood-tone (feelings of painful dejection), difficulty in thinking, and psychomotor retardation. The general retardation, however, may be masked by anxiety, obsessive thinking, and agitation in certain depressions. Depression is . . . "a pathological state of conscious psychic suffering and guilt, accompanied by a marked reduction in the sense of personal values, and a diminution of mental, psychomotor, and even organic activity, unrelated to actual deficiency."

Many of the facets of this complex disorder are associated with biological disturbances, including genetic factors that may predispose individuals to this illness, which affects many different systems of the body. It involves the way people eat and sleep, the way they feel about themselves, and the way they think about things. It is *not* a passing blue mood, *not* a sign of personal weakness and *not* a condition that can be willed or wished away. It can accompany or follow physical illness or some forms of medical treatment and may accompany other forms of mental illness as well.

Depression comes in various forms and, depending on whether a person is talking to a clinician, researcher or other mental health specialist, it is sometimes referred to by various terms. Not everyone agrees on the names and definitions given to the different kinds of depression. In fact, even psychiatrists disagree on the various terms used to describe its different forms. It has several different subtypes that require different forms of treatment (see TYPES OF DEPRESSION). Since the various terms overlap and are not mutually exclusive this can pose significant diagnostic challenges for physicians.

Some people experience only one depressive episode in a lifetime; others have several recurrences. Some depressive episodes begin suddenly for no apparent reason, while others can be associated with a situation or stress. Sometimes people who are depressed cannot perform even the simplest daily activities, such as getting out of bed or getting dressed. Others go through the motions, but it is clear they are not acting or thinking as usual. Some people suffer BIPOLAR DEPRESSION.

In *From Sad to Glad* Dr. Nathan S. Kline wrote:

All of us experience moments of sadness, loneliness, pessimism, and uncertainty as a natural reaction to particular circumstances. In the depressed person those feelings become all-pervasive. They can be triggered by the least incident or occur without evident connection to any outside cause. The level of psychic pain varies widely. Some patients are only vaguely aware that they feel blue most of the time. For such victims chronic depression is felt not so much as overt pain but rather as the inability to experience pleasure. For others the pain is acute. Some withdraw deeply into themselves, becoming dull and lethargic. Some become frightened and irritable.

Today we are much more alert to the disease than in the past, and we have much new information and better diagnostic methods for identifying and treating more depressed people. When recognized, the illness can be treated and appropriate treatment can help over 80% of those who suffer from depression. Without treatment, symptoms can last for weeks, months or years.

Unfortunately, many people with a depressive disorder do not seek appropriate treatment because their symptoms; (1) are not rec-

ognized; (2) are blamed on personal weakness; (3) are so disabling they cannot reach out for help; or (4) are misdiagnosed and wrongly treated. As a result depressive disorders cause inestimable pain to millions of people and hurt millions more whose lives are affected and disrupted. (See also COMMON SIGNS AND SYMPTOMS.)

Hinsie, L.E. and Campbell, R.J., *Psychiatric Dictionary*, 4th ed. (New York: Oxford University Press, 1970).

Kline, Nathan S., *From Sad to Glad* (New York: Putnam, 1974).

Nacht, S. and Racamier, P.C., *International Journal of PsychoAnalysis*, 41:481(1960).

depression pathology The study of the essential nature of depression and, especially, of the structural, functional and abnormal changes produced by the disease.

depressive The name given to a victim of depression.

Depressive Disorders in Different Cultures A World Health Organization (WHO) publication that describes progress in the first phase of a multicenter study coordinated by WHO. (See also WORLD HEALTH ORGANIZATION (WHO) COLLABORATIVE STUDY ON STANDARDIZED ASSESSMENT OF DEPRESSIVE DISORDERS.)

Depressive Disorders Self-help Group A Canadian organization of people from all walks of life who have joined together to provide support, education, sharing and caring to depressives and manic-depressives as well as to their families and friends. Formed in May 1987, the group has become a very active participant in the informal mental health system. It is based on a circular, rather than pyramidal, model of participation. Every member has an equal say in what occurs in the group, and what is discussed in the weekly meetings is held in confidence by the group members. For information: Depressive Disorders Self-Help Group, 9th Floor,

10050-112 St., Edmonton, Alberta T5K 2J1. Phone: 403-466-5253.

depressive neurosis (dysthymia) A depressive disorder in which symptoms similar to but not as severe as those experienced in major depressive disorder reoccur or persist over a long time, usually for at least two years. Any or all of the symptoms, except delusions, hallucinations or incoherence, may be present all the time or be interrupted by a normal mood for a few days or weeks.

Depressives Anonymous: Recovery from Depression A nonprofit organization headquartered in New York and founded in 1979 by DR. HELEN DEROSIS. As a self-help program for depressed persons, it provides information, training and public service programs designed to help depressed men and women of all ages change some patterns of living. It is directed to depressives in the general population and is for persons who are generally dissatisfied and distressed with certain areas of their lives and who are motivated to help themselves. It is not a substitute for professional treatment of depression, and the program is not designed for severely depressed persons, though many of the latter have attended its meetings and reported they benefited from them. For information contact Depressives Anonymous: Recovery from Depression, 329 East 62nd St., New York, NY 10021. Telephone: 212-689-2600

depressive spectrum disease (DSD) A serious depression occurring in a person with a family history of alcoholism. Such a person may or may not also have a first-degree relative with an unipolar depression. Often DSD patients suffer from social maladjustments, continuous dysphoric moods and unstable personalities. When compared to depressives who have no family history of alcoholism they are more likely to have received a clinical diagnosis of neurotic-reactive depression, more likely to have shown lifelong

characteristics of fear, demanding behavior, need for reassurance, dependence, nervousness, complaining and irritability, and more apt to show evidence of stormy life events such as divorce, separation and sexual problems.

In addition to the examples of instability cited above other characteristics can be drunkenness, excessive illness, throwing or breaking things, defaulting on obligations, phobias, histrionics, seductiveness, fainting, quitting jobs, getting fired, school difficulties and legal troubles.

Behar, David et al., "Familial Subtypes of Depression: A Clinical View," *Journal of Clinical Psychiatry*, 42:2 (February 1980).

Winokur, George et al., "Neurotic Depression: A Diagnosis Based on Preexisting Characteristics," *European Archives of Psychiatry and Neurological Sciences*, 236(1987), 343–348.

DeRosis, Helen, Dr. A psychiatrist, psychoanalyst, author, and founder and director of DEPRESSIVES ANONYMOUS. She is also an educator and has a leading role in the activities of the American Institute for Psychoanalysis and the affiliated Karen Horney Clinic. She believes there are many contributing factors to unhappiness, including environmental, interpersonal, physical and genetic ones. However, she also believes that individuals become the primary agents in the continuation of their own unhappiness and that they can become the agent for a shift to personal well-being. A prime philosophy behind her Depressives Anonymous program is that depressives are usually overwhelmed by the number of concerns they have, and she finds that when they focus on a very discrete item and function with that, they tend to be able to go on and progress to a number of items. Since this is the case, she has developed a Twenty-Step Program to help depressed and anxious individuals strengthen qualities that are lying dormant within them. In her Depressives Anonymous meetings she concentrates on the first four steps:

Step 1. Select a single troublesome issue that causes you to feel anxious, or that creates repeated tension, guilt, anger or conflict. (Identifying an item.)

Step 2. Determine how the troublesome issue is causing you or someone else to suffer. (Deciding on how you're going to work on that item.)

Step 3. State whether or not you have tried to disregard the issue. (Taking action on it.)

Step 4. State whether or not you have tried to deal with the issue. (Evaluating the results.)

"As you read over these steps," she wrote in *Women and Anxiety,* "I think you can tell that their main purpose is to keep your attention on only one trouble point at a time, rather than scattering it over several issues. That way you are left with some sense of accomplishment, for efforts directed at one point only are more likely to clarify something for you. When your efforts are scattered and you jump from one thing to another, you may come to feel that you can't deal with any of them."

DeRosis, Helen, *Women and Anxiety* (New York: Delacorte Press, 1979).

Desyrel See TRAZODONE.

developing countries, depression in
In 1975 the World Health Organization Expert Committee on Mental Health reported that in developing countries mental disorder caused severe disablement and incapacity in 10% of every population at some period in their lives. The disorders included schizophrenia, affective psychosis and organic brain syndromes. In that decade the cross-cultural aspects of diagnosis and outcome of schizophrenia were receiving attention but the identification of depression and anxiety with florid somatic symptoms had been ignored.

By 1987 Dr. S. Haroon Ahmed, College of Family Medicine in Pakistan and Depart-

ment of Neuropsychiatry at Jinnah Postgraduate Medical Centre in Karachi, reported that, in speaking for his country, the prevalence of psychiatric disorders in general practice was much higher among adult patients than the percentage reported by some studies and estimates.

As things stand in the early Nineties, the developing countries are depending heavily on the concepts and natural history of psychiatric disorders derived from the investigation of Western society. Some attempts were made in the past to generate data for the incidence and prevalance of various disorders in developing countries. But early Western observers failed to document the pattern of illness correctly, according to Ahmed. "The most likely cause of bias was that their frames of reference were those of Western classical psychiatry," he wrote in *Mental Disorders, Alcohol- and Drug-Related Problems.*

Now, however, groups of researchers are directing efforts toward greater documentation of mental disorder because of the importance of planning and developing mental health services on objective realities.

"The most significant contribution to clarity in this issue and to a new systematic approach has been that made by the World Health Organization [WHO] international collaborative study on schizophrenia," Ahmed wrote. "A striking finding has been that the course and outcome—and, on the average, the prognosis—are more favorable in developing than in the industrialized countries. Such studies have opened up new avenues of research and developed tools that can be used in different cultures."

According to Ahmed, one helpful tool that resulted from a multifaceted WHO research program on depression is the Schedule for Standardized Assessment of Depressive Disorders (WHO/SADD), an instrument that enables psychiatrists from different cultures to be consistent in assessing depressive symptomatology and applying specific diagnostic criteria.

Akhund, F., Khan, M., Mohsin, A. and Ahmed, S.H., "Psychiatric Disorders in General Practice," *Journal of the Pakistan Medical Association*, 37(January 1987).

Ahmed, S. Haroon, "Treatment Response and the Clinical Continuum of Illness," in *Mental Disorders, Alcohol-and-Drug-Related Problems* (Amsterdam: Excerpta Medica, 1985).

dexamethasone　A synthetic corticosteroid. (See also DEXAMETHASONE SUPPRESSION TEST.)

dexamethasone suppression test (DST test or DEX test)　A screening test that is used to see if people fall into the depressed category. Though this test alone cannot confirm or rule out depression, is not yet part of regular medical practice, and is still being studied and standardized, many physicians and hospitals are using it as a diagnostic tool. It was originally developed to screen for a rare medical disorder, Cushing's Syndrome, and is considered an interesting research tool because it is one of the first biological markers of a clinical dysfunction in the central nervous system.

In depression, many people secrete an excess amount of CORTISOL, a natural steroid stress hormone, from their adrenal glands into their blood stream. Why this happens is not clear, but when normal people are given another steroid, dexamethasone, the regulatory systems within the body seem to get the message that there is enough hormone circulating. Cortisol secretion is then suppressed, usually for about a day.

On the other hand, many depressed people have quite a different reaction to dexamethasone. Cortisol secretion is suppressed briefly, but then it bounds upward within less than a day, essentially escaping from the effect of dexamethasone. Somehow, the regulatory systems for cortisol secretion are altered.

"If dexamethasone escape does define a true 'biologic' type of depressive disorder, then the DST should provide a useful standard against which to validate alternative diagnostic and classification criteria," stated Dr. Sidney Zisook of the University of California at San Diego, who, along with other researchers, has been studying the DST and depression. In an attempt to validate several subtypes of affective disorders, Dr. Zisook and his colleagues studied 52 patients hospitalized at a clinical research center for the study of affective disorders. The subjects were comprehensively classified according to several diagnostic and phenomenologic (the study of the development of human consciousness and self-awareness) measurements. Cortisol levels of each patient were evaluated at baseline and after the administration of 0.5 and 1.0 milligrams of dexamethasone. None of the depressive subtypes responded significantly differently to the 1.0 milligram dose. However, the bipolar subtype was associated with significantly different DST responses to the 0.5 milligram dose. Patients with bipolar affective disorder, both manic and depressed, had higher postdexamethasone mean cortisol levels than all other groups. "Further studies with larger populations and other biologic markers are currently in progress to further assess the biologic distinctiveness of bipolar affective disorders and to delineate other biologically distinct subgroups of depressed patients," reported Dr. Zisook.

"Some of the various research data tends to indicate that about 15% of the people with treatable depression seem to have a positive response to the test," pointed out Dr. Ira Lipton, a colleague of the late Dr. Nathan S. Kline who is now continuing Dr. Kline's Manhattan private practice. "But the response varies depending on whose data one studies and the patient population that is sampled."

According to DST researchers the test is administered in the following manner:

1. The blood level of a patient's cortisol is measured.

2. A tablet of 1.0 milligram of dexamethasone (or sometimes 0.5 milligram as noted above) is then given to the patient.

3. On the next day the serum of cortisol is

drawn and another blood cortisol measurement is made.

4. If a patient is depressed the feedback mechanism between the hypothalamus and the pituitary will not be functioning correctly, and the person will have an elevated cortisol level—thus indicating the likelihood of a form of depression.

However, since other conditions (including other psychiatric conditions, recent alcohol abuse and recent physical illnesses) can also give abnormal results on the test, many physicians warn that a positive response must be interpreted cautiously. Similarly, normal results do not mean that depression is absent, and many physicians would not deny giving a patient antidepressant medication based on negative information from the DST test, since many patients with negative results are ultimately medication responsive.

Zisook, Sidney et al., "The Dexamethasone Suppression Test and Unipolar/Bipolar Distinctions," *Journal of Clinical Psychiatry*, 46:11(November 1985).

diagnostic interview schedule (DIS)
A highly structured interview designed for use by lay interviewers in epidemiologic studies of psychiatric disorders. The DIS elicits information about symptoms, their severity, frequency, distribution over time, and whether those symptoms are explainable by physical illness, use of drugs or alcohol, or the presence of another psychiatric disorder. The questions are precoded so that answers can be directly entered into a computer. The DIS is relatively economical because it does not require a clinician, external data, coders or a lengthy training program.

Zimmerman, Mark and Coryell, William, "The Validity of a Self-Report Questionnaire for Diagnosing Major Depressive Disorder," *Archives of General Psychiatry*, 45(August 1988).

***Diagnostic and Statistical Manual of Mental Disorders* (DSM-III-R)** Published by the American Psychiatric Association, this is the diagnostic bible used by vir-tually all mental health professionals. The initial edition—DSM-I—appeared in 1952 and was the first official manual of mental disorders to contain a glossary of descriptions of the diagnostic categories. A second edition—DSM-II—was published in 1968. In 1974 the American Psychiatric Association appointed a task force to begin work on the development of DSM-III, and this edition became official in 1979.

In 1983 a work group was appointed to revise DSM-III. During the process of developing the current volume—DSM-III-R—two successive drafts of the proposed revised diagnostic criteria were made available to interested professionals and widely distributed for critical feedback and review. In 1987 DSM-III-R was published. The diagnostic criteria for mood disorders published in this volume include separate criteria for manic episodes, major depressive episodes, bipolar disorders, cyclothymia and dysthmia.

diagnostic techniques and criteria
Physicians have traditionally used many types of information to diagnose depression, specifically: (1) the patient's current symptoms and the context in which they developed; (2) the patient's physical condition (as revealed by a physical examination); (3) a physical health and mental health history; and (4) the family's history of mental and physical health problems. Paper-and-pencil tests may also be used, often focusing on current symptoms, such as feelings of sadness and hopelessness, problems with sleeping and eating, or suicidal thoughts.

Some of the best-known and most widely-used inventories, criteria and scales are the DSM-III-R diagnostic criteria; SCID (Structured Clinical Interview For DSM-III-R); Beck Depression Inventory (BDI); Zung Self-Rating Depression Scale; Inventory To Diagnose Depression (IDD); diagnostic interview schedule (DIS); Hamilton Psychiatric Rating Scale for Depression (HRS); Global Assessment Scale; research diagnostic criteria (RDC); Schedule for Standardized Assessment of Depressive Disorders (WHO/

SADD), and Schedule for Affective Disorders/Schizophrenia (SADS).

The foregoing techniques, along with laboratory blood screenings and blood counts continue to be used as the foundation for diagnosis. But now there are also a number of new laboratory tests that have the potential to augment and refine these diagnostic techniques in the future. (See BLOOD TESTS; DEXAMETHASONE SUPPRESSION TEST [DST TEST OR DEX TEST]; DIURNAL CORTISOL TEST [DCT]; MHPG TEST; THYROTROPIN-RELEASING HORMONE TEST [TRH].) Though the TRH test is not as well known as the DST test, some clinicians and researchers feel there are patients who suffer from a subclinical hypothyroidism, indicating that subclinical hypothyroidism is a serious issue in the depressed person. As a result, these researchers consider monitoring for thyroid function an important diagnostic tool.

Many of the laboratory tests now being considered are currently being studied in research laboratories around the country and, as of this writing, are still regarded as highly experimental, while their clinically-useful diagnostic results are being established.

New tests assume that some types of depression are usually accompanied by abnormalities in brain or body function. These abnormalities can be detected through measurement of chemicals in the blood and/or urine (and, occasionally, in the cerebrospinal fluid) or by measuring brain waves. (See also BRAIN IMAGING.)

diazepam (Valium) A benzodiazepine derivative and one of the most widely prescribed drugs in the United States. It is a minor tranquilizer and sedative hypnotic that comes in tablet form and is used in the treatment of tension and anxiety and for alcohol withdrawal.

Its chief danger is that tolerance can develop, along with physical and psychological dependence on it. It has a significant potential for abuse when taken with alcohol or other central nervous system depressants.

diet There are conflicting views on the role of diet in depression. Some researchers believe that what people eat and when they eat it can have subtle and occasionally dramatic effects on their mood and behavior. They point out that studies have suggested that: (1) foods and nutrients might be used to treat depression; and (2) sometimes an episode can be controlled or lessened by eating the right foods because the consumption of certain nutrients can change the levels of brain chemicals that transmit messages between nerve cells. The nutrients are the chemical precursors, or parents, of the NEUROTRANSMITTERS, which regulate a wide variety of brain activities and can affect both mood and performance.

On the other hand, some researchers say that changes in neurotransmitters have no correlation with changes in behavior. Says Nancy Ryan, a nutritionist with the American Fitness Institute in Greenwich, Connecticut, "The whole issue is open to debate, the research is still going on, and in general, the jury is still out."

One researcher who is convinced food can control neurotransmitters is Judith Wurtman, a research scientist at the Massachusetts Institute of Technology who has researched the effect of food on the brain and studied the neurotransmitters DOPAMINE, NOREPINEPHRINE and SEROTONIN. Wurtman points out that the first two are the alertness chemicals, while the latter is the calming chemical. When the brain is producing dopamine and norepinephrine, people have a tendency to think more quickly, react more rapidly and feel more attentive. They are more motivated and mentally energetic. When the brain produces serotonin, stress and tension are eased and the ability to concentrate is enhanced.

Wurtman's husband Dr. Richard J. Wurtman, a professor in the department of brain and cognitive sciences at M.I.T. and director of M.I.T.'s Clinical Research Center, has also done studies on nutrition and depression. As part of their joint research the Wurtmans have focused on mood fluctuations among carbohydrate cravers.

When the Wurtmans asked carbohydrate cravers why they succumb to foods they know will exacerbate their obesity, they found that most said they do this to combat tension, anxiety or mental fatigue. After eating, the majority reported feeling calm and clearheaded.

This caused the Wurtmans to wonder whether the consumption of excessive amounts of snack carbohydrates leading to severe obesity might not represent a kind of substance abuse in which the decision to consume carbohydrates for their calming and antidepressant effects is carried to an extreme. To determine this, Judith Wurtman set out to test the relationship between carbohydrate snacking and mood. Forty-six volunteers, including both carbohydrate cravers and noncravers, were given standard psychological tests before and after eating a carbohydrate-rich, protein-free meal. The carbohydrate cravers were significantly less depressed after snacking, whereas noncravers experienced fatigue and sleepiness. These findings suggest that carbohydrate cravers may eat snacks high in carbohydrates in order to restore flagging vitality much as some people pour another cup of coffee when they feel their energy level or attention span is flagging.

In their research the Wurtmans also found that people who suffer from SEASONAL AFFECTIVE DISORDERS (SAD) experience episodic bouts of depression combined with profound cravings for carbohydrate-rich foods. In an article in *Scientific American* they wrote:

Why do patients with SAD have a tendency to crave carbohydrate snacks and how is it that the brain normally knows when carbohydrates have been or should be consumed? We now know the answer to these questions involves serotonin, one of the neurotransmitters (substances that are released from a neuron when it fires and that

convey the nerve impulse across the synapse to the next neuron). Serotonin is a derivative of tryptophan, an amino acid that is normally present at low levels in the blood stream. The rate of conversion is affected by the proportion of carbohydrates in a person's diet; carbohydrates stimulate the secretion of insulin, which facilitates the uptake of most amino acids into peripheral tissues, such as muscle. Blood tryptophan levels, however, are unaffected by insulin and so the proportion of tryptophan in the blood relative to the other amino acids increases when carbohydrates are consumed. Since tryptophan competes with other amino acids for transport across the blood-brain barrier, insulin secretion speeds its entry into the central nervous system where it enters, among other cells, a special cluster of neurons known as the raphe nuclei. There it is converted into serotonin. The level of serotonin in turn figures in a feedback mechanism affecting the amount of carbohydrate an individual subsequently chooses to eat. When the feedback mechanism is disturbed as we believe happens cyclically in patients with SAD, the brain fails to respond when carbohydrates are eaten, and so the desire for them persists longer than it should.

Only small amounts of carbohydrates are needed to produce the calming effects the carbohydrate cravers report, so Judith Wurtman advises consuming them in moderation, since they are fattening.

The list to choose from includes candy, cookies, pie, cake, ice cream, jams, jellies, preserves, syrups and soft drinks. In the starch category, there is bread, crackers, muffins, rolls, bagels, pasta, potatoes, rice, corn, barley, kasha, oatmeal and other cereals. Individuals who need a quick revival around 3:00 P.M. or 4:00 P.M. might combine a cup of caffeinated coffee with five graham crackers or a large bran muffin.

It is usually recommended that anyone

with a history of depression consume a diet high in protein since protein increases alertness and has an energizing effect on the mind. "The most beneficial proteins are those with small amounts of fats or carbohydrates such as shellfish, fish, chicken, veal, and very lean beef trimmed of visible fat," advised Judith Wurtman. "The group of proteins next in line are low-fat dairy products, including cottage cheese, milk, and yogurt; dried peas, beans and lentils; and tofu and other soybean-based foods. Eat sparingly of high-fat proteins, which include beef, lamb, pork, lunch meats, organ meats, hard cheese, whole milk and regular yogurt."

Some years ago some researchers felt that tyrosine, an amino acid from protein foods that is the precursor of the neurotransmitter norepinephrine, showed promise in combating depression. At that time Dr. Alan J. Gelenberg, associate professor of psychiatry at Harvard Medical School, and his group did a study of tyrosine for the treatment of depression. Preliminary results, published in two papers were favorable, but, according to Dr. Gelenberg, the results of a prospective double-blind trial against both placebo and the tricyclic antidepressant imipramine (Tofranil and others) failed to find antidepressant efficacy for tyrosine.

As far as diet precautions go, depressives taking lithium must avoid crash diets, since such diets may affect lithium levels. Also, to avoid excessive weight gain while on lithium, people should refrain from drinking excessive amounts of cola or other drinks with high sugar content to quench the increased thirst that may accompany lithium therapy. People on MAO inhibitors must watch what they eat, too, and be strict about avoiding certain foods because combining some foods with MAO inhibitors can trigger very high blood pressure, rapid pulse, headaches, vision problems and, sometimes, paralyzing or fatal strokes. Specific foods to avoid while on MAOs are chocolate, cheese, yogurt, pickled fish, soy sauce, pods of broad beans, canned figs, bananas, avocados, raisins, liver, yeast, meats prepared with tenderizer, sour cream, wine, beer, ale and alcohol. Caffeine should be used in moderation.

Much remains to be learned about diet and depression. But regardless of the conflicting views about it, all nutritionists and researchers agree that a well-balanced diet based on good nutrients is vital for good mental health. Depressives must be kept aware of this.

Wurtman, Judith, *Managing Your Mind and Mood Through Food* (New York: Harper & Row, 1989).

Foster, Valerie, "Foods That Set the Mood," *The* [Hackensack, N.J.] *Record*, May 24, 1989.

Wurtman, Richard J. and Judith J., "Carbohydrates and Depression" *Scientific American*, January 1989.

diurnal cortisol test (DCT)   The DCT is a test of the hypothalamic-pituitary-adrenal (HPA) axis; it identifies a different patient group than the DEXAMETHASONE SUPPRESSION TEST (DST). In a chapter in *Inpatient Psychiatry* Dr. A.L.C. Pottash et al. explain that in this test the DCT measures cortisol levels and endogenous diurnal rhythm. In normal patients at 8:00 A.M. normal levels are present, and cortisol falls by 4:00 P.M. and is significantly lower by midnight. In the test the patient goes to bed and arises at his or her regular time. Plasma samples for cortisol by radioimmunoassay (RIA) are taken at 8:00 A.M., 4:00 P.M. and midnight.

In patients with major depression, there is excessive secretion of cortisol, although sometimes this is seen only in the 4:00 P.M. or midnight samples. The hypersecretion may suggest major depression or Cushing's syndrome.

Pottash, A. et al., "The Use of the Clinical Laboratory," ch. 9 in 2nd ed. of *Inpatient Psychiatry–Diagnosis and Treatment*, (ed.) Lloyd I. Sederer (Baltimore: Williams & Wilkins, 1986).

dopamine   A biogenic amine that serves as a neurotransmitter and assists in the transmission of electrochemical impulses from one nerve cell to another in the brain by activating the "on" switches. At one time it was not considered an important factor in depression, but today it is regarded as a chemical that can play a key role.

Dostoevski, Feodor Mikhailovich A Russian novelist (1821–1881) whose own life experiences and bouts with depression and despair—plus his insight and understanding of the pathological conscience, depth and complexity of the human soul—have made his writings particularly relevant today.

History tells us that the brutal slaying of his father, a military surgeon of harsh, despotic temperament, by his own serfs haunted Dostoevski's entire life and perhaps accounted in part for his preoccupation with murder and guilt in his writings.

His first books were published in 1846 and shortly after that he became involved with a group of radical utopianists. The discovery of their illegal printing press brought about their arrest and sentencing to hard labor. As a result, Dostoevski lived for four years among the criminal dregs of society in a Siberian penal colony. During that time he suffered great physical and mental pain, including depression and attacks of epilepsy.

After his prison experience and several years of military service in Siberia he returned to St. Petersburg with a widow he had married and went into publishing with his brother. Subsequent financial troubles and a passion for roulette led to a nightmarish time in his life. In 1864 both his first wife and brother died, compounding his depression and despair.

double blind studies Experimental procedures that involve investigation or research in which neither the subjects nor the experimenters know who is a test patient and who is a control patient. A code for which one person has the master plan is set up and later broken to find out which patients were receiving what treatment. Throughout the research, however, those doing the investigation do not know which patient receives treatment substance and which receives control substance.

double depression See DYSTHYMIA.

dreams There is a new respect for dreams, as dream specialists stress that our emotional state influences what we dream about, and point out that dreams can tell us many things about ourselves and the unresolved issues of our lives. For example, many say that when we have a dream in which we are extremely anxious, we are often going through a time of depression, stress and insecurity.

"Until very recently dreams seemed like a vaguely disreputable way for a scientist to make a living," reported Sharon Begley in a *Newsweek* article, "The Stuff That Dreams Are Made Of." But what was once a fad is now a mainstream, and many dream researchers, psychotherapists and psychologists—who believe that dreaming is the collection of mental images that arise during "rapid eye movement" (REM) sleep—are disputing the notion that dreams are the meaningless epiphenomena of a firing of neurons.

According to Begley, even some scientists who tickle neurons and map brain chemicals have this newfound respect for dreams, in part because of the work of psychiatrists Dr. Robert W. McCarley and Dr. J. Allan Hobson of Harvard Medical School.

Begley writes:

The psychiatrists developed a theory to explain how dreams are generated by neurons during REM sleep and how the mind makes sense of the signals it receives. Dreams, they conclude, are born in the brainstem, which controls such basics as reflexes. In the brainstems are two kinds of neurons known to control sleep, each using a different chemical to communicate. One type uses acetylcholine; they are "on" during REM. The others use norepinephrine and serotonin; they are "off." Only when these latter neurons are turned off can the acetylcholine neurons turn on. Then a dream is born. The acetylcholine neurons send rapid bursts of electrical signals to the cortex, the seat of higher thought and vision. The cortex takes this information and weaves it into a coherent story, say Hobson and McCarley, interpreting the signals by referring to preexisting memories.

Begley goes on to report that such research draws bitter criticism from researchers who think it dismisses dreams as mere random products of REM sleep. But in *The Dreaming Brain* Hobson bends over backward to say dreams are *not* meaningless and that the brain is so "inexorably bent upon the quest for meaning" it takes essentially random automatic signals from the brainstem and imbues them with sense. What *kind* of sense reveals the dreamer's "drives, fears and associations."

In writing about depression and dreams in *Depression: How to Recognize It, How to Treat It, and How to Grow From It*, Wina Sturgeon wrote:

The dreams of the depressive often have unpleasant story lines. They are quite complete and can be very vivid. But it's the theme of the dreams which is the giveaway. The depressive will dream themes of masochism and defeat. A woman may dream that she is being reviled for her ugliness, a man that he has done something that makes him look like a sissy. There may be dreams of humiliation at work. Some of these dreams may come as perceptions only—there may be swiftly changing blurs of color, but the person is upset and frightened by them, or some meaningless sequence may leave an impression in the depressive's mind that it meant he or she had just done something terrible. In the dreams of the depressive, the masochistic theme is often constant.

There are never dreams which make the person feel triumphant or good.

There is still much research to be done on dreams since, as Sandra Blakeslee pointed out in "New Methods Help Researchers Explore the Dark World of Dreams," the proponents of today's dream research are convinced they have discovered new ways to explore mind and body relationships and assist people in psychotherapy. To this Bill Domhoff, a professor of psychology at the University of California, Santa Cruz, who has studied dreams and hosted an international conference on the subject, added: "The study of dreams is an important and serious endeavor that can aid in our general understanding of human behavior. In an age of great interest in cognitive psychology, a theory that can't encompass dreams is no theory at all."

Begley, Sharon, "The Stuff That Dreams Are Made Of," *Newsweek*, August 14, 1989.

Blakeslee, Sandra, "New Methods Help Researchers Explore the Dark World of Dreams," *The New York Times*, August 11, 1988.

Stewart, Walter A. and Freeman, Lucy, *The Secrets of Dreams* (New York: Macmillan, 1972).

Sturgeon, Wina, *Depression: How to Recognize It, How to Treat It, and How to Grow From It* (Englewood Cliffs, N.J.: Prentice-Hall, 1979).

Woods, Ralph L. and Greenhouse, Herbert B., *The New World of Dreams* (New York: Macmillan, 1974).

drug abuse   See ABUSE POTENTIAL OF DRUGS.

drug addiction   In 1957 the World Health Organization's Expert Committee on Addiction-Producing Drugs defined drug addiction as "A state of periodic or chronic intoxication, detrimental to the individual and society, produced by the repeated consumption of a drug (natural or synthetic). Its characteristics include: (1) an over-powering desire or need (compulsion) to continue taking the drug and to obtain it by any means; (2) a tendency to increase the dose; (3) a psychic (psychological) and generally a physical dependence on the drug.''

Although physical dependence is only one aspect of drug addiction, the term ''drug addiction'' is often used to refer to physical dependence. Because of the confusion surrounding ''drug addiction'' and physical dependence (and the term ''drug habituation,'' which came into use in the 1930s to define dependence on the psychological effect resulting from the repeated consumption of a drug), the World Health Organization recommended in 1964 that the term ''drug dependence'' be substituted for the term ''drug addiction.'' In 1965 the term was adopted to cover the physical and psychological aspects.

As indicated above, however, the term ''drug addiction'' is still used to refer to physical dependence. Sometimes there is a tendency among persons addicted to the repeated consumption of a drug to become depressed. There can also be a tendency among depressed people to seek drugs as a way of treating their own depression. If a drug's intake is reduced severely or stopped completely illness or withdrawal effects can occur. (See also DRUG DEPENDENCY; PSYCHOLOGICAL DRUG DEPENDENCE.)

drug dependency In 1965 the World Health Organization defined drug dependence as ''a state, psychic and sometimes also physical, resulting from the interaction between a living organism and a drug, characterized by behavioral and other responses that always include a compulsion to take the drug on a continuous or periodic basis in order to experience its psychic effects, and sometimes to avoid the discomfort of its absence. Tolerance may or may not be present. A person may be dependent on more than one drug.'' This dependency can take place after

periodic or prolonged use of a drug, and its characteristics vary according to the drug involved.

Most clinicians and researchers agree that whether or not it is common for drug dependent people to become depressed, and how likely it is that depressed people treated with drugs may become dependent, are two separate questions and are too complicated to answer with an all-or-nothing response. (See also DRUG ADDICTION; PSYCHOLOGICAL DRUG DEPENDENCE.)

drug interaction   see SYNERGY.

drug therapy   Even though many patients respond to a combined use of drugs and psychotherapy, a great many experts believe that drugs are our most hope-filled area for bringing people out of depression. In fact, one of the most important developments in recent years has been the improved diagnosis of depressive illness, allowing doctors to distinguish between patients who are likely to respond best to different drugs, according to Dr. Sidney Zisook of the University of California at San Diego, who is doing clinical research on some of the newest ANTIDEPRESSANTS.

The present approach to the pharmacotherapy of major depressive illness still relies mainly on the tricyclic antidepressants, which show efficacy in an estimated 60% to 70% of patients. But despite the large number of different antidepressant medications now available, there still remains a need for more effective, safer compounds, since current drug therapy remains unsuccessful for some 30% of depressed patients. Moreover, some available antidepressants also have the disadvantages of sedation, troublesome anticholinergic effects, occasionally dangerous and even lethal cardiovascular effects, and slow onset of antidepressant action. This slow onset—and the several weeks it sometimes takes to ease symptoms—can be a matter of life or death in patients whose depression brings them close to suicide. Because of the latter disadvantage much research is being aimed at finding new drugs that quickly counteract depression. However, as things stand now, many researchers feel that even the newest drugs have failed to act fast enough to make an important difference.

Right now the three basic groups of antidepressant drugs most widely used are the TRICYCLIC COMPOUNDS, the MONOAMINE OXIDASE INHIBITORS (MAOIs) and LITHIUM. The first two are generally used to treat unipolar illness (see UNIPOLAR DEPRESSION) in which the patient may be severely depressed but does not become manic. Lithium is used principally against bipolar, or manic-depressive, illness (see BIPOLAR DEPRESSION), but is also used to augment the action of tricyclics or MAOIs.

In addition to these drugs (which have been in general usage for some time) several newer ones are being tried with increasing frequency, and researchers hope that new ones, such as Fezolamine, studied by Dr. Zisook, will help patients who are not helped by established drugs. In the so-called newer generation (or second generation) of antidepressants, bupropion (Wellbutrin), trazodone (Desyrel), maprotiline (Ludiomil) and amoxapine (Asendin) are used.

Other newer-generation drugs are under investigation, and within the past few years, several drugs, such as Merital (nomifensine) have been introduced, marketed briefly, then later recalled for further investigation because of serious side effects. Merital was withdrawn because of reports of serious hypersensitivity reactions. A recently released drug, Prozac (fluoxetine), has been prescribed widely, primarily due to a side-effect profile quite different from the other commonly used agents.

Along with the above-cited drugs, the following drugs are also, at times, used for depressive disorders.

1. AMPHETAMINES—Prescribed for persons with mild or transient depression for the effect of self-worth and energy the drug can provide.

2. BENZODIAZEPINE derivatives— Used as TRANQUILIZERS. Valium, a minor tranquilizer, is one of most widely prescribed drugs. Xanax is also commonly used.

Along with finding drugs that quickly counteract depression, another major challenge facing researchers is to learn more about the chemistry of severe depression and discover drugs that make more of the key chemicals needed by the brain available to the nerve cells that require them. A way the brain normally regulates the chemical flow is to have some cells absorb the excess in a process called RE-UPTAKE. But since depressed people apparently need more of the chemicals than their brains allow them to use, drugs are used to block the re-uptake, thus leaving more of the chemicals available to work against depression. Each drug used for treatment presumably has a different chemical effect on the brain.

Currently scientists differ on how successful the search for new drugs has been. Some note that drugs discovered 20 years ago are still the main mode and standard of effective treatment. Others say there has been real progress, but it has been painstaking. In summing up the current status Dr. Zisook states: "Given the prevalence and morbidity of depression as well as the limitations of the currently available therapies, there is ample room for the development of newer antidepressants with even greater biological specificity, effectiveness and safety."

Because of the way some drugs, both old and new, have serious (or even fatal side effects) in some patients, all experts agree that it is imperative that, under all circumstances, drug therapy be used with care. In an already complicated picture of depression and drug therapy, Dr. Thomas A. Wehr and Dr. Frederick K. Goodwin of the National Institute of Mental Health noted in a Feb. 16, 1988, *New York Times* article, "Depres ion Studies Bring New Drugs and Insights," that evidence from many studies shows that antidepressant drugs can actually cause mania in some patients. Other researchers point out that, though drugs are in general usage as a treatment for depression, they can also at times worsen depression or be the cause of it, thus creating their own vicious circle.

The duration of drug therapy must be determined on an individual basis, depending on the previous pattern of episodes, degree of impairment produced, the adverse consequences of a new recurrence, and the patient's ability to tolerate the drug. However, keeping persons on an antidepressant long enough for the effects to be felt often proves difficult. During the first two to four weeks the patient can feel the side effects of the drug but may experience little relief from the depression. At that point physicians often make the mistake of taking their patients off the drug too soon for its antidepressive effects to be felt or of not raising the dose to an adequate level to be effective—though all experts in drug therapy would deplore a general rush to high dosages by doctors inexperienced in drug treatments.

Many physicians recommend that patients be kept on a drug regimen for six to eight months, and, sometimes, for as long as a year, since the relapse rate of patients taken off too early is high. Although firm data concerning the optimal duration of treatment are lacking, some clinicians feel that if a patient remains free of recurrences during a period equivalent to several of the previous cycle lengths, a decision may be reached to discontinue treatment, provided that a family member or friend of the patient is available to alert the patient and, if necessary, the physician to symptoms of recurrence. In general, the stronger the indications for initiating preventive treatment, the longer its duration should be.

When tricyclics are discontinued after long-term exposure to the drug, the process should be gradual to avoid symptoms that sometimes occur after sudden cessation.

In using lithium some patients interrupt their treatment when they find it takes away the feeling of well-being that they experienced when they were in a mildly manic state. Most patients resume taking their medication when they find that, if they do not, they will again have disabling manic episodes. Some patients discontinue lithium because they feel they no longer need the medication. It is understandable that, if one remains well week after week, there is a tendency either to forget to take medication or to believe that one is completely well and in need of no further treatment. However, if medication is stopped the probability of having another manic or depressive attack may be just as great as before taking lithium, no matter how long the medication has been used.

Zisook, Sidney et al., "Efficacy and Safety of Fezolamine in Depressed Patients," *Neuropsychobiology*, 17(1987), 133-138.

drug therapy, side effects Common side effects of antidepressants include dry mouth, constipation, bladder problems, sexual problems, blurred vision, dizziness and drowsiness. However, these adverse reactions are usually mild, occur early in treatment and subside as the body adjusts.

The National Institute of Mental Health (NIMH) suggests the following as ways to deal with common side effects:

Dry mouth	Drink lots of water, chew sugarless gum, clean teeth daily.
Constipation	Eat bran cereals, prunes, fruit and vegetables.
Bladder problems	Call a doctor if there is any pain. Emptying the bladder may be troublesome, and the urine stream may not be as strong as usual.
Sexual problems	Sexual functioning may change, so if worried discuss this with a doctor.
Blurred vision	This will pass without a need to get new glasses.
Dizziness	Rise from a bed or chair slowly.

Drowsiness   This, too, will pass, but do not drive or operate heavy equipment if feeling drowsy or sedated. Taking the medication at bedtime may be helpful.

In most cases the foregoing side effects are more annoying than serious. However, any other uncommon or unusual side effects that interfere with functioning should be reported to a physician immediately. In some uncommon cases drugs have caused damage to the kidney and heart.

DSM-III-R diagnostic criteria   The explicit criteria provided in the DIAGNOSTIC AND STATISTICAL MANUAL OF MENTAL DISORDERS (DSM-III-R) for use by clinicians making diagnoses for depression. The diagnostic criteria published in this volume include separate criteria for manic episodes, major depressive episodes, bipolar disorders, cyclothymia and dysthymia. Each of the foregoing categories is defined and symptoms to be used as guidelines for diagnosis are listed.

dst or dex test   See DEXAMETHASONE SUPPRESSION TEST.

duration of drug therapy   See DRUG THERAPY.

dysphoria   Derived from the Greek meaning "hard to bear," this is the medical term for the mood of sadness, worthlessness, guilt and helplessness of depression which seems as though it will never end.

dyspnea   Shortness of breath.

dysthymia   Generally a less severe type of depression that was once called neurotic depression. It involves long-term chronic symptoms that do not disable people but keep them from functioning at "full steam" or from feeling good. Some people with dysthymia also have episodes of major depression,

with their symptoms becoming dramatically more severe for a while and then returning to their usual reduced level. These people are said to have double depression (dysthymia plus major depression). Individuals with double depression are at a much higher risk for recurring episodes of major depression, so careful treatment and follow-up is very important.

According to Robert E. Becker, Ph.D., of the Department of Psychiatry, Medical College of Pennsylvania, there is little information available about the clinical treatment of dysthymia. Few studies have focused exclusively on patients diagnosed with a dysthymic disorder. Instead they have mixed this group with patients with major depressive disorder.

With Richard G. Heimburg, Ph.D., Becker conducted a study aimed exclusively at dysthymia disorder. The researchers' purpose was to combine treatments that offered promise of significant treatment effects and then to compare them in a controlled fashion. They chose to compare psychological treatments and pharmacological treatments in the hope that these combinations would produce synergistic effects. Their treatment combinations were: (1) nortriptyline plus social skills training; (2) placebo plus social skills training; (3) nortriptyline plus crisis supportive psychotherapy; and (4) placebo plus crisis supportive psychotherapy. Patients were randomly assigned to treatment. The 39 patients had a mean age of 38.17 and 13.87 years of education. Their occupations included such work as computer programmer, librarian, engineering technician and office manager. Assessments were done by blind evaluators, and treatments were monitored for integrity.

Although all four treatment combinations were significantly effective, the results suggested that the pharmacological combinations (nortriptyline plus social skills training and nortriptyline plus crisis supportive psychotherapy) tended to be the most effective treatment.

"The diagnosis of dysthymic disorder is

difficult and not without controversy," stated Becker in "Treatment of Dysthymic Disorder." "This study was an attempt to find and treat such patients by a very careful psychiatric and medical screening. The screening appears to have been successful. Previous work suggested that patients diagnosed with dysthymic disorder were not highly responsive to treatment. Yet, this group of 39 has shown significant improvement by the end of any of the treatments employed here. By implication, it may mean that carefully selected dysthymic disorder patients are much more responsive to both psychological and pharmacological treatments than previous work has suggested."

Becker, Robert E. and Heimberg, Richard G., "Treatment of Dysthymic Disorder," to be published in a professional journal.

E

Eagleton, Thomas F. In 1972 Thomas F. Eagleton of Missouri was George McGovern's running mate for vice president of the United States on the Democratic presidential ticket. When it was disclosed that Eagleton had been hospitalized for "nervous exhaustion" in the 1960s and had received electric shock therapy he was forced to withdraw from the campaign. In 1988 during the George Bush (Republican)/Michael Dukakis (Democrat) campaign, history attempted to repeat itself when rumors began circulating in the media that Dukakis, governor of Massachusetts, had once been treated for depression. To nullify the rumors that he had sought treatment Dukakis had to release his detailed medical history, and his campaign managers had to follow this with a strong statement that Dukakis had never had any kind of professional therapy. The 1988 incident caused mental health professionals, the media and many enlightened members of the public to examine and reexamine the ongoing stigma attached to high-level government officials who need to (or who seek) mental health counseling or therapy and to debate the fact that all too often public knowledge that a top official has sought therapy can mean at least a temporary setback or stumbling block in a high-level government career.

eating disorders See ANOREXIA NERVOSA; BULIMIA.

economic impact See WORKPLACE, DEPRESSION IN.

elderly Estimates for occurrence of depression among the elderly vary according to the sources that report them. This variation attests to the difficulties of diagnosing depression in the older population.

Statistically speaking, fewer people over 65 (as opposed to younger age groups) are affected by it. But it is nevertheless both common and serious among the elderly.

Symptoms of depression are often misdiagnosed as senility (organic brain syndrome) or mistaken for the everyday problems of the aged. For example, the memory loss, confused thinking or apathy symptomatic of senility actually may be caused by depression. On the other hand, early awakening and reduced appetite typical of depression are common among many older persons who are not depressed.

To further complicate a diagnosis, elderly persons rarely admit feelings of depression, even though they may have much to be depressed about. Among the reasons for their depression are poor health, physical ailments and waning strength; a general feeling of uselessness; a growing anxiety about what they have to live for; an awareness of mortality; emotional problems such as loneliness and boredom; lower incomes, financial problems and poverty; the death of a spouse or other beloved family members or friends.

Often they incorrectly attribute these symptoms of depression to physical ailments, and either ignore them or seek inappropriate treatment. This is understandable, too, because depression does accompany many of the illnesses that afflict older persons, such as Parkinson's disease, cancer, arthritis and the early stages of Alzheimer's disease.

Medications taken by older persons can also cause depression as a side effect. Sometimes the misuse or abuse of medication and drugs is involved.

Careful observation by a knowledgeable person, in addition to sophisticated medical evaluation, may be necessary to recognize the depressed older person. A physician attempting to differentiate between senility and depression may call on family members or longtime friends for information on the patient's history, since the onset of depression is usually more sudden than the slow and gradual process of senility. Also the individual with organic problems typically minimizes loss of mental function such as memory, while the depressed person exaggerates the loss.

Treatment of the elderly, if antidepressants are indicated, can be complicated by physical problems in addition to diagnostic problems. The older person is more apt to have a complex set of physical ailments for which various drugs are taken. Before prescribing an antidepressant, a physician must carefully consider all other drugs used by the patient, particularly those for heart conditions, to avoid unwanted side effects. Also, because the elderly metabolize drugs more slowly than younger people, the prescribing physician needs to carefully consider and monitor the dosage of antidepressants.

Because drug therapy may not be appropriate for some elderly depressed patients, an important area of research is the role of psychotherapies. One of several studies conducted by Dolores W. Gallagher, Ph.D., and Larry W. Thompson, Ph.D., of the Geriatric Research, Education and Clinical Center at Palo Alto V.A. Medical Center examined whether or not older adults in a major depressive episode would improve systematically when treated with short-term psychotherapies, and whether or not they would respond differentially to treatment approaches emphasizing the importance of either cognitive, behavioral, or relational/insight therapy. (The latter is the more traditional psychodynamic approach that fits within a brief treatment framework.)

In this study, 30 elderly outpatients were assigned to one of the three individual treatment programs mentioned above for 16 sessions over a 12-week period. Evaluation occurred before and after therapy, and at four times during a one-year follow-up. According to the researchers, comparable improvement in depressive symptoms was seen from pre to post for clients in all three treatment conditions. As a result, the researchers believe psychotherapy may be an effective alternate method of treatment for major depressive disorders in the elderly.

The results of the above study showed that improvement during the one-year follow-up was maintained more effectively by clients treated with behavioral or cognitive therapy than with relational/insight therapy, indicating to researchers that structured therapies may be more beneficial than nonstructured, relationally-oriented therapy during a treatment-free follow-up period. "This may be due in part to the skill acquisition focus of these (cognitive or behavioral) therapies," stated Gallagher in "Treatment of Major Depressive Disorder in Older Adult Outpatients with Brief Psychotherapies." "In fact, during the various follow-up interviews, questions were asked to determine what skills (if any) were still being used by clients in their everyday lives. Approximately two-thirds of those in cognitive or behavioral treatment indicated that specific skills they had learned in therapy (e.g., mood monitoring, recording dysfunctional thoughts, etc.) were used on a regular basis. In contrast, only one-third of the relational/insight therapy clients reported use of knowledge or skills acquired in therapy."

Ongoing studies by Gallagher and other

researchers continue to offer encouragement that short-term therapies, in some cases, can be an effective alternative to drugs. But researchers point out there are still a number of unanswered questions and that a major challenge for the future is being able to pinpoint specifically who is more likely to benefit from one kind of treatment than from another.

Despite this and other difficulties in finding appropriate treatments for depressed older people, evidence clearly points to the fact that—as with younger individuals—effective treatment can reduce unnecessary suffering, help afflicted individuals cope with the medical problems they may also have, and offer a new lease on life and renewed productivity. (See also BEHAVIORAL DISORDERS; COGNITIVE THERAPY.)

Gallagher, Dolores E. and Thompson, Larry W., "Treatment of Major Depressive Disorder in Older Adult Outpatients with Brief Psychotherapies," *Psychotherapy Theory, Research and Practice*, 19:4(Winter 1982).

Thompson, L., Gallagher, D. and Breckenridge, J.S., "Comparative Effectiveness of Psychotherapies for Depressed Elders," *Journal of Consulting and Clinical Psychology*, 55:3(1987).

electroconvulsive therapy (ECT)

With the availability of psychoactive drugs, use of ECT (which began in 1938) has declined. Nevertheless, it remains a very effective treatment for major ENDOGENOUS DEPRESSION and mania (it is not effective for dysthymic depression, see DYSTHYMIA), and new techniques make it safer, producing less of the temporary confusion and memory loss that once resulted from it. These improved techniques and judicious use of ECT are changing negative attitudes caused by early abuses. Many researchers feel that until a fast-acting drug is developed ECT remains the most effective emergency treatment and is particularly effective when the individual is severely depressed; severely malnour-

ished; has severe delusions; is at high risk for suicide; does not respond to drugs (or can't tolerate their side effects); or, as often happens among the elderly, cannot take drugs because of a medical problem.

Although most persons can take ECT, people who are *not* candidates are those with a damaged heart or recent coronary attack. Other exceptions are persons with an active infection or unusual debility, and extremely young children. Studies on animals suggest that antidepressants and ECT alter the same chemicals and receptors in the brain.

Current ECT practices are designed to bring symptomatic relief with minimal discomfort. It is usually administered three times a week for up to eight treatments. The patient is briefly put to sleep with an intravenous anesthetic, ensuring that the procedure is painless and not consciously experienced or remembered. A muscle relaxant is administered to minimize muscular response when the electric current is applied.

Electrodes are placed either on both sides of the scalp (bilaterally) or on one side of the scalp (unilaterally), on the "non-dominant" side of the brain (usually the right side). There is substantial evidence that unilateral electrode placement over the "non-dominant" hemisphere produces less temporary memory loss and confusion. However, there is also some evidence that unilateral "non-dominant" placement may be less effective or require more treatments than bilateral placement.

The age of the patient and the length, spacing, number of treatments and intensity of electric current administered influence the above-mentioned memory loss and confusion. (The lower the intensity of electric current administered, the better.) However, even under optimum conditions, patients experience transient memory loss of events surrounding the treatment—most often for those occurring six months to a year before the ECT treatments.

In an article in *The New York Times*, "Experts Say Treatments Affect Recall," Dr.

Larry R. Squire of the Veterans Administration Medical Center in San Diego, who has studied memory loss from electroshock therapy, said the treatment can cause loss of memory for current and past events. But the loss gradually recedes.

Several months after the treatments patients remember new events, as shown on psychological tests. They are left with a gap covering a few weeks before, during and after their treatments. Dr. Squire stated that some patients will also have some spotty memory loss going back months before their treatment.

The ability to learn new information during and immediately after ECT can be temporarily affected, but is typically regained after several weeks.

Kolata, Gina, "Experts Say Treatments Affect Recall," *The New York Times*, October 19, 1988.

electroencephalogram (EEG) The oldest and simplest brain imaging technique. It records the brain's electrical activity with electrodes pasted on the scalp. The signals come from the firing of billions of cells in different parts of the brain.

Romney, Elizabeth, "Breaking Through," *NARSAD Research Newsletter*, 1 (Spring 1988).

electroshock treatment See ELECTRO-CONVULSIVE THERAPY.

Elizabethan England (1558–1603) During the Elizabethan period England passed through one of its greatest times in history as it rose from a comparatively minor nation to become both a first rate European power and a world power. It was also a period that produced such celebrated persons as William Shakespeare, Edmund Spenser, Francis Bacon, Walter Raleigh and Francis Drake.

However, the change from minor-nation status to world-class status was accompanied by tumult and strife, the abandonment of old

social moorings, and the restless groping toward an uncertain future. The period became known as the great age of melancholy.

In keeping with this, Elizabethan England produced a great outpouring of melancholic literature. Depression was brought out in the open and, to the Elizabethans, it was a much-discussed subject. Dr. Nathan S. Kline wrote in *From Sad to Glad:* "Many even preened themselves on being melancholy for they came to consider it a superior malady, a mark of refined sensibility among those deeply touched by the pathos of life. Some advertised their elegant suffering by adopting a sad, languid air and ostentatiously dressing all in black."

Kline, Nathan S., *From Sad to Glad* (New York: Putnam, 1974).

Ellis, Albert A New York psychologist (1913–) and president of the Institute for Rational/Emotive Therapy, Dr. Ellis believes that people's thinking patterns can strongly affect their moods. He is the author of over 50 books on mental health, and in his book *Reason and Emotion in Psychotherapy* he discusses the history of his view of mood disorders. Ellis believes people may inadvertently undermine what they attempt by driving themselves with so many "oughts," "shoulds" and "musts" they drain themselves of any desire to get moving. Ellis describes this mental trap as "*must*erbation," and two of his slogans to live by are "*I Will Not Should On Myself Today*" and "*MUSTurbation Means Self Abuse.*" (See also RATIONAL EMOTIVE PSYCHOTHERAPY.)

Ellis, Albert, *Reason and Emotion in Psychotherapy* (New York: Lyle Stuart, 1962).

Emotional Health Anonymous (EHA) A California-based self-help program and fellowship of men and women who meet to share their experience, strength and hope with one another so they may help each other with such common emotional and mental problems as depression, anxiety, anger and fear. With the permission of Alcoholics Anonymous, members use the Twelve Steps of A.A., slightly modified. At meetings members relate their personal experiences with their emotional problems and tell how they have improved with the help of the Twelve Steps and the program. Meetings are non-professional and are led by an EHA member. Professional people in the mental health field, members of the clergy or anyone in the helping professions are invited to attend as visitors. Some participate in EHA as active members on a non-professional basis. Many people are referred to EHA by mental health and social service professionals, doctors, judges and members of the clergy.

EHA (originally named Emotional Health Groups) was started in 1970 by a man in Rosemead, California. In 1972, the original group became the Fellowship of Emotional Health Anonymous. Since that time, EHA's growth has continued, first in Southern California, then throughout the United States and subsequently to other countries. There are no dues or fees for membership. The groups are self-supporting through their own contributions. For information on EHA or to find a group meeting near you consult your telephone directory or contact: Emotional Health Anonymous, General Service Office, 2420 San Gabriel Boulevard, Rosemead, CA 91779. Phone: 818-573-5482.

empty nest syndrome   The "empty-nest syndrome" has been offered to explain change-of-life depression. The theory is that when children grow up and leave home, women who have devoted their lives to raising children feel no longer needed and bereft of ego-supporting activities, much in the way that some men respond to RETIREMENT. However, the lack of increased rates of depression among women at this stage of life suggests that most do not get seriously depressed, even though changes of any kind can trigger depression in vulnerable people.

(See also INVOLUTIONAL MELANCHOLIA; MENOPAUSE; MID-LIFE.)

endogenous depression   A term that has been used to designate forms of depression thought to come from within, in contrast to EXOGENOUS or reactive DEPRESSIONS, which were thought to be caused by factors external to the depressed person. This category has been abandoned in recent classifications of psychiatric disorders.

Endogenous depressions involved a cluster of symptoms long thought more likely to have biological origins, such as sleep disturbance, weight loss, psychomotor retardation, severe depression, diurnal variation, difficulty in concentration, and lack of response to environmental changes that would enhance the mood of most people. More recent classifications have taken to using "with melancholia" to refer to such depressions.

England   The burdens imposed by depression, anxiety, dementia and psychotic illnesses are heavy and weigh on those suffering from these disorders—as well as on their families and the services that offer treatment and support. But, according to *On the State of the Public Health,* an HMSO publication (Her Majesty's Stationery Office), dramatic changes in treatment have taken place over the last 40 years. The development of a wider range of services outside of hospitals, together with the advent of new treatments such as the major tranquilizers, lithium and antidepressant drugs, has led to a marked fall in the number of patients who reside in mental hospitals and units—specifically from 149,480 in 1956 to 60,280 in 1986. Most people, even those with serious mental illness, will show a good response to modern treatment. However, it remains an unpalatable fact that many mentally ill people require support and treatment on a long-term basis.

In discussing depression and anxiety the above-mentioned publication states:

Very considerable numbers of people suffer long-term distress as a result of depression and anxiety. They are looked after mainly by the general practitioner (GP) and the primary care team. GPs identify some 14% of the patients attending their surgeries as having a significant psychological disorder. The use of validated screening tests show that a further 9% of general practice attenders have a similar degree of disorder but are not identified as such. These groups are therefore termed "conspicuous" and "hidden" morbidity. There is evidence that if hidden morbidity can be detected by the GP, then its prognosis improves. Research has shown that depression is associated with an increased risk of physical illness (and hence increased mortality), increased risk of suicide and parasuicide, marital breakdown, and with considerable occupational problems, such as sickness absence, labour turnover, problems with colleagues, poor performance and accidents. It also results in emotional and cognitive impairment in the children of depressed parents, which in turn can predispose to adult mental illness when the children grow up, as well as having an adverse effect on the children's ultimate intellectual attainment. Children may come into care as a result of neglect and abuse from a depressed parent.

A number of researchers are involved in studying the lifetime risk of depression for people up to age 65. One study conducted by Dr. Paul Bebbington of MRC Social Psychiatry Unit, Institute of Psychiatry, and his colleagues was based on a population survey in the area of Camberwell, South London. The study consisted of a two-stage survey of the general population in Camberwell. Trained interviewers from a reputable social survey agency interviewed a random sample of 383 men and 407 women aged 18 to 64. The interviewers used the 40-item version of the Present State Examination (PSE), a semi-structured interview schedule designed to elicit symptoms experienced in the last month. This was followed with a question-

naire eliciting basic social facts about each subject.

A second interview was carried out four to six weeks after the first one. It included items from the PSE plus a Clinical History Schedule. The latter is a semi-structured interview that concentrates on key symptoms such as persistent and depressed mood to elicit a history of possible previous episodes of depression (and other psychiatric disturbance). When it appears that the subject may have had a previous episode, more free-ranging questions are asked to determine the presence of accessory symptoms, the duration of the episode, the presence of associated social impairment and whether treatment was sought. The included episodes were characterized by persistent and unalleviated depression of mood, usually lasting more than a month and in a majority of cases leading to treatment at least by the family doctor.

The results of the two-stage survey showed that the risk of Camberwell subjects suffering an episode of depressive disorder by the age of 65 was 62%. Using this survey and the method cited above it was 46% for men and 72% for women. However, the researchers pointed out that, using another method based on (untenably) conservative assumptions, the statistics became 16% and 30% respectively.

In summing up their work the researchers believe their results suggest that the risk of experiencing a clinically noteworthy depressive episode up to age 65 may be very high indeed. In their view the high estimated risk of depression by age 65 is the natural corollary of the high prevalence of depressive conditions commonly found in a community survey. But they believe the results of their survey must at least form a caveat for genetic research workers who seek to use non-referred episodes of depression in relatives as an indication of concordance. Relying on such episodes to define a history of depression, say the researchers, results in such a high rate in the community that a direct comparison of lifetime risk would have little hope of demonstrating dramatic genetic effects. This may be because non-referred disorders, which are typically less severe than referred cases of depression, are relatively uninfluenced by genetic differences.

"Alternatively, the effects of a genetic predisposition towards affective disorder may be to increase the number of episodes and reduce the age of onset," concluded the researchers in "The Risk of Minor Depression Before Age 65."

If so, it requires to be quantified in a manner other than the relatively crude measure afforded by lifetime risk. Finally, it may be *resistance* to minor depression that is the interesting (and possibly inherited) trait. The genetic effects that have been clearly demonstrated in affective disorders are based on the more severe cases that reach the clinic or hospital ward, and it would seem most secure to rely on a history of psychiatric contact in establishing the existence of episodes of depression in the relatives of probands.

The Medical Research Council (MRC) headquartered in London was originally set up in 1913 as the Medical Research Committee to administer funds provided for medical research under the terms of the National Insurance Act of 1911. In 1920 MRC was incorporated under its present title by royal charter. Its function is to promote the balanced development of medical and related biological research in England.

Along with its membership, which serves as an advisory board, MRC employs its own research staff and also provides grants for other institutions and for individuals who are not members of its own staff, thus complementing the research resources of the universities and hospitals. In addition the council advises government on matters relating to medical research and cooperates with government departments and with other organizations in England and overseas.

Though not a government department the council receives an annual grant-in-aid from Parliament via the Department of Education and Science and also receives funds for specific projects from a number of other government sources. Because of the terms of its charter, the MRC is able to receive and administer funds or other properties entrusted to it by grant, gift or bequest, either for the general purposes of research or for research on specific diseases. As such it is involved in funding research for depression.

Some of the work and studies with which it has been involved are: possible viral infection in schizophrenia, manic-depressive illness and dementia; the adult outcome of depressive and non-depressive disorders arising in childhood; genetic family investigation into child and adult depressive disorders; basic and clinical studies of the mechanisms of action of ECT, antidepressant drugs, anxiolytics and lithium, with emphasis on the role of 5-hydroxytryptamine; clinical psychopharmacology of depression and anxiety; alcohol and depression; depression in community and hospital populations; neurochemical pathology of neurodegenerative disorders and major depression; clinical neuroendocrine and biochemical investigations in dementia and depression; factors associated with depression in young married women; the effects of maternal depression postpartum on infant development; and determinants of recovery and relapse in depression.

Bebbington, P., Katz, R. et al., "The Risk of Minor Depression Before Age 65: Results from a Community Survey," *Psychological Medicine,* 19(1989).

HMSO, *On the State of the Public Health, 1987* (London: HMSO, 1988).

Medical Research Council, *MRC Handbook 1987* (London: MRC, 1987).

environmental/psychosocial factors

Some researchers theorize family environment may play a role and believe that a person brought up in a household with a depressed or manic individual may learn by example to handle stress in an abnormal manner. Also, other environmental as well as biochemical influences may represent a genetic vulnerability set in motion by prolonged stress, trauma, physical illness or some other condition.

Financial problems, midlife crises, sex role expectations, and such psychosocial phenomena as personality, upbringing and a negative thinking style have been cited as contributors to depressive disorders.

Any changes, serious loss or stress—a divorce, the death of a loved one, the loss of a job or a move to a new home—can trigger depression, usually temporary but sometimes requiring treatment to alleviate symptoms. (See also CAUSES OF DEPRESSION.)

enzymes Numerous complex proteins that are produced by living cells and catalyze specific biochemical reactions at body temperatures. The action of enzymes is an important area of study in biochemistry since they are involved in the metabolism of living things, and many diseases are known to exist that are caused by the deficiency or malfunction of certain enzymes.

epidemiologic catchment area study (ECA) To answer the questions (1) "What is the prevalence of depression in America?" (2) "Are there male/female differences?" and (3) "Are there age differences?" the National Institute of Mental Health conducted between 1980 and 1983 an Epidemiologic Catchment Area (ECA) Project, a probability sample of over 18,000 adults aged 18 years or older from five United States communities. The communities studied were New Haven, Connecticut; Baltimore, Maryland; St. Louis, Missouri; Piedmont County, North Carolina; and Los Angeles, California. The surveys in the five communities used comparable interview schedules and study designs. In 1984 the preliminary results from three of the five ECA sites were published in the October issue of *Archives of General Psychiatry*. And in 1988 "Affective Disorders in Five United States Communities," a paper published in *Psychological Medicine*, pre-

sented the first findings on the epidemiology of affective disorders in the five communities.

According to the paper, the epidemiologic findings on the age/sex specific prevalence rates and age of onset of three affective disorders—MAJOR DEPRESSION, BIPOLAR DEPRESSION and DYSTHYMIA—are reasonably consistent across geographic areas in the United States and are reasonably consistent with findings reported from clinical studies. There is some suggestion in a 1985 publication based on these data, "Psychiatric Disorders: A Rural Urban Comparison," that rates of major depression are lower in the rural than in the urban or suburban areas. The ECA findings on prevalence rates and sex ratios support the separation of bipolar disorder and major depression. These findings also suggest that the onset and highest risk periods for these disorders are in young adulthood, with a residual of dysthymia in middle and older ages.

In speaking of the researchers' findings (up through the 1984 preliminary results from three sites) Dr. Martin E.P. Seligman of the University of Pennsyvania pointed out in "Why Is There So Much Depression Today" (G. Stanley Hall Lecture Series in Washington, D.C.) that the results published in 1984 showed that if people were born around 1960 (about 20 to 25 years old) their probability of having had at least one episode of major depressive disorder was 5% or 6%. If they were 25 to 44 years old, their risk went up to about 8% or 9%. For people born around 1925 (even though they had had much more opportunity to experience depression) the rate plummeted to little more than 4%. And people born around World World I had a rate of only 1%.

In his lecture Seligman stated that in a second epidemiological study reported in 1985 researchers looked at close relatives of people who had a major depressive disorder. In this study 523 people were diagnosed as having a major affective disorder. The 523 people had 2,289 first-degree relatives—fathers, mothers, brothers, sisters, sons and daughters—who all received the same structured diagnostic interview to determine their risk for major depressive disorder. In discussing the findings of this study Seligman said:

Consider just people who were born before 1910, the generation of your grandmothers or great-grandmothers. By the time your grandmothers' generation reached age 20 only 1% or 2% of those who later had a depressed relative themselves had a depressive disorder. By the time they reached age 70, perhaps 10-15% had a depressive disorder. That is a much larger prevalence than the ECA sample, because, of course, these women are at a genetic risk for depression. Now look at 1950 for age 20 and 30. If you are 30 years old and you were born around 1950 your risk is about 60% whereas your great-grandmother's risk for depression was about 3% by the time she reached 30.

In summing up the Epidemiologic Catchment Area Study (ECA) the ECA researchers point out that the accurate determination of prevalence rates may require more probing and the use of more informants than those in five community surveys. Further analysis will examine the rates and risks of subtypes of major depression. The American Medical Association points out that for the United States, this program is a landmark in psychiatric epidemiology and psychiatric research generally. For the first time, mental health epidemiology is linked to ongoing biological, nosological, genetic, familial and clinical research on mental disorder. (See also NATIONAL INSTITUTE OF MENTAL HEALTH EPIDEMIOLOGIC CATCHMENT AREA (ECA) PROGRAM.)

Weissman, Myrna et al., "Affective Disorders in Five United States Communities," *Psychological Medicine*, 18(1988).

Blazer, D., "Psychiatric Disorders: A Rural Urban Comparison," *Archives of General Psychiatry*, 42(1985).

Freedman, Daniel X., "Psychiatric Epidemi-

ology Counts," *Archives of General Psychiatry*, 41(October 1984).

Seligman, Martin E.P., "Why Is There So Much Depression Today?" The G. Stanley Hall Lecture Series, Washington, D.C., 1988.

epidemiology The medical science that studies variations, occurrences and prevalences (epidemiologic studies) in the distribution of diseases in populations. As opposed to the clinician who deals with individual cases, the epidemiologist deals with large numbers of people in a community.

In "Epidemiology of Depression," W.O. McCormick, M.D., professor of psychiatry at Dalhousie University in Halifax, Nova Scotia explained: "Epidemiology consists of counting the number of cases of some disorder in a defined population over a defined time and looking at a sub-grouping of that population who may have different frequencies of the disorder from the population as a whole."

McCormick, W.O., "Epidemiology of Depression," *Psychiatric Journal-University of Ottawa*, 14:2(1989).

etiology A branch of knowledge that deals with the causes of a disease or abnormal condition. As a science, it investigates the origin of a condition.

euphoria A psychological, and sometimes pathological, condition in which people feel thriving and well off, cheerful and optimistic, and jubilant and elated. In addition, they can be hyperactive. It accompanies the manic state in a manic-depressive illness.

exogenous depression A term sometimes used to describe a type of depression that's associated with life events or environmental factors, as opposed to ENDOGENOUS DEPRESSION, which comes from within. Exogenous depression can vary from case to case and overlap other forms caused by the two above factors.

F

failure Therapists have frequently reported seeing failure as a factor likely to cause depression, and today new research—after rigorous laboratory experimentation—supports the belief that some people read the worst into even the most trivial setback. This trait is now being implicated directly by some psychotherapists as an important factor in a wide range of emotional turmoil, including depression. Researchers have also noted a tendency among patients with this trait to minimize the importance of their successes.

In "Depression and the Magnification of Failure," published in the *Journal of Abnormal Psychology,* Dr. Richard Wenzlaff, a psychologist at the University of Texas in San Antonio, stated that when people continually exaggerate the importance of their failures, it sets up a downward spiral of disappointment that can end in depression.

With Sherilyn Grozier, also a psychologist at the University of Texas, Dr. Wenzlaff researched how people interpret a setback. In their experiment volunteer undergraduate students were given a series of psychological tests, including one they were told was a new test of social perceptiveness. The finished tests were collected by a researcher who then went into the next room, purportedly to score them. Five minutes later the researcher returned and gave the volunteers their scores on the social perceptiveness test. In fact, each volunteer was arbitrarily given a score that placed the subject either in the bottom half or in the top 7% on the new scale. As part of the other psychological tests, the volunteers rated the relative importance of 15 personality traits, including social perceptiveness.

The subjects' ratings of their social perceptiveness were analyzed using depression (depressed vs. nondepressed) and feedback (success vs. failure) as a measure factor. The analysis indicated that depressed subjects generally believed they were less socially perceptive than did nondepressed subjects.

"The present findings indicate that there are specific differences in the way depressed and nondepressed individuals respond to success and failure," reported Dr. Wenzlaff.

Wenzlaff explains that the depressed and nondepressed subjects differed in terms of the importance they assigned to social perceptiveness after receiving the success vs. failure feedback. The depressed subjects judged social perceptiveness to be more important after they had failed on a test presumed to assess that trait. In contrast, nondepressed subjects ascribed more importance to social perceptiveness after they had succeeded on the test. Non-depressed subjects' inflated view of the importance of social perceptiveness following success is consistent with a growing body of research suggesting that nondepressives have selfenhancing biases.

In earlier research on failure, led by Dr. Martin E.P. Seligman of the University of Pennsylvania, researchers found that the ability to take setbacks in stride was fundamental to success in endeavors ranging from sales to presidential elections. Similarly Dr. Aaron Beck, who developed COGNITIVE THERAPY, found that magnifying the importance of a failure is one of several such cognitive distortions that have been described as being at the root of depression.

Recommended treatment for people whose depression is caused by failure requires helping them learn to assess setbacks more realistically and take them in stride. It also involves helping them see that there are things that they succeed in and convincing them that being less than perfect is acceptable and does not mean they are a failure.

Wenzloff, Richard and Grozier, Sherilyn, "Depression and the Magnification of Failure," *Journal of Abnormal Psychology,* 9:1(1988).

familial pure depressive disease (FPDD) A term used to categorize the depression of persons who have a first-degree relative with depression.

fatigue See CHRONIC FATIGUE.

fezolamine A relatively new non-tricyclic antidepressant agent. In research reported by Dr. Sidney Zisook of the University of California at San Diego, 42 outpatients with major depressive disorder were treated with oral fezolamine in a six-week pilot study at three study sites. Therapy was initiated at 100 mg/day. Thereafter dosage was increased based on the response of the patient. Maintenance dosage usually ranged between 100 and 450 mg/day. Clinically significant improvement relative to the patient's prestudy state was observed after two weeks in both patient and physician-rating scales. The median dose associated with a clinically significant response was 245 mg/day. Five of the six patients who dropped out did so because of adverse gastrointestinal effects. The most common adverse effects were nausea, headache, constipation and dry mouth. Despite differences in the depressed outpatient populations in the three-center study, each study site, to varying degrees, found fezolamine to be an effective, safe and relatively well tolerated antidepressant medication. Consequently, the results from these three pilot studies singly and together indicate that fezolamine may be an effective antidepressant with minimal anticholinergic, sedative and cardiovascular effects.

Zisook, Sidney et al., "Efficacy and Safety of Fezolamine in Depressed Patients," *Neuropsychobiology*, 17(1987), 133–138.

fluoxetine (Prozac) One of the newest antidepressant drugs. As a compound that seems to affect primarily the SEROTONIN system (see NEUROTRANSMITTERS, BIOCHEMICAL FACTORS) it was first used in Europe where experience indicated it helped some people who did not respond to standard drugs. Under research, roughly half of the persons who respond poorly to older drugs seemed to benefit from fluoxetine. As a pure serotonin reuptake blocker, it does not have the drawbacks and side effects that some of

the other tricyclic antidepressants do—e.g., dry mouth, constipation, blurred vision. It also causes fewer problems with blood pressure than some of the earlier antidepressants do. Although every drug that has positive effects can also have negative ones, clinicians who prescribe fluoxetine feel that the frequency of these side effects is much less than that of some of the other tricyclics.

food, effects of See DIET.

Freud, Sigmund See FREUDIAN THEORY OF DEPRESSION.

Freudian theory of depression Some early psychoanalysts, such as the Austrian psychiatrist and founder of psychoanalysis, Sigmund Freud (1856–1939), felt that persons who were depressed were trapped by some unresolved trauma or anger from a phase of childhood development. Thus Freud was strong in his belief that internalized anger was the cause of depression, and his treatise *Mourning and Melancholia* became the basis for the orthodox psychoanalytic approach to treating depression. As a result, some therapists urge depressed patients to understand and accept their anger and externalize it more often. Others believe there is no real evidence to support Freud's belief.

Though this aspect of Freud's approach to depression was never totally accepted, it was a strong force in medical thinking through the first half of the 20th century. In the last half, however, it has been increasingly challenged by people who believe depression's basic cause, in at least some cases, is a biochemical disorder.

Interestingly enough, early in his career Freud himself was a victim of depression. In *The Interpretation of Dreams* he wrote: "I am now experiencing myself all the things that as third party I have witnessed going on in my patients—days when I slink about depressed because I have understood nothing of the day's dreams, fantasies or mood, and other days when a flash of lightning brings coherence into the picture, and what has gone before is revealed as preparation for the present."

Freud was so depressed at times that he tried cocaine, on which he was doing research, and widely recommended its use before it was realized how habit-forming and dangerous the drug could be. When one of his friends to whom he had recommended cocaine became an addict, Freud grew so opposed to it that from that time on he avoided cocaine and any other drug that affected mental processes.

From Sad to Glad In 1974, when Dr. NATHAN S. KLINE, a pioneer in drug research for depression, published this work, it was considered a breakthrough book on the subject. As it outlines the social history of depression, the detective-like medical research involved in tracing causes and cures, and the pharmaceutical methods of treating the problem, it is still considered a popular masterwork on depression.

Kline, Nathan S., *From Sad to Glad* (New York: Putnam, 1974).

funerals Funerals are part of the GRIEF and MOURNING process, and the symbolism and ritual of both the funeral ceremony and the burial of the dead are supposed to provide psychological comfort and solace to the bereaved. As the rituals make the universality of death a formal and collective ceremony in which survivors participate, the funeral custom is meant to fill important emotional needs that help survivors express feelings and discharge grief. For many people these events symbolize a passage from one life to another. They are often referred to as a "rite of passage" and are generally religious.

Throughout history, people of all cultures have regarded the disposal of the dead as an act requiring group concern accompanied by certain ceremonies. The ceremonies and practices take varied and diverse forms, and in some societies a death vigil is practiced. Some old funeral and burial customs are still practiced. Others have become more modern in concept and procedure.

Some societies have disposed of their dead in ways other than burial or cremation. The Sioux Indians of North America placed their dead on high platforms. Some groups of aborigines, e.g., the original inhabitants of Australia, left dead bodies in trees. In Tibet bodies have been sunk in water. The Parsis, a religious group who live mainly in India, have been known to take their dead to special enclosures called "towers of silence." There, birds picked the bones clean.

The Hindus and Buddhists burn the deceased's body. Fire taken from the deceased's home is carried to the cremation ground in a black earthen pot. This is carried in front of the deceased. At the cremation site a lighted torch is handed to the eldest son or grandson who ignites the pyre. According to Moslem funeral customs, relatives wearing mourning bands look on as the body wrapped in a seamless shroud is entombed on its side facing the holy city of Mecca. Ancient Roman funeral processions were notable for the parade of ancestors' death masks. And in Islamic countries friends carry the corpse on an open bier, generally followed by women relatives and hired mourners.

In writing about burial customs for suicides in *The Encyclopedia of Suicide,* Glen Evans and Dr. Norman Farberow describe how, starting with the mid-1500s, punishment was meted out on the corpse of a suicide. The cadaver was subjected to various indignities and degradations. A common practice in England was to bury the suicide at a crossroad by night with a stake driven through the heart. Some suicides were buried in this manner as late as 1811, and the bizarre practice was not discontinued until 1823.

Evans and Farberow relate that Tacitus, the Roman historian, reported on so-called "bog burials," the practice of pinning down the body with a stake. This practice, confirmed by numerous authorities, seems to antedate Christianity among the Germanic people of Europe. The purpose was to ensure that the spirit of the dead person would not return to haunt or otherwise do harm to the living.

In the 18th century in France and England a suicide's body was dragged through the streets, head downward on a frame or sledge, similar to what was used for dragging criminals to their place of execution. Then the corpse was strung up to hang from public gallows. Because of the popular revulsion at the practice of dragging the corpse, the penalty was not carried out after 1768. Evans and Farberow quote Dr. George Rosen, in a historical essay on *A Handbook for the Study of Suicide,* as saying, "In general, the penalties against the body of a suicide tended to lapse by the latter part of the seventeenth century." Today the funeral rites accorded to the suicide differ only in a relatively few instances from the rites accorded those who have died a natural death.

In *The Body Snatchers* Daniel Cohen wrote that as late as the mid-19th century the chiefs of some African tribes were buried along with the sacrificed bodies of servants and, occasionally, wives. In the East Indies widows were buried alive with their dead husbands as recently as a hundred years ago. The best-known practice of sacrifice in connection with death, though not in this case with burial, is the Indian custom of "suttee," according to which the widow climbs upon the funeral pyre of her dead husband. This custom so horrified the British conquerers of India that they made it illegal in the 19th century and expended a good deal of energy attempting to stamp it out.

The great wish of the ancient Egyptians was to live forever. They believed that after they died a new life began and that they would live in their tombs as they lived on earth. To do this, they mummified or embalmed the bodies. Coffins were painted inside and out with gods, goddesses and magic spells of protection, and a long and solemn funeral procession took the mummy to the tomb. Priests, family, servants and mourners who were paid to weep followed. Porters car-

ried the food, jewels and other possessions that would be buried with the mummy. The Egyptians believed the deceased's spirit would someday return to inhabit the body. Therefore, the body had to be preserved to prevent the soul from perishing.

According to Georgess McHargue, author of *Mummies,* mummification was also common among Native American Indians. Dried mummies have been found in the southwestern United States where the climate offers some of the same advantages as that of the Egyptian desert. Mummies from this area were always in a flexed position, bundled with fiber rope. The early Floridians are said to have dried the bodies before a fire, dressed them in their best clothes, and set them in caves. In Kentucky the procedure was supposed to be to fill the body with sand, wrap it in skins, and bury it in a cave or under the floor of a hut.

The people of China have historically believed in immortality. The previously-mentioned book by Evans and Farberow gives an account of the Chinese custom of burning paper money so the survivors could provide the deceased with spending money in the other world. In the past Chinese children would sell themselves as slaves in order to give a parent a good funeral. When the time came to cover the casket, the living would always turn their backs toward the casket, so evil spirits that might hover around the dead would not follow them home.

According to the early folklore depicted in *The Book of Negro Folklore,* edited by Langston Hughes and Anna Bontemps, a league appropriately named the Bury League was a cooperative society that grew out of the Negro desire for an elaborate and respectful funeral. Negroes believed a proper funeral ceremony would be of great help in enabling a soul to find the right road to heaven and God or to hell and Satan. Otherwise, they thought the soul would haunt houses and burial grounds and frighten the very people it loved best on earth.

All members of the Bury League paid a

small sum each week to a common fund, which provided for the next funeral. As the folklore goes, every neighborhood had a local chapter headed by a "Noble Shepherd" who kept the treasury until, when it was heavy with dues, he turned it over to the "Leader of the Flock" who owned and drove the automobile hearse and provided coffins and white gravestones. Bury League members were required to attend every burial unless hindered by providence. The women carried white paper flowers, and the officers who carried the banners of the organization wore large badges.

Before the Bury League was organized, coffins were simple pine boxes made by the plantation carpenter, and hearses were farm wagons drawn by mules. The services were long, with much mourning, praying and singing. Lightwood torches gave light for the burial and for marching around the grave.

Turning from older customs to more modern ones, military funerals seem to bridge the gap, since the older traditions are still carried on. In describing military rituals Edgar N. Jackson wrote in *Understanding Grief*: "Military funerals have their own special rituals. The caisson is symbolic of the last lonely ride; the firing of the volley illustrates the energy that is spent and gone; and the playing of taps marks the ending of the day of life. Each part of the military service urges the facing of stark reality."

"An interesting custom has been prevalent in New Orleans," added Jackson. "After days of intense and visible emotional displays of mourning, the family returns from the cemetery with the stirring music of a brass band playing lively tunes to which the mourners dance and sing. Symbolically the mourning is left behind at the grave, and the future is faced with a song."

Mexico also has a jubilant ritual in which each year, with the arrival of the Day of the Dead on November 2, burial places come alive with festivities. The Mexicans celebrate that day by going to their cemeteries to relax, talk and drink, while children play tag and run among the graves. Outside the cemetery gates, vendors sell such things as tortillas, pork rinds, flowers, balloons and candy. Writing in the *New York Times* Larry Rohter explained that, according to anthropologists and sociologists, modern Day of the Dead celebrations are a direct outgrowth of Mexico's Aztec past. To the Aztecs, death was not the end of life, but "merely another phase of an endless, repetitive cosmic process of destruction and regeneration, and some of that system of belief survived the destruction of the Aztec empire." For the Day of the Dead, Mexicans eat skulls made of sugar candy and bread baked in the shape of bones. Many adorn their homes with tissue-paper skeletons. When someone dies in Mexico, survivors usually have the choice of buying a perpetual plot or burying the deceased in a temporary cemetery plot where after seven years the bones are reinterred, often in a mass grave.

Today's Irish wakes are the outgrowth of the medieval custom of sitting up with the dead. This custom of holding an all-night watch—or a wake—beside the corpse was rooted in the belief that the wake comforts the spirit of the dead or protects the body from evil spirits. Early wakes were enlivened by what was termed "rousing the ghost," and many wakes became spirited farewell parties with a funeral feast and much heavy drinking. In fact, historians have commented that in earlier days rich and poor alike felt that funeral arrangements were as incomplete without liquor as without a hearse or coffin.

Today an Irish wake is much more subdued. Funeral customs follow the now common practice of "viewing" the body in a funeral home prior to the funeral mass. Following the church mass and burial, however, there is a celebration, or a festive party at an inn or in a home, during which there is laughter, fun, drinking and food. Often as many as 50 to 75 relatives and friends gather to, among other conversation, remember and talk about the deceased.

In the Jewish culture, the members of the immediate family solemnize a time of mourning following the death and prior to the burial. During that period they are freed from conforming to the precepts of the Torah and are not to be consoled by others. The funeral is followed by seven days of mourning (called *shivah*). At that time the bereaved remain at home, except for the Sabbath when they may attend the synagogue for worship. After the seven days and until the 30th day from the time of burial, the mourning customs are eased and the family members begin their return to normal life. As they return to normal—and for the next 10 months—it is customary for the bereaved to recite the mourner's prayer, which concludes every congregational service of worship.

In most Christian faiths throughout the United States the usual custom (as mentioned in Irish custom) is to place the body, prior to the funeral, in an open or closed casket so that during special visitation hours friends and relatives may pay their respects to the family and deceased. The funeral service, which is held in the funeral home, church or sometimes a private home, usually includes prayers, hymns, other music and eulogies. After a funeral procession to a cemetery there is a brief graveside service as the body is committed to the grave. Sometimes, rather than the foregoing procedure in which the body is at the funeral, some families hold memorial services in a church.

The burial of the body in the ground is the most common practice. However, the practice of cremation is increasing in the United States. But Orthodox Jews, Roman Catholics and some Protestant groups do not favor this practice.

Funerals are generally planned and supervised principally by a professional funeral director. However, for the past few decades, many people have begun to view North American funeral practices more and more critically, and a great many say they are needlessly elaborate and expensive. One of the strongest critics is Jessica Mitford, author

of *The American Way of Death.*

Rohter, Larry, "In Mexico, This Is Not the Day to Bury Mirth," *The New York Times,* November 2, 1988.

Jackson, Edgar N., *Understanding Grief* (Nashville: Abingdon Press, 1957).

"Funeral Customs," *The World Book Encyclopedia* (Chicago: World Book, 1988).

Evans, Glen and Farberow, N.L., *The Encyclopedia of Suicide* (New York: Facts On File, 1988).

"Funerals," *Encyclopedia Brittanica,* 15th ed. (Chicago: University of Chicago, 1986).

"Funerals," *Encyclopedia Americana* (New York: Grolier International, 1985).

Hughes, Langston and Bontemps, Anna (eds.), *The Book of Negro Folklore* (New York: Dodd Mead, 1959).

Mitford, Jessica, *The American Way of Death* (New York: Simon and Schuster, 1963).

Cohen, Daniel, *The Body Snatchers* (Philadelphia: Lippincott, 1975).

McHargue, Georgess, *Mummies* (Philadelphia: Lippincott, 1972).

G

Gallup survey on depression In a 1986 Gallup study on depression done for the Christian Broadcasting Network and released by the Princeton Religion Research Center, 1,007 adults, 18 and older, were interviewed by telephone. According to the survey, 81% felt depressed or discouraged at least on occasion, while 19% said never. Women were slightly more likely than men to say they found themselves depressed or discouraged most of the time or quite often. Young adults (18 to 19) were more inclined than older persons to give these responses.

Income and level of formal education were strong factors. Persons in lower income groups and those with little formal education were the most likely to feel depressed or discouraged on a frequent basis.

Money and bills, one's job and problems at work, family problems and worry about health were volunteered most frequently as some of the things that caused feelings of discouragement or depression by the 81% who at least on occasion have a period of feeling depressed or discouraged. Next most frequently cited were life-in-general frustrations, problems with children, state of the economy, world affairs and one's social life.

The 81% who were "ever" depressed or discouraged were asked how frequently they engage in a variety of activities as a way to deal with their depression or discouragement. Cited most often was a hobby, television, reading, or listening to music. Next was seeking out friends or family members with whom to talk.

Princeton Religious Research Center, "Prayer, Bible Reading Cited Often As Ways to Beat Depression," *Emerging Trends*, 9:7(September 1987).

gastrointestinal tract The gastrointestinal tract is the part of the digestive system that is comprised of the stomach and the small and large intestines. The digestive tract itself includes the complete food canal from the mouth to the anus.

Digestion begins in the mouth, and drugs taken by mouth begin to enter the blood through the walls of the stomach or through the upper portion of the small intestine. Generally, the moderate use of prescribed drugs for depression appears to have little or no unfavorable effect on the gastrointestinal tract. However, the abuse of these drugs can cause such side effects as nausea and vomiting.

The secretions and enzymes of the gastrointestinal tract make it possible for food—as it is processed through the digestive tract—to be transformed into soluble or emulsified material that can be absorbed by the blood, circulated for distribution and then used by the various tissues of the body.

Barbiturates and other sedative drugs are quickly absorbed into the body through the upper portion of the small intestine. When food is in the stomach the absorption of these drugs is retarded.

gene/environmental connection See CAUSES OF DEPRESSION; ENVIRONMENTAL/PSYCHOSOCIAL FACTORS; GENETIC FACTORS.

generic With regard to medications, this term refers to the chemical description of a drug's class as opposed to any commercial, brand or trade name for the same compound.

genetic factors "I inherited a vile melancholy from my father, which has made me mad all my life, at least not sober," wrote Samuel Johnson, English lexicographer and author (1709–1784).

Today, two centuries after Johnson, increased evidence shows that at least some forms of depression seem to run in families. To date, the exact mechanisms by which depressive disorders are transmitted from one generation to another are not yet known. But there is growing evidence that a genetic factor is involved, especially in manic-depressive disorder. There is still much to investigate, so much that Dr. Sidney Zisook of the University of California at San Diego has said that scientists are just now entering the next phase of research into depression—its genetics.

Although some scientists have identified genes that they say are common to patients with depression, geneticists continue to search for a depression gene or marker that could identify potential victims through a laboratory test that would show who has the trait and who hasn't. In an article on depression research in *The New York Times* Harold M. Schmeck Jr. reported that in some families, markers for suspected faulty genes had been found on chromosome 11 (see OLD ORDER AMISH STUDY). In other families, clues to a genetic abnormality have been found on the X CHROMOSOME.

By late 1989, however, new evidence cast serious doubt on the conclusion of the original study that linked chromosome 11 to manic-depressive illness. At that time Dr. Steven M. Paul, the senior scientist for a National Institute of Mental Health (NIMH) study involving new data and painstaking re-analysis of the original evidence, said the new data collected by the study team drastically reduced the probability that such a gene was at the location suspected. Alternative explanations are that more than one gene plays a role or that there is a single faulty gene at a different location.

Other studies reported by the National Institute of Mental Health (NIMH) have shown that if one identical twin suffers from depression or mania there is a 70% likelihood that the other twin will also be afflicted. Among nonidentical twins, however, as with siblings, parents or children of the afflicted person, the risk decreases to about 15%.

Among second-degree relatives, such as grandparents, uncles or aunts, the risk of affliction drops to about 7%. Since identical twins have all their genes in common, and siblings and other first-degree relatives have only half in common, and second-degree relatives even fewer, the affliction rates attest to genetic involvement.

Even more suggestive of a genetic factor are studies of adoptees carried out in New York, Brussels and Denmark. The New York and Brussels researchers identified adopted individuals who had been diagnosed as having a depressive disorder and then compared the incidence of diagnosed depression in biological and adoptive parents. They found higher correlations between depressed adoptees, particularly those with bipolar depression, and their biological parents than with those who adopted and raised children from early childhood.

The Denmark study, which included first- and second-degree relatives of both biological and adopting families of depressed individuals, found a higher concentration—three times higher—of depressive disorders among biological relatives than were found among the adopting families. (See also CAUSES OF DEPRESSION.)

Schmeck, Harold M., Jr., "Depression: Studies Bring New Drugs and Insights," *The New York Times*, February 16, 1988.

————, "Scientists Now Doubt They Found Faulty Gene Linked to Mental Illness," *The New York Times*, November 7, 1989.

geriatric depression Many of today's researchers believe the proper diagnosis and treatment of depression in the ELDERLY may be the most important task of modern psychiatry and that all physicians treating elderly patients should screen for depressive illness, whether or not concurrent medical illness exists.

Although we know that a high percentage of persons under 40 are susceptible to depression and that some researchers feel fewer people over the age of 65 are affected by it, geriatric depression—from an overall view—is indeed a challenge for the 1990s.

This is the case because of the tremendously wide range of estimates for the occurrence of depression among older populations. For example, according to the National Institute of Mental Health (NIMH), the range is so wide that it varies from 10% to 65%. Other estimates and epidemiologic studies report that 20% of the geriatric outpatients are clinically depressed and that up to 75% of nursing home patients have some type of psychiatric disorder.

In one archival study done by Dr. Robert B. Wesner and Dr. George Winokur of the University of Iowa 58 patients with unipolar depression who were 55 years of age or older were compared to 155 depressed control patients age 54 years or less. The older patients with unipolar depression had a significantly worse outcome, with only 51.7% experiencing a period of full remission during follow-up.

These data, say the researchers, indicate

that the overall outcome for older depressed patients is significantly worse than that for younger patients. The reasons for this are not clear, but having an ongoing medical problem may in some way increase a subject's risk of developing a chronic affective illness or, perhaps, increase the probability of receiving inadequate treatment.

The researchers' data, however, also indicate that ELECTROCONVULSIVE THERAPY (ECT) has had a substantial impact on the outcome of depression in older patients. Without ECT less than 20% of depressed patients have a period of recovery during follow-up, while nearly 75% have a period of full recovery after ECT treatment, despite the high rate of concurrent medical disorders.

Wesner and Winokur found that the clinical presentation of depression in older patients is very similar to that seen in young patients. The major findings involved concurrent medical disorders, response to treatment and overall outcome. Ongoing medical problems were common in the elderly population, and older depressed patients showed a clear excess of cardiovascular disorders. As a result of these ongoing medical problems the researchers feel physicians may be led away from making the diagnosis of depression in an elderly subject, even though older depressed patients may have the same depressive symptomatology as younger patients.

But because some patients with geriatric depression have been responsive to treatments such as ECT the Iowa researchers support the premise that the proper diagnosis and treatment of depression in the elderly is one of the most important challenges in modern psychiatry and that clinicians should and must be aggressive in the treatment of elderly patients. (See also AGE FACTORS.)

Wesner, Robert B. and Winokur, George, "An Archival Study of Depression Before and After Age 55," *Journal of Geriatric Psychiatry and Neurology*, 1(October-December 1988).

Gestalt therapy   A school of psychology and a major force in psychotherapeutic approaches. It takes a humanistic view of man's existence in the here and now and states that the whole is more than the sum of its parts. Its existential approach proposes that we are occupied not just with dealing with symptoms or character structure but with the total existence of a person.

Begun in Germany the movement was transferred to the United States in the 1930s. The term had been coined by Charles von Ehrenfels in 1890 and stemmed from the premise that Gestalt psychologists perceived the world in unitary wholes or "Gestalts" (from the German *gestalten*, which roughly translates as "whole" or "pattern"). After 1895 investigation was carried out along lines suggested by von Ehrenfels. In 1912 the movement was given further impetus by Max Wertheimer, Wolfgang Kohler and Kurt Koffka.

FRITZ PERLS was a main proponent and developer of Gestalt therapy, and today the influence of the Gestalt ideas remains strong in some areas of psychology. Some of its most popular perspectives are: (1) power is in the present; (2) experience counts most; (3) the therapist is his own instrument; and (4) therapy is too good to be limited to the sick. As Erving and Miriam Polster say in *Gestalt Therapy Integrated* (Vintage, 1974): "The therapy experience is an exercise in unhampered living now, where topics or past and future activities are no longer of prime consequence. The famous prayer in Gestalt therapy is:

I do my thing, and you do your thing,
I am not in this world to live up to your expectations
And you are not in this world to live up to mine
You are you, and I am I
And if by chance, we find each other, it's beautiful
If not, it can't be helped.

Global Assessment Scale (GAS)   Developed by Robert Spitzer, Jean Endicott and their associates, GAS is a single rating scale for recording judgments about the health-sickness level of psychiatric patients. Ratings can be based on direct interview, case records or a reliable informant. The GAS reflects current state without regard to prognosis. Serial uses of the scale can demonstrate progress or lack of progress during a hospitalization. It can be used for depressed patients, but is not specifically designed for them.

Gold, Dr. Mark As author of *The Good News About Depression* and countless other writings on the subject, Dr. Gold is a leading authority on this affective disorder. He is director of research at Fair Oaks Hospital in Summit, New Jersey, a nationally-known psychiatric, diagnostic, therapeutic and clinical research facility, and also director of research of Psychiatric Diagnostic Laboratories of America, in Summit. In his work he has applied his background in neuroanatomy and neurochemistry to develop diagnoses and treatments for both substance abuse and related depression.

grief The link between depression and grief has been well established. By definition the latter is the human experience that follows a LOSS (or pending loss) and the process through which individuals disengage from significant attachments. People react to grief differently at different levels, so grief patterns are not the same. The main ones are anticipatory grief, normal grief, pathological grief, suppressed grief.

Anticipatory grief is the process of starting the disengagement of one's life from another prior to the actual separation taking place. This can happen to a person who will be bereaved by death; a person confronting death; or a person facing surgery and loss of a limb or other body part. When loss impends or threatens, people need to do some advance disengaging rather than denying or tightly holding in check the feelings involved in grief.

The normal grief that follows a loss is characterized by intellectual and emotional awareness of the loss. It's a time of emotional distress but in its normal state (see BEREAVEMENT) it allows people to express their feelings openly and to discover and develop the inner capacities that can keep them going as they reorganize their lives and discover meaning and purpose again. It's a healing process, which is essential for the restructuring of one's life, and generally most people work through it and grieve to completion without requiring GRIEF THERAPY/TREATMENT.

Pathological grief is an illness or disease in which persons who have suffered a loss exhibit severe dissociation, behavioral or psychiatric symptoms. The complex symptoms and emotions, often subclinical, can increase in severity if unresolved. In some cases pathological grief can even be fatal, if the grief-stricken do not seek professional treatment.

In suppressed grief people conceal their emotions and try to avoid mourning by appearing to be so controlled that no sense of loss is apparent. Some are quiet in the midst of crowds, stoically not talking about the feelings of loss. Others are constantly busy with neurotic hyperactivity. In either case, their behavior is detrimental to them. If their grief remains unresolved, they may get physically or mentally ill. In fact, it is not unusual to become a recluse or an alcoholic.

In any grief pattern a feeling of depression is almost universal, so the symptoms of grief are often many of the same signs and symptoms experienced by people in a depressed state.

The natural and normal physical symptoms are—primarily—an empty feeling in the stomach; headaches; heaviness in the chest; insomnia (or a need to sleep too much); lethargy; loss of appetite or altered eating habits; numbness; skin eruptions; shortness of breath; tears; tendency to hyperventilate; and tightness in the throat.

Psychological symptoms run the gamut of aimlessness; anger; anxiety; difficulty in finishing things; disorganization; dreams of the loved one; forgetfulness; guilt; hostility; inability to concentrate; indecisiveness; loneliness; mood changes; persistent weeping, crying at unexpected times or inability to cry at all; resentment; restlessness; self-doubt; self-pity; and unreasonable worry. Some people experience an intense preoccupation with the life and death of the deceased and a need to tell, retell and remember details. Others refuse to accept the loss is real and live with a sense that the loved one is present and that they can hear his voice and see his face. Psychologists note that some people even take on the symptoms of the deceased and feel the same kind of stomach and chest pains their loved one had. And, as still another symptom, albeit an extreme one, grief-stricken people sometimes assume even the mannerisms or traits of the person who has died.

Along with all the symptoms of depression and the physical and psychological symptoms of grief (often occurring in their most excessive forms) the symptoms of suppressed grief include feelings of craziness and disorientation; nightmares; and possible hallucinations. The bereaved may sell possessions or, in fits of generosity, give everything away; seal off the room and possessions of the deceased; have anniversary grief experiences. (See also GRIEF, CAUSES AND EFFECTS OF; LENGTH OF GRIEVING PROCESS; MOURNING; STAGES OF GRIEF.)

grief, causes and effects of   The causes of GRIEF and depression are often interrelated and as varied as the people who experience them. A prime cause, however, is the LOSS that touches many of us at one time or another, not only loss by death but also many other losses and separations that cause tears, sadness, bitterness, self-reproach and similar emotional reactions.

In addition to the very major loss of friends or loved ones because of death, alienation or other reasons, researchers cite the following as the most usual causes of grief: loss of health, eyesight, hearing, home, job, money, status, faith and hope.

Additional causes are marital and family

problems; separation and divorce; moving and uprooting of families; departure of children from home; elimination of work due to retirement; major illnesses or accidents; notification of a loved one's unfavorable prognosis; financial, personal and on-the-job troubles; disappointments; and, as in depression, an inability to live up to one's expectations.

There are many psychosomatic side effects to grief and to the situations it creates. Consequently, the effects are not the same for everyone. These effects on the survivor's health are not new to medicine; a 1657 document classifying the causes of death in London lists "Griefe" as fifth, between "Gout" and "Griping and Plague in the Guts." But only in recent years have the unhealthy effects of grief moved from the realm of medical folklore into that of scientific research.

Along with such effects as depression, weeping and sorrow, grieving people often experience: (1) a difficulty in returning to normal activities; (2) a sense of functioning mechanically; and (3) a fear for their own survival. In addition, when someone close dies, it's common to feel not only loss but also regret and guilt for things people had not done but wish they had—or felt that they should have. According to experts in the field, normal guilt is the guilt they feel when they have either done something—or neglected to do something—they ought to do, by the standards of society. Pathological guilt (or neurotic guilt) is feeling guilty out of all proportion to their real involvement in a situation.

Some individuals, unable to grasp the full significance of their loss, embrace a sense of unreality that temporarily provides the false belief that the loved one is "just outside the door." Some look forward to dreams that permit interaction with the deceased, and some have an urgent wish to contact the dead through seances. However their grief affects them, they can think of nothing but their loss.

Moreover, it is not uncommon for people

to become ill and even hospitalized as they work out their hurt in illness and substitute sickness for grief. In "The Hospital Chaplain Looks at Grief" Robert B. Reeves Jr. writes:

When no grieving is done it is likely to be accomplished through sickness. The frequency with which people who have suffered loss subsequently have to be hospitalized surely suggests a connection. The recently bereft, the divorced, those who have lost job, fortune, or reputation, those who have lost a cause they had been fighting for, or have lost a following, such people as these enter the hospital daily. Often because of our preoccupation with physiology we fail to relate their symptoms to their loss. Inquiry almost always discloses that at a conscious level they had handled their loss successfully, they had not broken down, they had kept functioning, they had borne up well. Unable to grieve in any other way, their only course was to work out the hurt in illness. The ones I see are those whose ego structure and controls are too strong to permit "nervous breakdown." They somaticize instead. There is almost no physiological disease that they cannot come up with if they need the disease as a substitute for grief.

In an article in *American Health*, L.H. Lang reports on various studies in which patients hospitalized with problems ranging from heart disorders to severe skin problems had reported the loss of a loved one. The loss was accompanied by feelings of helplessness and hopelessness just before their illnesses, and some researchers felt those losses may also have triggered traumatic recollections of earlier loss of parents.

Many researchers believe that grief can be a death-provoking factor, and some studies have indicated it can lead to premature death. Other researchers doubt that this effect is so. But regardless of the controversy, premature death from grief is attracting more and more attention and research. For example, in his book *The Broken Heart* Dr. James J. Lynch stressed that human relationships are desperately important to people's mental and physical well-being and that social isolation, the lack of human companionship, death or absence of parents in early childhood, sudden loss of love, and chronic loneliness are significant contributors to premature death.

As things stand now, scientists know that young people 20 to 35 are at a higher risk for premature death after a spouse's death than older people; that women are at highest risk in the second year; that men are at highest risk in the first six months following BEREAVEMENT; and that men are at a higher risk overall than women, except in the case of young widows with children.

Over and above that, an epidemiologist at Yale University School of Medicine, Dr. Adrian Ostfeld, puts grief among the top 15 causes of death in the United States. In one study he and his colleagues conducted he found that depressed men, those who had poor morale, didn't like themselves, or expected life to be rough, had more than twice the rate of cancer over the succeeding years as their more cheerful counterparts.

On the other side of the controversy on premature death from grief, a study conducted by Dr. Itzhak Levav and others from Hadassah Medical Organization and Hebrew University in Jerusalem noted that parents who had lost a son to war or accidental death did not face a greater risk of dying, and the study cast at least some doubt on the idea that people may die of a broken heart after the death of a child or spouse. Even though studies have also found that when a spouse dies, the surviving husband or wife is also at risk of an untimely death, other researchers believe that the survivor's death could result from a lifetime of sharing the same hazards, such as smoking or poor diet, rather than the effects of grief. (See also GRIEF THERAPY/ TREATMENT; LENGTH OF GRIEVING PROCESS; MOURNING; STAGES OF GRIEF.)

Lang, L.H., "A New Prescription: The Family," *American Health*, Fall 1980.

Lynch, James J., *The Broken Heart* (New York: Basic Books, 1977).

Reeves, Robert B., Jr., "The Hospital Chaplain Looks At Grief," *Horizons*, New York (date unknown).

grief, stages of   See STAGES OF GRIEF.

grief therapy/treatment   Treatment of normal grieving must allow some degree of distress. Consequently, grief-stricken people need to ventilate and express their feelings, and GRIEF needs such legitimate outlets as tears, sadness and self-reproach. People must be given a lot of room for doubts and relapses. Latent feelings of anger, bitterness, guilt and regret must be extinguished if health is to be restored emotionally and spiritually.

Some psychologists and psychiatrists believe that one good therapeutic measure for helping rid oneself of latent destructive emotions is each day to set aside time alone to reflect on the memories and thoughts of the loved one. During that time alone the bereaved can dwell on all the negative thoughts that haunt them. But when that time alone is over it is then "time" for the bereaved individuals to put those thoughts behind them and start reentering life's mainstream, as they reach out to other relationships and get on with their lives. Often this time-alone therapy helps people gain some control over grief.

In addition to time alone it's equally important for grieving persons to have a support system of friends who will listen to them talk about their LOSS, their life together and the details of the death. Friends can help them restore confidence in themselves, make decisions, handle day to day affairs, possibly do things differently than they did in the past, resolve self-doubts and expand their social network. For many people it is also beneficial to seek help from COUNSELING and support groups (see SELF-HELP/SUPPORT ORGANIZATIONS) that provide an opportunity to talk about experiences and losses, tell and retell stories, and remember things about loved ones.

As in depression, unresolved, pathological, suppressed or excessive grief may justify counseling and PSYCHOTHERAPY if daily life becomes so impaired at home or at work that people realize their conduct is hurting themselves and others. Although there are varying opinions (and rushing into therapy is not generally suggested) many professionals advise seeking treatment if deep grief lasts more than twelve months, since treatment in the early stages can prevent a more serious progression. Help is available from a psychologist, psychiatrist or social worker who has experience with similar problems; a local health or mental health clinic; a general hospital department of psychiatry or outpatient psychiatric clinic; a state hospital outpatient clinic; a university or medical school-affiliated program; a family service or social agency; and private clinics or facilities.

Excessive sedation and drug therapy are not recommended as a treatment for grief because of the potential that with too much sedation individuals will lose the impact of their grief and end by suppressing or prolonging it. (See also BEREAVEMENT; GRIEF, CAUSES AND EFFECTS OF; LENGTH OF GRIEVING PROCESS; MOURNING; STAGES OF GRIEF.)

group therapy   See COMMUNITY MENTAL HEALTH SERVICE; COUNSELING; PSYCHOTHERAPY; SELF-HELP/SUPPORT ORGANIZATIONS.

H

Haldol   See HALOPERIDOL.

hallucination   An abnormal mental state and unreal experience that is common in some psychotic states. It is a sensory perception with no external stimulus to account for it. It can occur in any of the sensory modalities, but auditory hallucinations and visual hallucinations are the most common. Usually hallucinations are caused by a disorder of the nervous system or a response to drugs.

hallucinogens   Drugs that act on the CENTRAL NERVOUS SYSTEM and produce mood changes, which may range from euphoria to depression, and pleasant or unpleasant perceptual changes, which can vary from sensory illusion to HALLUCINATIONS. In low doses the drugs commonly alter moods and perceptions, though they do not necessarily produce hallucinations or other psychotic-like reactions. In high doses the drugs may produce hallucinations.

"Because some of the drugs have the ability to 'mimic' psychotic reactions—loss of contact with reality, hallucinations, mania and schizophrenia—they are sometimes called psychotomimetic drugs," explain Robert O'Brien and Sidney Cohen in *The Encyclopedia of Drug Abuse*. "The term psychotogenic, which refers to the production of a psychotic-like state, is also applied. In addition, because of their mind-expanding qualities, the hallucinogens are sometimes called psychedelics."

According to O'Brien and Cohen, the federal Controlled Substances Act, aimed at reducing the consumption of illicit drugs, sets forth the following findings for hallucinogens: (1) they have a high potential for abuse; (2) they have no currently accepted medical use in treatment in the United States; (3) there is a lack of accepted safety for use of the drugs under medical supervision. Because of these findings and federal regulations, the hallucinogens are basically research substances. They can be manufactured only in federally-regulated laboratories for research purposes and cannot be sold by prescription.

It has been hoped that hallucinogens could be beneficial in the research and treatment of various mental illnesses. But while many therapeutic claims have been made for them, none has proven safe or effective in the treatment of mental disorders to date.

Hallucinogens include LSD, mescaline, peyote, DMT, psilocybin, marijuana and tetrahydrocannabinol.

O'Brien, Robert and Cohen, Sidney, *The Encyclopedia of Drug Abuse* (New York: Facts On File, 1984).

haloperidol (Haldol)   A major tranquilizer, a highly potent neuroleptic drug prototypic of the butyrophenone class. It is used extensively in the treatment of psychosis and a variety of other neurological diseases.

Hamilton Psychiatric Rating Scale for Depression   Commonly referred to as the Hamilton Rating Scale (HRS). Developed in England, it provides a method for systematically recording observations based on conventional clinical interviews. Seventeen items are rated on a 3- or 5-point scale: depressed mood, feelings of guilt, suicide, early insomnia, middle insomnia, late insomnia, work and interests, psychomotor retardation, agitation, psychic anxiety, somatic anxiety, gastrointestinal somatic symptoms, general somatic symptoms, genital symptoms, hypochondriasis, loss of weight, and insight. For the quantitative assessment of depressive symptoms, it can be used repeatedly throughout a longitudinal period of study, although Hamilton does not recommend its use for diagnostic purposes.

Hamlet   A legendary prince and hero of Shakespeare's most famous play, *Hamlet*. Stories of the prince and the complexity of his character were recorded and passed down centuries before the early 1600s when Shakespeare wrote his version of the earlier stories and legends.

In the years since Shakespeare wrote his play in 1603, Hamlet has been portrayed differently in the various interpretations of the play. But the prince's complexity and melancholy are always part of the portrayal. Hamlet knows his reactions are irrational. But thought and will are both powerless against the emotions he feels. One of his famous lines is:

How weary, stale, flat, and unprofitable
Seem to me all the uses of this world.

Harvard Study According to a 1983 Harvard Medical School study, a sudden death can make grief and MOURNING especially difficult for widows and widowers. Those whose spouses died with little or no warning were more anxious or depressed two to four years after the death than those whose spouses died from long illnesses.

Dr. Robert Weiss, a social psychologist now with the Work and Family Research Unit at the University of Massachusetts in Boston, who did the study while at Harvard, found that 40% were still anxious and depressed for two to four years after the death of their spouses. Compared with non-bereaved controls they were rated as showing moderate to severe anxiety. Those with brief or no warning of their spouse's death did much more poorly than those with at least two weeks to prepare themselves for the loss. (See also LENGTH OF GRIEVING PROCESS.)

head trauma and depression Researchers are increasingly studying the relationship between head trauma and psychiatric illness. According to *Perspectives in Psychiatric Care* (24:2), a Neurosciences Information Center statement published by Upjohn Company reported studies that show that 10% of people with severe head trauma go on to develop a psychosis at some time in their lives. Schizophrenia, obsessive-compulsive disorder and manic-depression are all more likely to occur among the head-injured than among the general population. Recently epidemiologists have been looking at the relationship between head injuries and Alzheimer's disease. Studies have shown that head injuries may be a risk factor, but nothing is conclusive at this point.

Depression following closed head injury can be indistinguishable from a major depressive episode unrelated to external factors. Risk of suicide increases significantly—up to 14% of all deaths among people with severe head trauma—compared with the general population.

health insurance programs There is no single answer to "What will health insurance pay?" when a person is afflicted by depression. In fact, the Health Insurance Association of America (HIAA) reports that coverage for depression may vary from generous to non-existent.

As most holders of health insurance know, insurance is a contract between two entities, usually an insurance company and an employer. The level of benefits agreed upon by the two parties is the amount paid when a claim is made. Some states mandate minimum or maximum benefit levels for group contracts in their state, usually a specified number of visits or inpatient days per person, year or lifetime. State laws vary considerably. Large employers often self-insure, exempting themselves from state mandates.

A person purchasing individual insurance may or may not be offered mental health coverage, depending on the insurance company contacted and the person's medical history. The coverage offered will probably have the same deductible/copayment as the physical health coverage, but may have some inside limits on annual or lifetime maximum payments for mental health services. Most states do not require that individual contracts provide mental health coverage.

The Blue Cross and Blue Shield Association also points out that benefits are mandated by each state and that each of its own 73 separately incorporated Blue Cross and Blue Shield Plans operates under state laws. Blue Cross/Blue Shield spokespersons say that although each plan is a locally governed autonomous corporation, a plan must meet national standards promulgated through the association. Local environments vary, resulting in different approaches by which each plan covers and pays for services rendered for depression.

Blue Cross/Blue Shield reports that, in general, services rendered in conjunction with depression for the most part will be covered under a psychiatric/mental health benefit package. What a plan covers varies and will depend primarily on the type of coverage the subscriber purchased or what an employer purchased for its employees. Consequently, what is covered will be subject to the provisions of the subscriber certificate annual or lifetime dollar maximum and/or maximum number of outpatient visits and inpatient days. Other certificates may not specify limits and instead provide for "service benefits"—that is, guarantee the service in full rather than a fixed dollar amount—for the mental health services. Some certificates may reduce benefits depending on whether a subscriber goes to a plan-participating provider. Further, coverage is affected by state mandates. According to Blue Cross/Blue Shield, some states mandate that plans make available psychiatric and mental health benefits, the coverage of certain services, the type of providers that may render the specific services and the level of coverage (e.g., primary versus tertiary).

Two factors govern what and how much Blue Cross/Blue Shield Plans pay: the type of coverage purchased and the participating agreement between the plan and the provider. Some plans, because of their agreements with providers, pay the providers directly unless the subscriber pays for the services at the time of discharge or service. Plan contracts with providers specify the rates a plan will pay the providers, and in many instances will protect the subscriber from the provider, billing the subscriber for the difference between the amount charged by the provider and the amount paid by the plan. Other than the applicable copayments and deductibles, a provider may be prohibited from collecting any money from the subscriber.

Medicare currently limits mental illness treatment to 190 inpatient days per lifetime. Hospital outpatient visits are subject to the normal 80/20 copayment with a maximum payment of $1100 in 1989. However, Medicare rules can and do change. You can check with the Health Care Finance Administration for more information.

Hemingway, Ernest American novelist and short story writer (1899–1961) who suffered from severe depression. With the publication of his early novels in the 1920s he became known as the spokesman of the disillusioned "lost generation." His father was also a victim of depression, and Hemingway referred to his own bouts with the affliction as his "black-assed" days. An ardent hunter, he committed suicide by shooting himself in 1961.

herbals and herbalism Before the days of modern medicine a variety of plants were dried and used as medicinal agents. Today, along with the movement toward natural food, there is a revived interest in herbal teas and other herbal potions. Some herbals are used for physical and psychological ailments, including such affective disorders as depression. Some have psychoactive effects, and some are potentially toxic.

The Professional Herbal Formula Handbook by F. Joseph Montagna, a herbalist and author of several other volumes on herbal medicine, is a 100-page handbook that contains a complete listing of 70 professional herbal formulas along with an ailment index that provides access to both essential and supplementary herbal formulas for each ailment. In addition, each herbal formula listing provides readers with the specific ingredients in both English and Latin botanical names, as well as each formula's physiological action and compatible combinations. For further information on this handbook contact the Alternative Medical Association, 7909 S.E. Stark St., Portland, OR 97215.

heredity See CAUSES OF DEPRESSION; GENETIC FACTORS.

high blood pressure Also referred to as hypertension, high blood pressure affects about 60 million Americans—25% of all adults—and becomes more common with age. Among those between 65 and 75, nearly two-thirds have blood pressure that is considered "high." Generally, high blood pressure is defined as blood pressure higher than 140/90 (systolic/diastolic). Systolic pressure is recorded when the heart contracts during a beat. Diastolic is recorded when the heart is at rest. Drugs are often used in treating high blood pressure, and in persons predisposed to mood disorders some drugs used to lower high blood pressure appear to bring on attacks of a secondary depression as a side effect. This is not true of all hypertension drugs, but experience has shown that some have a tendency to deplete the brain of the amine chemical transmitters. As a result, the lowered amine levels may trigger the depressed mood. Reserpine is one high blood pressure regulator that is known to cause a secondary depression.

Henig, Robin M., "Beyond The Beat: Doctors Take New Look At Hypertension," *AARP BULLETIN*, July-August 1989.

Hippocrates A Greek physician-philosopher (460?–377 B.C.) and the father of Western medicine. Even in antiquity it was felt that the state of a person's health was influenced by both psychological and physical aspects. From a psychological point of view Hippocrates believed that behavior was related to the brain and that from the brain come joys, delights and laughter, as well as grief, despondency and melancholy. He assumed that different types of secretions caused mania and depression and attributed madness to dryness of the brain.

In blaming depression on different types of secretions he placed special emphasis on a surplus of *melan chole*, the Greek term for BLACK BILE. Our word "melancholy" comes from this. The black bile theory was a forerunner of today's theory of imbalances in the body chemistry, and was used to explain depression for many years after Hippocrates.

Hippocrates' theory was later expanded to include four bodily substances called HUMORS, whose ebb and flow supposedly determined physical and mental health. Each of the humors was considered vital, but an excess of any one upset the balance and created disturbance.

Hoffman, Abbie A chronic manic-depressive (1937–1989) who was nationally known for his political activism and radical protests in the 1960s. In the 1970s he went underground, and in the 1980s emerged, graying and middle-aged, to spend his time writing and giving speeches. In 1986 he was arrested with Amy Carter, daughter of former President Jimmy Carter, during an anti-CIA demonstration.

Some of Hoffman's friends and followers said Hoffman found life in the 1980s irrelevant, had problems coping with middle age, and was always on the edge of a nervous breakdown because he felt bypassed by history. At the time of his death he reportedly was taking lithium for his manic depression. It was also reported that he was writing a book on depression when he committed suicide with a huge dose of barbiturates combined with alcohol.

holiday depression The holiday blues syndrome is a form of depression that most adults have experienced at one time or another in varying degrees around Christmas, Hanukkah and other holidays as a result of frenzied activity or post-holiday letdown. For most people these moments of depression are short-lived, but for some the holiday blues become debilitating, destroying the joy of the season and making the holidays a time of dread. For those who live alone the holidays can be extremely stressful.

Researchers say that holidays can bring conflicts and dashed hopes and be particularly difficult because expectations are unreasonably high. The idyllic family gatherings, pictured by the media, of laughing, happy children, beaming grandparents and lovingly attentive spouses may make people wonder what is wrong in their own lives, which often seem to consist of bickering children, quarrelsome relatives and irritable spouses. Dr. George Benson, a psychiatrist and author of

What to Do When You're Depressed, relates Christmas depression to certain factors, which include:

1. Individuals holding on to fantasies and unachievable expectations of Christmas;
2. Older people reliving memories of earlier Christmases;
3. Christmas being terribly strained by the pre-Christmas build-up and the exhaustion of Christmas;
4. Teenagers experiencing ambivalence about growing up;
5. People being consumed by the frantic quality of Christmas shopping, which is fraught with anxiety.

Marjorie Baier, who is an instructor at the School of Nursing, Southern Illinois University, suggests in "The 'Holiday Blues' as a Stress Reaction" that holiday depression and stress can be reduced by planning ahead in several areas: gifts and other expenditures; time schedules; food and menu preparation; and arranging for social contacts (even if one feels like being alone at the beginning of December, the season of Christmas is highly social and one's feelings are likely to change by the time the holiday arrives).

Another area to consider in stress reduction, says Baier, is the interpersonal, which would include anticipating possible family conflicts, allowing for reminiscing at appropriate times, and maintaining a consistent daily schedule, especially for children, throughout the holiday period. Also, it is important for individuals to examine their personal expectations and priorities and for family members to examine their feelings of responsibility and discuss which members feel responsible for holiday festivities and for providing a happy holiday season.

If depression lingers it can and should be treated. Often, a few sessions with a qualified, professional counselor is all that is needed.

Baier, Marjorie, "The 'Holiday Blues' as a Stress Reaction," *Perspectives in Psychiatric Care*, 24:2(1987/1988).

Benson, George, *What to Do When You're Depressed* (Minneapolis: Augsburg, 1975).

holistic medicine Holistic medicine emphasizes the relation between parts and the whole. It considers man as a functioning whole, and the goal of its practitioners is to emphasize personal responsibility and lead patients toward optimal attunement of body, mind, emotions and spirit.

As it stresses the integration of physical, mental, emotional and spiritual concerns with environmental harmony, its nine basic areas are: (1) acupuncture, (2) behavioral medicine, (3) biomolecular therapies, (4) environmental medicine, (5) neuro-muscular integration, (6) nutrition, (7) physical exercise, (8) self-regulation and (9) spiritual awareness. It is a medical care system of interaction and growth, rather than "treatment only," because of the way it fosters a cooperative relationship among all those involved and focuses upon patient education in the healing process.

Patients choose a holistic practitioner who works with them in obtaining optimum health and maximum attunement of body, mind, emotions and spirit by: (1) viewing the patients as being ultimately responsible for decisions relating to their well-being; (2) fostering and maintaining a partnership with the patients, using therapies with which all feel comfortable; and (3) evaluating and treating the cause of an illness as well as the symptoms.

The practice of holistic medicine encompasses all safe and appropriate modalities of diagnosis and treatment. All active members of the American Holistic Medical Association are fully licensed physicians, but not all holistic practitioners are physicians. For further information write: American Holistic Medical Association, 2002 Eastlake Ave. E., Seattle, WA 98102. Phone: 206-322-6842.

home, support-therapy in See ROLE OF FAMILY AND FRIENDS.

homeopathy　A system of medical practice that treats a disease by the administration of minute doses of a remedy that would—in healthy persons—produce symptoms of the disease being treated. Founded by Dr. Samuel Hahnemann, a German physician, early in the 19th century, it is based on the theory that "like is cured by like." When a drug is found to produce the same symptoms as an illness practitioners of homeopathic medicine then use that drug to alleviate the illness. Schools of medicine teaching this system are recognized in the United States and Europe. Hahnemann Medical College and Hospital in Philadelphia was first chartered as the Homeopathic Medical College of Pennsylvania. For further information: National Center for Homeopathy, 1500 Massachusetts Ave., NW., Suite 41, Washington, DC 20005.

hormone　Chemical messengers produced by tissues or organs to regulate or modulate effects on other tissue or organs. Hormonal effects on mood and behavior have long been recognized, so deciphering how hormones work is especially important for understanding the affective disorders. The fact that some show circadian rhythmicity (see CIRCADIAN RHYTHMS) of activity and are phasically related to each other over longer cycles is intriguing to investigators. Some hormones produce internal adjustments of the different systems of the body, while some respond to external events and provoke behavioral reactions.

Neurohormones (a hormonal output of the brain) are produced by neurons called neuroendocrine transducers, which release a hormone in response to activation at the synapses by neurotransmitters. These neurons transduce a neural signal into a hormonal one. Most neuroendocrine transducers are located in the hypothalamus and release their hormones either into the hypophyseal portal system (a fine capillary system leading to the anterior pituitary) by transport along axons to the posterior pituitary and other brain regions, or into the third ventricle and the cerebrospinal fluid communication pathway. These multiple avenues allow quick, powerful, flexible neurohormone influence.

The neurohormone is the chemical messenger by which the brain influences endocrine function outside the brain, particularly by regulating pituitary hormone output. The neurohormone is also one important means for the brain to integrate its own activity. Thus, hypothalamic neuroendocrine transducers can release neurohormones into the cerebrospinal fluid or by axon transport to influence activity of brain neurons at sites distant from the hypothalamus. An example of a neurohormone influencing brain function is the secretion of vasopressin from hypothalamic neurons into the cerebrospinal fluid. [Vasopressin has been shown to alter memory function in experimental animals and man. It is assumed that as vasopressin circulates in the cerebrospinal fluid, it activates clusters of neurons, which are involved in the consolidation and retrieval of information.]

Corfman, Eunice, *Depression, Manic-Depressive Illness, and Biological Rhythms* (Rockville, Maryland: Alcohol, Drug Abuse and Mental Health Administration, 1982; DHHS #82-889).

Horney, Karen　See KAREN HORNEY CLINIC.

hospitalization　Only a small percentage of depressed persons need hospitalization. However, hospitalization may be required if the depressive person is so ill that a doctor believes he or she cannot be treated on an outpatient basis. There are several types of hospitalization.

Private psychiatric hospitals. Some private psychiatric hospitals admit both voluntary (the patient signs a written application at the hospital for admission at his or her own request and/or on the advice of a physician) and involuntary (a patient cannot be persuaded to cooperate and is hospitalized against his will). Other private hospitals take voluntary admissions only.

Generally, private psychiatric hospitals offer highly efficient and intensive care and treatment for short-term illnesses and, sometimes, long-term illnesses. All are licensed facilities that use every type of treatment. The standards of treatment in general are higher than those in many other psychiatric facilities. These hospitals are also better staffed than government facilities. They tend to attract the cream of the crop in personnel. They offer lounging rooms for daytime living and socializing, dining halls and areas for recreational and other activities, and psychotherapy and physical treatments.

General hospitals. Many general hospitals offer a psychiatric service. Treatment for depression is oriented to the acutely disturbed patient who will benefit from intensive care, with the result that a fairly accurate limit of one to two months can be set for the hospital stay. Many of these hospitals concentrate on a comprehensive program of care, which combines inpatient psychiatric treatment with an outpatient clinic.

State, county and municipal facilities. Most methods of psychiatric treatment as well as medical and surgical care are administered at state hospitals. However, because these hospitals tend to be overcrowded and insufficiently staffed the use of drugs as the least expensive treatment (and a form of treatment that requires the smallest number of trained personnel) dominates over other methods. When enough skilled personnel are employed, the depressed person will probably be given electroshock therapy (see ELECTROCONVULSIVE THERAPY). Psychotherapy is generally limited to group procedures. State hospitals take patients suffering from acute disorders that are expected to improve quickly with treatment, as well as long-term patients with chronic illnesses.

The psychiatric divisions of county and municipal hospitals are identical in purpose with those of the general and state hospitals. As a rule, county and municipal hospitals are equipped not only with psychiatric facilities but are also capable of all types of medical and surgical care. Like state hospitals, county and municipal hospitals tend to be over-

populated and understaffed. Whenever possible, though, the depressed person who is already there is treated intensively.

Veterans Administration Hospitals. The VA facilities are general hospitals. Most of them have a psychiatric service. They are located in many communities throughout the United States. Eligibility is based on active service in the Armed Forces of the United States, and admissions are governed by a priority system, with veterans needing hospitalization because of injuries or diseases incurred or aggravated in active service receiving top priority.

hot lines Through their continuing support systems that permit individuals suffering from depression, grief and other problems to express their feelings, hot lines provide people with instant and encouraging help. Across the United States hotlines cover a wide range of mental health and related problems. The numbers that can be called for information and help are often toll-free, and generally operate on a 24-hour basis. For easy reference, the front pages of county and city telephone directories provide a list (with phone numbers) of some of the available hot lines. Individuals and families in need of help can also call organizations listed under "Community Services Numbers" in the front pages of county and city telephone directories. *The Self-Help Sourcebook* ($8.00 via book rate postage), published by St. Clares-Riverside Medical Center, Dept. P, 1 Indian Road, Denville, NJ 07834, is a national directory of self-help groups and contains a listing of toll-free national 800 helplines. (See also COMMUNITY MENTAL HEALTH SERVICES; SELF HELP/SUPPORT ORGANIZATIONS; Appendix 6.)

humor Most persons who are depressed lose their sense of humor. As they withdraw from people and keep to themselves they appear sad and ready to cry at a moment's notice. Few things can make them smile or laugh.

However, there are numerous reports that

laughter can ease medical symptoms and possibly speed healing. For example, some Swedish researchers tried injecting humor into the treatment of six outpatients, ages 26 to 48, with painful muscular problems linked to minor depression.

Three good-humored nurses met with this group for 13 weeks at a health care center and supplied the patients with comedy books, records and videos. They also encouraged the patients to find humor in everyday life. Doctors logged results, and the findings were enough to provoke more research. In fact, the researchers said the Swedish patients often laughed enough to stop hurting.

In the United States, Lila Green, an Ann Arbor, Michigan consultant who sometimes bills herself as the University of Michigan Hospital's "Good Humor Lady," has suggested that instead of off-white walls, hospital rooms should be decorated with landscape posters and cartoons.

Laitner, Bill, "Laugh Until It Stops Hurting," *The* [Hackensack, N.J.] *Record* (Knight-Ridder News Service), September 17, 1989.

humors The ancient Greeks believed there were four bodily substances, called humors, whose ebb and flow supposedly determined physical and mental health. Each of the humors was considered vital, but an excess of any one upset the balance and created disturbance. Depression was blamed on a surplus of *melan chole*, the Greek term for BLACK BILE. Our word "melancholy" derives from this." (See also HIPPOCRATES.)

hypertension See HIGH BLOOD PRESSURE.

hypnosis A process that is sometimes used in combination with other therapies for a broad range of psychosomatic and psychophysiological disorders. Hypnotherapy was used for a time by Sigmund Freud, and in 1958 the American Medical Society recommended its use by qualified physicians as an aid in medical practice.

Hypnosis superficially resembles sleep and is generally induced by the monotonous repetition of words and gestures while people are completely relaxed. While in a hypnotic state subjects experience heightened suggestibility. According to Dr. Milton V. Kline, director of the Institute for Research in Hypnosis and Psychotherapy, the utilization of hypnosis as a therapeutic modality in relation to depression has a definite role in the treatment and management of depressive disorders.

Although a variety of problems appear to respond effectively to hypnosis, the process must be used correctly. As Robert O'Brien and Dr. Signey Cohen warn in *The Encyclopedia of Drug Abuse:* "The recent popularity of hypnosis has led to an increase in untrained and incompetent practitioners entering the field, which has caused the American Society of Clinical Hypnosis and the International Society of Hypnosis to take a strong stand against unskilled hypnotists since without training there can be untoward and possibly dangerous consequences."

O'Brien, R. and Cohen, S., *The Encyclopedia of Drug Abuse* (New York: Facts On File, 1984).

hypnotherapy See HYPNOSIS.

hypnotics Drugs that produce sleep. They slow down the action of the CENTRAL NERVOUS SYSTEM and include BARBITURATES and nonbarbiturates.

hypochondriacal complaints A neurotic reaction and an over-concern and preoccupation with one's (sometimes imaginary) health problems. Hypochondriasis with its accompanying morbid anxiety is often a complicating factor in a psychopathological condition.

hypomanias Mild manic episodes that can cause an elevated, expansive—or irritable—mood. Some hypomanias last for weeks or months. The elevated feelings and need to be overactive that accompany hypomanic periods can sometimes occur during the summer in SEASONAL AFFECTIVE DISORDER (SAD) and REVERSE-SAD (SUMMER DEPRESSION). In an article in *Perspectives in Psychiatric Care* Norine J. Kerr points out that during hypomanias there are at least three of the following 11 symptoms: (1) decreased need for sleep; (2) more energy than usual; (3) inflated self-esteem; (4) increased productivity, often associated with unusual and self-imposed working hours; (5) sharpened and unusually creative thinking; (6) uninhibited, seeking hypersexuality, without recognition of possibility of painful consequences; (7) excessive involvement in pleasurable activities with lack of concern for painful consequences; (8) physical restlessness; (9) more talkative than usual; (10) overoptimistic attitude toward the future or exaggeration of past achievement; (11) inappropriate laughing and joking.

Kerr, Norine J., "Signs and Symptoms of Depression and Principles of Nursing Intervention," *Perspectives in Psychiatric Care* 24:2 (1987/88).

hypotension   Abnormally low blood pressure. It is also one of the main features of shock, although it is not necessarily indicative of that. In some cases it may be caused by drugs, especially narcotics, sedatives or diuretics.

hypothalamic-pituitary-thyroid (HPT) axis   One part of the neuroendocrine system is known as the hypothalamic-pituitary-thyroid (HPT) axis. Classically, glands of the endocrine system—the pituitary, thyroid, parathyroid, pineal body, adrenals, pancreas and gonads—secrete hormones directly into the bloodstream to target organs that they regulate.

The importance of this HPT axis has emerged during the past decade or so of hugely expanded insight into its functions. But the close relation of endocrine diseases to mental disorders was noticed over 200 years ago. Consequently, for a long while the brain has been recognized as one of the most important target organs influenced by the "peripheral" hormones, those produced outside the brain. Through the years, however, the function and mechanisms of the action of the endocrine system have become more fully understood. Today the emphasis is on exploring the influence of substances produced by the brain on the peripheral hormones, and on the brain itself. This has created the field of neuroendocrinology. This new perspective sees the brain not only as a target but also as an endocrine organ in its own right, able to synthesize and secrete its own hormones and transport them by several pathways to both nearby and distant targets.

The thyroid gland is one link in the HPT axis. Within this axis, circulating thyroid hormones are tightly regulated by both central nervous system input and peripheral feedback control. In a chapter in *Handbook of Psychiatric Diagnostic Procedures*, Mark S. Gold and Michael H. Kronig explain that the hypothalamus secretes thyrotropin releasing hormone (TRH) into the portal system of the adenohypophysis. TRH stimulates the pituitary thyrotrope cells to release thyroid stimulating hormone (TSH), which in turn increases the rates of iodide uptake, hormone synthesis, and release of thyroxine and triiodothyronine. Hypothalamic input is essential for normal thyroid function. Experimental lesions that destroy or disconnect the hypothalamus from the pituitary result in HYPOTHYROIDISM. Most psychiatrists routinely include hypothyroidism in the differential diagnosis of depressive states. As an aid in diagnosing depression and assessing thyroid status, a test known as the THYROTROPIN-RELEASING HORMONE TEST is sometimes used.

Gold, Mark S. and Kronig, Michael H., "Comprehensive Thyroid Evaluation in Psychiatric Patients," ch. 2 of Hall, R. and Beresford, T. (eds.), *Handbook of Psychiatric Diagnostic Procedures* (Jamaica, New York: Spectrum Publications, N.D.).

Corfman, Eunice, *Depression, Manic-Depressive Illness, and Biological Rhythms*

(Rockville, Maryland: Alcohol, Drug Abuse and Mental Health Administration, 1982; DHHS #82-889).

hypothalamus   A basal part of the posterior subdivision of the forebrain. It lies beneath the thalamus on each side and is considered to include vital autonomic regulatory centers.

hypothyroidism   A deficient activity of the thyroid gland resulting in a lowered metabolic rate and general loss of vigor. Depression and hypothyroidism share several clinical features, such as weakness, lack of energy, lack of appetite, weight changes and constipation.

As an aid in diagnosing depression and assessing thyroid status a test known as the THYROTROPIN-RELEASING HORMONE TEST (TRH) is sometimes used. Though this test is not as well known as the DST test, clinicians and researchers who feel there are patients who suffer from a subclinical hypothyroidism consider monitoring for thyroid function an important diagnostic tool. In this test the thyroid-stimulating hormone (TSH) response is measured following the infusion of protirelin (thyrotropin-releasing hormone [TRH]). Researchers have discovered that manics seem to have a blunted response compared with that of normal controls. Proponents of the test believe it can be useful for both diagnosis and treatment planning. At this writing DSM-III-R does not list it as a routine diagnostic tool.

In one study reported by Dr. Mark S. Gold et al. of the Psychiatric Diagnostic Laboratory and Clinical Research Facilities at Fair Oaks Hospital in Summit, New Jersey, 250 consecutive patients referred to the psychiatric hospital for treatment of depression were studied. Twenty of the 250 patients had some degree of hypothyroidism. Two patients (less than 1%) were identified with grade 1 (overt); nine patients (3.6%), grade 2 (mild); and 10 patients (4%), grade 3 (subclinical) hypothyroidism. These results suggest that a significant proportion of patients with depression may have early hypothyroidism, the cases of about half of which are detected only by thyrotropin-releasing hormone (TRH) testing.

Because of studies such as this many researchers believe that both depressed inpatients and outpatients (and especially individuals with a poor response to traditional psychiatric treatments) may be appropriate candidates for a comprehensive thyroid evaluation, including the TRH test. This evaluation is especially important if the patient is taking or being considered for treatment with lithium carbonate, which is known to cause hypothyroidism in some individuals.

Sternbach, Harvey A. et al., "Thyroid Failure and Protirelin (Thyrotropin-Releasing Hormone) Test Abnormalities in Depressed Outpatients," *Journal of American Medical Association*, 249:12(March 25, 1983).

Gold, Mark S., "Hypothyroidism—Or Is It Depression?" *Psychosomatics*, 24:7(July 1983).

——, "Hypothyroidism and Depression" *Journal of the American Medical Association*, 295:19(May 15, 1981).

hysterectomy   The surgical removal of the uterus. For some time a widespread belief among health professionals in America has been that women who have hysterectomies are especially vulnerable to depression afterward. However, in early 1990 new research findings from Europe contradicted the risks of depression that women face after a hysterectomy and found that women who were depressed before a hysterectomy often recover from the depression after the operation. According to the studies of Dr. David Gath, a British psychiatrist, in 156 women who had hysterectomies unrelated to cancer, the rates of anxiety and depression among the women six months after surgery were just half what they had been before surgery. Earlier studies, which seemed to show higher rates of depression in women after hysterectomies, primarily involved cancer patients, but later studies have shown that the depression in those studies was related to having cancer, not to the hysterectomy.

Goleman, Daniel, "Wide Beliefs on Depression in Women Contradicted," *The New York Times*, January 9, 1990.

I

imipramine hydrochloride (Tofranil) One of the most widely used and effective antidepressants on the market. Since it was the first of the important tricyclic antidepressants it is often referred to as the parent drug of the tricyclics that block the RE-UPTAKE PROCESS. In addition to being used for depression, it is prescribed for serious anxiety and attacks of panic. It can have serious side effects if used with alcohol.

immune system   Studies done in the last decade based on tying depression and bereavement into changes in the immune system suggest that a person's psychological state may influence either susceptibility to illness and/or its course and prognosis—though research in this field is an ongoing project as researchers continue to seek firm conclusions concerning the clinical implications of data suggesting immunocompromise during stress, bereavement and depression.

One prime researcher is Dr. Joseph R. Calabrese of the Department of Psychiatry at the Cleveland Clinic Foundation, who has found that there is clear evidence that stress, bereavement and depression can compromise specific components of the immunological apparatus. Dr. Calabrese explains that a major function of the immune system is to distinguish "self" from "nonself." This capacity must occur in the context of an ability to respond to invasion by foreign antigens without disrupting central homeostatic mechanisms. The accomplishment of this task has

required the evolution of an exceptionally complex system of cellular and humoral components.

According to Dr. Calabrese: "Classically, immunologists have subdivided the immunologic apparatus into systems subserving 'cellular' and 'humoral' immunity. 'Cellular' immunity is now believed to be principally mediated by lymphocytes acting directly on an invading antigen, while 'humoral' immunity is thought to be rendered by lymphocytes which produce antibodies that circulate systemically." A growing body of evidence suggests that the humoral concomitants of the immune response can gain access to and affect central nervous system function and possibly behaviors that might be adaptive during illness.

The following material on evidence for interactions between the central nervous system and the immunological apparatus is quoted from *Alterations in Immunocompetence During Stress, Bereavement, and Depression: Focus on the Interplay Between the Immunologic Apparatus and Neuroendocrine Regulation*, written by Dr. Calabrese and his colleagues:

A specific mechanism by which stress and depression influence the immune system seems to be via neuroendocrine secretion, mediated by the hypothalamic-pituitary-adrenal axis. However, it should be emphasized that there are a variety of mechanisms by which the centeral nervous system could influence immune function, and any of these could theoretically contribute to the alterations in immune function noted in stress and depression. For instance, the recently demonstrated presence of neuroendocrine APUD cells (amine precursor uptake and decarboxylation) within various lymphoid organs suggests a further link between the neuroendocrine and immune systems. Moreover, hormones of the hypothalamic-pituitary-gonadal axis depress lymphocyte responses to antigen challenge via specific receptor-mediated mechanisms. Conversely growth hormone, insulin and thyroxine enhance cellular immunity.

In addition to the Cleveland Clinic Foundation research, other research also indicates that depression, bereavement and stress have specific effects on the body's immune system. In 1983 a Mount Sinai Hospital team directed by Dr. Steven Schleifer and Dr. Marvin Stein found a pattern of diminished activity of lymphocytes while researching the impact of stress on the immune system. In one phase of their study, in which 18 patients hospitalized for severe depression were examined before they were treated with medication, they found suppression of lymphocyte cells. The researchers noted, however, that the impact on the lymphocytes might have been partially the result of the stress of entering the hospital rather than an effect of the depression itself.

When they expanded the study to include 16 depressed patients in outpatient treatment they found a less severe effect on their lymphocytes. A study of 15 patients diagnosed as schizophrenic found no change in lymphocyte activity. Nevertheless Dr. Stein believes the depression had an independent effect on lymphocytes and that major changes apparently depend on how depressed you are. According to Dr. Stein, the actual impact on an individual varies according to who you are and whether you have a sensitivity or immunity, which allows dealing with stress without great depression or anxiety.

There is still much research to be done on the actual process of linking the experience of depression, bereavement and stress with the apparent effects on lymphocytes, but eventually, scientists say, exploration of the delicate interaction between the brain and the body on the cellular level might provide significant clues to dealing with recalcitrant forms of mental illness.

Dietz, Jean, "Study: Sorrow May Weaken Body," *Boston Globe*, February 1, 1984.

Calabrese, Joseph R. et al., *Alterations in Immunocompetence During Stress, Bereavement, and Depression: Focus on the Interplay Between the Immunologic Apparatus and Neuroendocrine Regulation* (Cleveland: Cleveland Clinic Foundation, N,D.; paper).

insomnia See SLEEP AND SLEEP DISORDERS.

Institute for Rational/Emotive Therapy See ELLIS, ALBERT; RATIONAL-EMOTIVE PSYCHOTHERAPY.

International Commission for the Prevention of Alcoholism and Drug Dependence (ICPA) Founded in 1952, ICPA is a nonsectarian, nonpolitical organization of the United Nations operated exclusively for scientific and educational purposes. It seeks to reveal the impact of alcohol and other drug dependencies upon the economic, political, social and religious life of nations, and to point up effective preventive actions. The commission is made up of 250 prominent men and women from around the world. The number of invited representatives is based on the population of a country.

Interpersonal psychotherapy (IPT) Interpersonal psychotherapy is based on the theory that depression is associated with disturbances in relationships and that depression can either predispose a patient to problems in relationships or that relationships can bring on the depression. Its developers—Dr. Gerald Klerman, Dr. Myrna Weissman and other researchers in the New Haven-Boston Collaborative Depression Project—believe that even if a person has a genetic vulnerability to depression it is usually a crisis in relationships that precipitates the episode.

"The depression is assumed to arise in the context of grief (loss of a partner through divorce or death), role disputes (I love him more than he loves me), normal life changes and transitions (the youngest child leaves home) and the lack of or unfulfilled relationships (the inability to develop or maintain steady relationships)," wrote Judy Folkenberg in "Multi-Site Study of Therapies for Depression."

By focusing on current issues (rather than delving into the basic character of a patient), the interpersonal therapist tries to help patients understand their illness and their feelings and how life events and interpersonal problems and conflicts relate to their depression. The therapist's first step is examining the interplay between the patient's relationships to other people and his depression. Next, the therapist uses the relationships as vehicles for improving the patient's life.

In turn, the patient is encouraged to identify and try to understand his relationship problems and to develop more adaptive ways of relating to others. The therapist also helps him deal with the connection between important events and the associated depression. "For example, after a divorce, the individual's guilt about real or imagined neglect or lack of communication may be a factor in depression," wrote Folkenberg.

In addition, interpersonal therapists teach patients better communication techniques, improved social skills, and more effective ways to deal with the important people in their lives.

Folkenberg, Judy, "Multi-Site Study of Therapies for Depression," *ADAMHA News* [Alcohol, Drug Abuse, and Mental Health Administration], August 1986.

Inventory to Diagnose Depression (IDD) A self-report scale developed by Mark Zimmerman, William Coryell and their colleagues at University of Iowa College of Medicine, Department of Psychiatry. It is a paper-and-pencil questionnaire designed to diagnose major depressive disorder according to DSM-III-R criteria. The IDD assesses depression with 22 groups of five statements. One symptom of depression is assessed by each group, and the statements are arranged in order of increasing symptom severity. The

IDD differs from other self-report depression scales in several important ways, First, the IDD covers the entire range of symptoms used to diagnose DSM-III-R a major depressive disorder. Inadequate symptom coverage reduces a scale's diagnostic sensitivity (i.e., ability to identify individuals with the disease). Second, thresholds are used to determine the presence or absence of symptoms. Each item is graded in severity from 0 to 4, so the IDD can be used to quantify the severity of depression. An item score of 0 represents no disturbance, a score of 1 suggests subclinical severity and a score of 2 through 4 indicates that the symptoms are present. Third, the IDD assesses symptom duration by asking the respondent to indicate whether the symptom has been present for more or less than two weeks.

Zimmerman, Mark et al., "The Validity of a Self-Report Questionnaire for Diagnosing Major Depressive Disorder," *Archives of General Psychiatry*, 45(August 1988).

involutional melancholia A term once used to define a depressive disorder that was commonly believed to affect people (especially women) at mid-life and beyond. The term is now obsolete.

Iowa 500 Study The "Iowa 500" was a large, blind family and follow-up study of 200 schizophrenic, 100 bipolar (manic), 225 unipolar depressed and 160 control subjects hospitalized in the 1930s and 1940s. Some of these patients (about 10%) who initially had experienced only depression eventually experienced both depression and mania and changed from having unipolar depression to having bipolar depression. In the follow-up study done by Dr. George Winokur and others at University of Iowa 30 to 40 years after the subjects had first been hospitalized between 1934 and 1944 the researchers found that bipolar subjects and unipolar subjects had more affective illness in their families than did control subjects. Although more relatives of bipolar subjects than of unipolar subjects had bipolar illness, the difference in risk for affective illness between relatives of bipolar subjects and of unipolar subjects was not significant. In general, there were more female than male depressed relatives among the unipolar depressed relatives but equal numbers of men and women among the bipolar relatives.

Winokur, George et al., "The Iowa 500: Affective Disorder in Relatives of Manic and Depressed Patients," *American Journal of Psychiatry*, 139:2(February 1982).

iproniazid (Marsilid) While researching a drug given to schizophrenics to lower extreme excitability, a New York physician, Dr. NATHAN KLINE, reasoned that if there was a drug that lowers the brain's activity, there must also be another to heighten it. With other researchers he came up with a theory of how this drug would work, despite the fact that he knew of no such drug in existence at that time.

Not long afterwards, Dr. Kline became aware of a drug called Marsilid (the trade name for iproniazid), which was first used to treat tuberculosis. As a side effect, it created a feeling of well-being, almost euphoria, in patients who took it. While that effect had been noted, its potential was practically ignored, even though, at the time, biochemists were researching a possible relationship between Marsilid and brain function.

In *Depression: How to Recognize It, How to Treat It, and How to Grow From It* Wina Sturgeon details how Dr. Kline decided to do some experimental work based on that research. In his experiment he gave the drug to a number of severely depressed patients in his practice. A little more than a month after treatment began, he noticed improvements in most of the patients. As his work continued, he saw that many of those treated with Marsilid completely recovered from depression in a relatively short time.

Today the drug is no longer used in the United States, since it was withdrawn from the market when it was found to be toxic to the liver in some patients. Evidence also showed it might produce high blood pressure. However, its history is important because it was a first-generation MONOAMINE OXIDASE INHIBITOR (MAO) and forerunner of MAO inhibitor drugs.

Sturgeon, Wina, *Depression: How to Recognize It, How to Treat It, and How to Grow From It*. (Englewood Cliffs, N.J.: Prentice-Hall, 1979).

Iran The city of Teheran was one of the five selected study areas for the WORLD HEALTH ORGANIZATION (WHO) COLLABORATIVE STUDY ON STANDARDIZED ASSESSMENT OF DEPRESSIVE DISORDERS—a study designed: (1) to develop and test simple instruments for clinical description of depressive states: (2) to examine with these instruments series of "average" depressive patients in different cultures; and (3) to set up a network of field research centers. Teheran came into being as an urban settlement and a capital not more than 200 years ago. It has developed quickly during the past 50 years, and now is a rapidly expanding city. Roozbeth Hospital, the field research center of the study, is the psychiatric teaching hospital of the University of Teheran and is located in one of the densely populated sectors of the city. It admits patients from all parts of Teheran, as well as from the provinces, including remote parts of the country. The hospital has 100 beds, 80 psychiatric and 20 neurological. The researchers stated that in the absence of demographic data on the population seeking mental health care in Teheran and the surrounding area, it is difficult to estimate whether the patients screened and selected for the study deviate from the general trends. There is no reason to expect that the patients with depressive disorders selected for the study were in any way unusual or different from patients suffering from depressive illnesses seeking care at Roozbeth Hospital at any other time in the last decade or so. (See also Appendix 1, Tables.)

Sartorius, N. et al., *Depressive Disorders in*

Different Cultures (Geneva: World Health Organization, 1983).

Ireland   Psychiatric hospital admissions in Ireland have been increasing steadily in recent decades, according to a report on the activities of Irish Psychiatric Hospitals and Units. Statistics for 1986 published in 1989 (the latest available at this writing) show there were 29,392 admissions to hospitals and units in 1986, as compared to 28,830 in 1984 and 29,082 in 1985. However, as first admissions in 1986 at 8,251 were down on the 8,441 of 1985 and the 8,749 in 1984 it is evident that the admission increase is entirely due to readmissions. First admissions now constitute 28% of all admissions in comparison with 34% in 1976 and 40% in 1966. Depressive disorders, alcohol abuse and schizophrenia constitute three-quarters of all admissions.

Two-thirds of all admissions for depressive disorders were women. In fact, depressive disorders accounted for 40% of all female admissions in 1986. In contrast, 80% of admissions for alcohol disorders and 59% of admissions for schizophrenia were for men. Overall, alcohol disorders accounted for over one-third of all male admissions in comparison with 10% of female admissions. The difference was much less for schizophrenia, which accounted for 22% of male and 19% of female admissions.

There was little change in the number of admissions for organic psychoses and other psychoses, between 1985 and 1986. Admissions for mania decreased by 8%. Numbers of admissions for personality and nervous disorders also decreased.

In private hospitals 35% of the admissions were for alcohol disorders, 34% for depressive disorders and 11% for schizophrenia. Thirty-four percent of all admissions to general hospital units were for depressive disorders, 21% for schizophrenia and 17% for alcohol disorders.

Ireland's Health Board area hospitals receive the majority of all psychiatric admissions in the country. In 1986 this proportion was 69%. The most commonly occurring diagnosis in Health Board area hospitals was depressive disorders, at 27%.

O'Connor, A. and Walsh, D., *Activities of Irish Psychiatric Hospitals and Units 1986* (Dublin: Health Research Board, 1989).

J

Japan   Nagasaki and Tokyo were the two Japanese selected study areas in the WORLD HEALTH ORGANIZATION (WHO) COLLABORATIVE STUDY ON STANDARDIZED ASSESSMENT OF DEPRESSIVE DISORDERS, designed: (1) to develop and test simple instruments for clinical description of depressive states; (2) to examine with these instruments series of ''average' depressive patients in different cultures; and (3) to set up a network of field research centers. Nagasaki occupies the northwestern tip of the island of Kyushu. Ethnically, the population is homogeneous. The percentage of Koreans, Chinese and other nationalities is negligible. The three most important sources of employment are shipbuilding, fishing and agriculture.

The Department of Neuropsychiatry of the Nagasaki University Hospital was the field research center for the study. A comparison of the age distribution of the patients screened for the study and the general population of the area showed minor deviations except for an under-representation of younger age groups (15–34) among the persons screened for the study.

The area around and including Tokyo is approximately in the middle of Japan and is also at the center of Japanese politics, economy and culture. It has a very high population density since it is the biggest industrial region of Japan, producing more than one-third of the nation's industrial ouput. The main industries are metals, machinery and chemicals. The most important agricultural product of the area is rice.

The field research center participating in the present study, the Department of Psychiatry and Neurology of Jikei University Hospital, is located in the center of metropolitan Tokyo. The types of people screened and included in the study did not deviate from the average patient with depressive illnesses seen at the Department of Psychiatry and Neurology of the Jikei University Hospital. Comparisons, even in general terms, were extremely difficult because of the vast population and the large number of psychiatric services in the area.

In comparing Toyko and Nagasaki, the researchers pointed out that the indices of standard of living and "modernity" are all higher in Tokyo than in Nagasaki. However, over-populated Tokyo suffers various corresponding disadvantages. The researchers noted that, on the whole, the natural environment in Tokyo has deteriorated to a much greater extent than in Nagasaki. (See also Appendix 1, Tables.)

Sartorius, N. et al., *Depressive Disorders in Different Cultures* (Geneva: World Health Organization, 1983).

Jensen, Jim   A well-known, former television anchorman; in early 1989 at the completion of 25 years with WCBS-TV he took an extended leave for treatment for severe depression at St. Mary's Hospital in Minnesota. It was reported at that time that Jensen had been fighting drug and alcohol abuse as well as depression.

Unidentified friends who discussed his depression stated he had never gone through a real grieving process and had been unable to get over the death of his only son who died in a hang gliding accident in 1979, at the age of 26. He had also had two divorces, before and after his son's death.

Since so much of Jensen's energy was needed for his recovery process, his physician, the station and Jensen himself agreed that when he was able to return to work he would come back as a senior correspondent rather than an anchorman. After four months of treatment he was able to return, apparently fully recovered, though on his return he stated he was still seeing a psychiatrist and taking an antidepressant, which he didn't expect he'd have to continue for the rest of his life.

Job   Some theologicans identify Job as a victim of reactive depression caused by severe personal setbacks. Early in Job's life he was considered the greatest of all people in the land of Uz, with his seven sons and three daughters, 7,000 sheep, 3,000 camels, 500 yoke of oxen, 500 she-asses and many servants.

At the instigation of Satan, however, he was struck by a succession of calamities and misfortunes. For a long time he tried to ward off his feelings of despair and despondency over his numerous afflictions. However, he finally succumbed to despair and longed for death: "Let the day perish wherein I was born" . . . "Let that day be darkness" . . . "Why died I not from the womb" . . . "Why did I not give up the ghost when I came out of the belly" . . . "For the thing which I greatly feared is come upon me and that which I was afraid of is come upon me" . . . "If I wait the grave is my house" . . . "I have made my bed in the darkness." His mood of constant sadness and anxiety was a prime sign of reactive depression, since people suffering from this type feel a keen loss of an external factor in their lives. Although this form of depression can engulf people for a time it is not usually interminable. So it was with Job who, during his considerable misery and suffering, ultimately sought counsel and acceptance from the Lord, and who after his blessings were restored (in greater abundance than before) lived a full and long life with his reactive depresssion behind him.

Johnson,   Samuel   A British author (1709–1784) who, despite his eccentricities, ungainly appearance and often uncouth manners, was known as an arbiter of England's literary tastes and the most influential conversationalist of his age.

Johnson experienced a lifetime battle with melancholy moods, and periodically feared a melancholy insanity. He wrote in his diary: "Since the Communion of last Easter I have led a life so dissipated and useless, and my terrours and perplexities have so much increased, that I am under great depression and discouragement."

journal keeping Research shows that keeping a journal and writing down one's feelings and thoughts can sometimes provide an emotional release for depressives. In one study conducted by Dr. James W. Pennebaker, professor of psychology at Southern Methodist University in Texas, Dr. Janice Kiecolt-Glaser, an Ohio State University psychologist, and Dr. Ronald Glaser, an immunologist, the researchers found that, among other things, people who shared a traumatic event by writing about it reported feeling less depressed, as though a weight had been lifted off their shoulders.

Squires, Sally, "How to Help Yourself," *Parade Magazine*, March 26, 1989.

K

Kahlbaum, Karl L. A German psychiatrist (1828–1899) who used the word CATATONIA in 1874 to name a clinical condition, which subsequently became the 20th-century diagnostic category of catatonic schizophrenia. Although his name is associated primarily with catatonia he used the word PARANOIA in 1863 to designate various persecutory and grandiose states of depression and psychosis.

Kaluli of New Guinea A society or tribe in New Guinea, dating back to primitive

times, that does not seem to have despair, hopelessness or depression in the way we know it. Instead they have a ritual based on the premise that if a member of the tribe loses something valuable (such as his pig) he has a right to recompense through a ritual such as dancing and screaming at the neighbor who he thinks killed his pig. This ritual is recognized by his society, and when he demands recompense for the loss, either the neighbor or the whole tribe takes note of his condition and usually recompenses him in one way or another. Dr. Martin E.P. Seligman of the University of Pennsylvania hypothesizes that this reciprocity between the culture and the individual when loss occurs provides strong buffers against loss becoming helplessness and hopelessness. He suggests that a society that prevents loss from becoming hopelessness prevents sadness from becoming despair, and in so doing breaks up the process of depression. In contrast to this, Seligman believes, modern Western culture promotes depression through a transition from loss to helplessness to hopelessness.

Seligman, Martin E.P., "Why Is There So Much Depression Today?" G. Stanley Hall Lecture Series (Washington, D.C., 1988).

Karen Horney Clinic A nonprofit psychiatric clinic that opened its doors in 1955 to offer outpatient mental health services to all people regardless of race, religion, social and intellectual levels, or ability to pay. It is named for Dr. Karen Horney (1885–1952), a German-American pioneer in the field of psychoanalysis, who believed that individuals have the potential to be warm, joyful, spontaneous and unafraid human beings. Her humanistic philosophy is the foundation of the clinic, which is dedicated to the psychoanalytic and psychotherapeutic treatment of persons with psychoneurotic and emotional problems. The clinic is funded through a combination of private contributions, foundation and government grants, and sliding scale fees for service, based on the patients' ability to pay. Address: 329 E. 62nd St., New York, NY 10021. Phone: 212-838-4333.

Kiev, Ari One of the leading authorities (1933–) on depression in America and a practicing psychiatrist who has received world-wide recognition for his research, writings and teachings in the field of depression. He is medical director of the Social Psychiatry Research Institute in New York and clinical associate professor of psychiatry at Cornell University Medical College. He is also originator of the Life Strategy Workshops, which are offered in major metropolitan centers and the author of more than a dozen books, including *Recovery from Depression* and *A Strategy For Daily Living* (Free Press, 1973).

killing potential of grief See GRIEF, CAUSES AND EFFECTS OF.

Klerman, Gerald L. A winner in 1986 of one of the most prestigious research awards in psychiatry, the Anna-Monika Prize, for his work over a 20-year period as part of a group that developed a brief psychotherapeutic treatment for depression called interpersonal psychotherapy or IPT. Klerman (1928–) is associate chairman for research and professor of psychiatry at New York Hospital-Cornell Medical Center. He is researching environmental factors and gene/environmental factors that are underway in pathogenesis (origin and development of a disease) that may affect the changes in the rates of depression and its age distribution in the United States. He was also the presenter of the Third Eli Lily Lecture to the Royal College of Psychiatrists in London and has written several books, including the chapter on "Affective Disorders" in *The Harvard Guide to Modern Psychiatry.*

Kline, Nathan S. A pioneer (1916–1983) in the use of both tranquilizers and antidepressant drugs. For over three decades he was director of the Research Center at Rockland State Hospital. Located in Orangeburg, New York the center is now named for him and known as the NATHAN S. KLINE INSTITUTE for Psychiatric Research. In recognition of his work the Nathan S. Kline Medal of Merit is awarded annually to a person or organization that has made significant humanitarian contributions to the field of mental health.

Dr. Kline was also a clinical professor at Columbia University Hospital and attending physician at Lenox Hill Hospital, in addition to maintaining a private practice in New York in which he treated thousands of patients suffering from depression. *New York* magazine called him "the ultimate specialist" on depression, and he was honored by two Albert Lasker Clinical Research Awards for his role in the development of antidepressant medications. His book FROM SAD TO GLAD is considered a classic in the field.

Kraepelin, Emil A German psychiatrist (1856–1926) who was concerned mainly with diagnostic classification and who helped introduce scientific methods of investigation.

In the 1880s Kraepelin began using the term "depressive insanity" to name one of the categories of insanity, and he included a "depressive form" as one of the categories of paranoia. He continued to use "melancholia" in a manner in keeping with his times and to use "depression" to describe affect. He considered the melancholias to be forms of mental depression. By the turn of the century he identified manic-depressive illness as a separate entity.

Kubler-Ross, Elisabeth A psychiatrist and noted authority (1926–) on death and dying—and the stages of depression and grief that accompany a terminal illness. Before coming to America she practiced medicine in Switzerland. After coming to the United States, she began her work with the dying while teaching psychiatry at the University of Chicago. She is the author of *On Death and Dying, To Live Until We Say Goodbye* and *Death: The Final Stage of Growth*. Her breakthrough work offers new insight for the management of the terminally ill as she focuses on people confronting death as human beings and provides those who face bereavement and grief with a new understanding for dealing with both the dying and their own impending loss.

L

laboratory tests   All of today's tests assume that some types of depression are accompanied by abnormalities in brain or body function. These abnormalities can be detected through measurement of chemicals in the blood and/or urine (and occasionally, the cerebrospinal fluid) or by measuring brain waves. A variety of different tests are now being studied in research laboratories around the country. Most must still be regarded as highly experimental, while their capacity to provide clinically useful diagnostic results is being established. In some cases, some of the experimental tests may never reach a stage in which their usefulness as diagnostic tools is proven. (See also BLOOD TESTS; COMPUTERIZED AXIAL TOMOGRAPHY; DEXAMETHASONE SUPPRESSION TEST; ELECTROENCEPHALOGRAM; MAGNETIC RESONANCE IMAGING; PET SCAN.)

laughter   See HUMOR.

L-dopa   See LEVODOPA.

length of grieving process   The time required to complete the grieving process and resolve the psychological impact resulting from the death of a loved one remains largely unexplored. Research indicates, however, that the time-consuming healing process, which is essential for the restructuring of a

person's life, can take weeks, months or even years. According to a study at the University of Illinois at Chicago as many as one in four people who lose a spouse to death may need some professional help to cope with their grief and avoid clinical depression.

In the study, 130 individuals who lost spouses were interviewed at five weeks after the death and then nine or 10 months later. While signs of depression were common shortly after the spouse's death, most people felt much better after the second interview. But about one in four still had significant problems at the second interview. "A significant proportion of the population might be miserable for years after their spouse's death unless given some kind of help and support," reported Dr. Joseph Flaherty, professor of psychiatry and community health at the university.

In many cases the main signs of grieving, such as overwhelming sadness or anger, typically decrease noticeably after six to nine months, and signals of the end of MOURNING come after a year or so. But researchers say that mourning for two or three years is not unusual, and in some people signs of GRIEF can linger for years.

In an Ann Arbor study on individuals who lost a spouse or child in a motor vehicle crash, Darrin R. Lehman and Camille B. Wortman of the University of Michigan and Allan F. Williams of the Insurance Institute for Highway Safety in Washington, D.C. found that four to seven years after an accident, bereaved spouses and parents reported marked depression and a failure to resolve their LOSS.

This study, reported in *Science News*, points out that emotional recovery from loss is longer and more difficult than has often been assumed in the past and indicates that, following the traumatic loss of one's spouse or child, lasting distress is not a sign of individual coping failure but rather a common response to the situation.

The researchers used state records to identify every motor vehicle fatality in Wayne

County, Michigan between 1976 and 1979. Potential subjects were then located and asked to be interviewed in 1983 in their homes. The spouse study included 39 bereaved individuals (most of them women) and 39 non-bereaved controls matched for sex, age, income, education, and number and ages of children. The parent study was conducted with 41 pairs of bereaved parents and 41 matched pairs of non-bereaved parents. Though individual responses varied, responses to structured interviews generally showed bereaved spouses to be doing significantly poorer than controls on several indicators of general functioning, such as depression, anxiety and other psychiatric symptoms, social contacts, satisfaction with current life situations, apprehension about the future and confidence in the ability to cope with serious problems. Among those who had lost a child significant differences in functioning, especially depression, were observed between bereaved and control parents, but these were not as pervasive as differences in the spouse study. Part of the reason, suggest the researchers, may be that a spouse is a more critical source of support and security than a child. Nearly all of the bereaved subjects said the deceased continued to occupy their thoughts and conversations, often making them feel hurt and pained.

The question of when a person needs psychological treatment depends on distinguishing between normal grief and pathological or suppressed grief. Though a person who has experienced a loss may be extremely disturbed at various times he may not need GRIEF THERAPY/TREATMENT. But when the sorrow is constant and excessive and seems to have no end therapists say that mourners may need help. For whatever time it takes, however, (and regardless of whether the grief is normal or pathological or suppressed) people who have suffered a loss need to vent their feelings during times of emotional distress. (See also BEREAVEMENT; GRIEF, CAUSES AND EFFECTS OF; HARVARD STUDY; STAGES OF GRIEF.)

Bower, B., "Bereavement: Reeling in the Years," *Science News*, 131(February 7, 1987).

levodopa Abbreviated as L-dopa, this drug is used in the treatment of PARKINSON'S DISEASE (PD), a disorder in which depression is a common symptom. Late in the course of PD some patients develop a combination of depression and DEMENTIA. The powerful therapeutic effects of combining levodopa and carbidopa (known as SINEMET) for the treatment of Parkinson's were demonstrated 20 years ago in initial, large-scale clinical trials and considered a historic advance in the treatment of Parkinson's disease.

In the early 1970s the side effects seen in the early course of high-dose levodopa treatment were reduced with the introduction of dopa decarboxylase inhibitors (carbidopa and benserazide). Since then the combination of levodopa and a dopa decarboxylase inhibitor rapidly became, and remains, the most widely used treatment of idiopathic Parkinson's disease.

With most patients, though, the initial response to levodopa diminishes with prolonged use, and a common side effect is fluctuating motor performance. This is so common that researchers have found that approximately 50% of patients treated with levodopa for five or more years develop fluctuations in motor response. In these patients the length of therapeutic benefit derived from each dose is diminished.

Traditionally the approach employed to control this is to reduce dosage level of levodopa and increase dosage frequency. However, the effectiveness of this approach is limited, so the challenge is to develop controlled-release and longer-acting preparations of levodopa. To achieve this researchers have been studying other agents that will be released in the body over time and have advantages over the currently available, standard Sinemet.

According to Dr. Thomas Hutton, professor and director of the Parkinson's Disease Information and Referral Center at Texas Tech University, Madopar (known as Madopar HBS) is another drug that shows some promise in the treatment of Parkinson's disease. As a combination of levodopa and. the peripheral dopa decarboxylase inhibitor benserazide, it is the mainstay of treatment for Parkinson's in many countries. Although it is not available in the United States, a controlled-release form of Madopar has been developed and, at this writing, is undergoing clinical investigation. (See also SINEMET CR.)

Hutton, J.T. and Morris, J.L., "Long Acting Levodopa Preparations," *Neurology* Supplement, October 1989.

Librium   See CHLORDIAZEPOXIDE.

light therapy   The effects of light therapy (exposure to bright artificial light) have reduced depression in some patients, so for the past few years scientists throughout the world have been testing full-spectrum electric lighting (also known as phototherapy) to artificially lengthen the day of persons who suffer from SEASONAL AFFECTIVE DISORDER (SAD), a condition in which winter depression and summer HYPOMANIAS (a milder form of mania) alternate. An outstanding characteristic of SAD is reactivity to changes in environmental lighting in which the changes in day length are important. This knowledge has stimulated attempts to modify winter depressive symptoms by extending the day with bright artificial light.

Scientists do not know at this time exactly how phototherapy exerts its antidepressant effects. However, it seems likely that light, entering via the eye, modifies brain chemistry and physiology in such a way as to correct the abnormalities resulting from light deficiency in vulnerable individuals. This modification seems reversible, and when light is withdrawn, a relapse can occur. It also appears that the photochemical effect of light requires that the light be of sufficient intensity and administered for a sufficient duration. The hypothalamus seems a likely site of action because it mediates many of the vegetative functions that are disturbed by SAD and reversed by phototherapy.

In research studies at the National Institute of Mental Health (NIMH), Dr. Norman E. Rosenthal, chief, Unit of Outpatient Services, Clinical Psychobiology Branch, and Dr. Thomas E. Wehr, chief, Clinical Psychobiology Branch (CPB), have found that extending the day with five to six hours of bright, full-spectrum light has had significant antidepressant effects whereas dimmer control light treatments have not. This finding has been replicated by other groups.

In reporting on their findings in *Psychiatric Annals* the NIMH researchers stated that even though it is generally accepted that bright artificial light is a viable treatment for SAD the properties of phototherapy that are necessary or optimal for achieving an antidepressant effect continue to be a focus of interest and research. According to Dr. Rosenthal and Dr. Wehr, it appears that two hours of light treatment in the morning may be more effective than two hours in the evening. However, other studies have shown that light treatment may be quite effective if administered only in the evening or even during the day.

"Although most studies have used full-spectrum light," report the researchers, "there is evidence that it is not necessary to achieve an antidepressant effect, and we do not know at this time which spectral properties of light are necessary for its antidepressant effect. Although early studies used five to six hours of light per day, more recent studies suggest that two hours of treatment per day may be effective. However, there does seem to be some relationship between duration and efficacy with greater effects occurring as duration is increased."

In discussing their methods for treating patients, Dr. Rosenthal and Dr. Wehr strongly recommend that light therapy (and any treatment for mood problems) be supervised by a qualified therapist or psychiatrist. They also emphasize that antidepressant effects have been shown only in certain people with seasonal depression. Despite its success rate in the treatment of SAD, this therapy has been less successful in the treatment of non-seasonal depressions. At this point its wide-spread usefulness has yet to be demonstrated, but as the treatment continues to be used experimentally the results of future research look promising.

The NIMH researchers suggest using a metal box containing six power-twist Vitalite tubes, behind a translucent plastic screen, when administering light therapy for SAD victims. This light box has been built to meet research and safety specifications. It should be placed either vertically on the floor or horizontally on a level surface like a desk or table, and people using it are advised to sit in front of the light for two to five hours per day. Rather than staring directly at the light for this period people can read, watch TV or pursue other sedentary activities while glancing at the light from time to time. Some anti-depressant effect usually occurs within the first week.

The researchers have no reason to suspect that the treatment, administered as described above, is detrimental to the eyes, and they have documented no visual problems in the time during which they have used light treatment, but, understandably, they cannot rule out the possibility of visual problems following long-term usage of lights in some people. They do believe, however, that in some cases the light may make people feel uncomfortably energized or irritable, and patients sometimes complain of eyestrain, fatigue, nausea and headaches. In some patients the light treatment can induce migraine headaches. If insomnia occurs it is most likely to take place when patients use lights late at night.

Generally, these side effects are uncommon and can be reversed easily within a few days by decreasing the duration of treatment, increasing the distance from the light source or discontinuing the treatment temporarily. At a later date the treatment can at times be increased in duration or strength. If light treatment is judged to be unsuitable for a victim of SAD, antidepressant drugs can often be effective.

Suitable light fixtures can be obtained from several sources, and the NIMH does not endorse any particular light company. However, they have had the most experience with the SunBox Company, 1132 Taft St., Rockville, MD 20850. Phone: 301–762-1786. This company ships to any location via UPS.

limbic system A group of subcortical structures of the brain that comprise the center of emotional response.

Lincoln, Abraham Historians believe the Illinois lawyer (1809–1865) who became the 16th president of the United States had a predisposition to clinical depression, which triggered his lifetime of bouts with it. In today's political climate, when everything regarding a presidential candidate's past is uncovered and examined microscopically, chances are good that Lincoln, like vice presidential candidate Thomas Eagleton in 1972, would never have made it to Washington.

As a young man Lincoln brooded so much his friends feared he might take his life. Subsequently he met Mary Todd, a vivacious 21-year-old Kentucky belle and daughter of a wealthy banker who appeared to be fascinated by politics. At the time Mary gave no indication of her future mental problems. But now researchers who believe depression can be contagious feel Lincoln's depression was compounded by Mary's bouts with it.

In 1841 when Lincoln broke his engagement with Mary because of the vigorous objections of her family, who considered Lincoln beneath her, Lincoln plunged into the worst emotional crisis of his life. According to one Lincoln biographer, Russell Freedman, for a week he refused to leave his room.

People said "he had thrown two cat fits and a duck fit and gone crazy for a week or two."

To his law partner John Stuart he wrote: "I am now the most miserable man living. If what I feel were equally distributed to the whole human family, there would not be one cheerful face on earth. Whether I shall ever be better, I cannot tell. I awfully forbode I shall not. To remain as I am is impossible. I must die or be better."

Fifteen months later the couple resumed their courtship, married and had four sons. But throughout their marriage Lincoln's manners and homespun ways bothered Mary. Freedman writes that when she lost her temper at him the neighbors would hear the furious explosions of anger.

Lincoln himself, however, was not easy to live with, with his moodiness and long lapses of brooding silence. During his blackest moments he could assuage his depression somewhat in the company of his sons. But when the Lincolns' second son, Eddie, died in 1850 (before he was four years old), things took a turn for the worse for the Lincolns. Mary collapsed in shock, shut herself in her room and stayed there for weeks. Lincoln brooded and buried himself in work. In their house, draped in black, the silence was broken only by Mary's uncontrolled sobbing.

In 1862 while Lincoln's oldest son Robert was at Harvard University, eight-year-old Tad and eleven-year-old Willie lived with their parents in the White House. Early that year both boys fell ill with a fever, and when Willie died Mary was so overcome with grief and depression she could not attend the funeral. For three months she refused to leave the White House, and the depression and imaginary fears she experienced were to stay with her for a long time to come. Lincoln himself plunged into the deepest depression and grief he had ever known.

The Civil War years took their toll, too, and Freedman writes that the summer of 1864 was the most dismal period of Lincoln's presidential career. He faced problems with corruption in the War Department and increasing criticism for his handling of the Union commanders. He even felt his Gettysburg Speech was a failure when opposition newspapers criticized the speech as unworthy of the occasion and when some papers didn't mention it at all. Throughout his presidency he lived with rumors of abduction and assassination, too. In fact, he received so many threatening letters he had a file labeled "Assassination."

History and Lincoln's biographers give no indication that the president whose face has been described as "a portrait in melancholy" ever really recovered from his bouts of depression. Perhaps his closest step toward overcoming them is recorded by Freedman, who wrote that on the fateful day of his assassination Lincoln told Mary before going to the theater, "We must both be more cheerful in the future. Between the war and the loss of our darling Willie we have been very miserable."

Freedman, Russell, *Lincoln: A Photobiography* (New York: Clarion Books, 1987).

Kline, Nathan, *From Sad to Glad* (New York: Putnam, 1974).

Lincoln, Mary Todd See LINCOLN, ABRAHAM.

Lipton, Ira D. A New York psychiatrist (1941–) who worked with the late Dr. NATHAN S. KLINE, the noted pioneer in the use of antidepressant drugs, and who has continued Dr. Kline's Manhattan practice in the psychopharmacology of depression.

lithium In medicine lithium is the name commonly applied to lithium carbonate and lithium citrate, chemicals that are used as ANTIDEPRESSANTS. Pure lithium is one of the 103 chemical elements that occur in nature. An electrolyte, it is similar to ordinary table salt. Because of its high chemical reactivity, however, it is almost never found in a free or uncombined state. Rather, lithium compounds, such as lithium oxide or lithium chloride, are found in certain rocks in the sea and in minute amounts in mineral springs and plant and animal tissues.

In 1949 an Australian psychiatrist, JOHN CADE, noted that lithium caused sedation in guinea pigs. When he observed this and tried administering lithium to patients with manic symptoms he discovered it had a calming effect on humans. For some years his discovery—and lithium treatment—was largely ignored, but gradually lithium caught on as drug of first choice for treating manic-depressives, and the Food and Drug Administration approved it for psychiatric use in 1969.

Without causing the drugged feeling that sometimes accompanies the use of tranquilizers, lithium can stabilize extreme mood swings, smooth out destructive mood cycles and reduce the frequency and severity of cycles. In a National Institute of Mental Health (NIMH) study at least 70% of the manic-depressive patients maintained on lithium stopped having episodes or had fewer, shorter or less severe ones. Studies have also indicated that some persons experiencing depression (particularly those who have a family history of mania) also respond favorably to lithium. Most of the manic-depressive patients who do not respond to lithium have rapidly changing cycles and can generally be helped by the addition of carbamazepine.

The effects of lithium are complex and it is not known for certain how one drug can have two opposite effects—bringing down the euphoric highs of mania and, at the opposite end of the pole, working against the depressive phase. How lithium also effectively controls depressive episodes and can prevent both manias and depressions is not yet known. This paradox is one of many challenging puzzles that psychiatric researchers are trying to solve.

Research evidence suggests lithium affects a variety of functions in the body, including the distribution of major electrolytes such as sodium and potassium, which regulate impulses along the nerve cells. It also appears to affect the activity of NEUROTRANSMITTERS

as well as other biological systems in a number of ways. The relationship between these effects and lithium's impact on mania and depression, however, is not completely understood. Several theories have been suggested, but none has provided a satisfactory explanation for all of lithium's biochemical and clinical effects. The use of the drug in the treatment of recurrent depressions in the absence of manic mood swings is still at the research stage.

Another effect can be memory deficits and a slowing of mental processes. In a *New York Times* article Dr. Richard Jed Wyatt, chief of the neuropsychiatry branch of the National Institute of Mental Health (NIMH), stated: "Depending on the dose, it does, at times make memory more difficult." He added that the drug could also "blunt the thinking processes and make it difficult to concentrate." But doctors usually try to adjust the dose to minimize the effects.

Lithium's major drawback is that it is relatively slow acting and may require four to 10 days (or even three weeks) before achieving full effectiveness. If the patient is severely manic, physicians often start with a major tranquilizer such as haloperidol or chlorpromazine to achieve rapid control of the mood swing until lithium has a chance to act. When taken for a prolonged period of time, lithium's effectiveness seems to increase. The dose must be carefully monitored through frequent blood testing and other evaluations by a physician.

Maintenance on medication is essential for persons with recurrent forms of depression, particularly manic-depressive disorder and recurring episodes of major depression. Such continuous treatment can offer essentially normal functioning to those whose lives might otherwise be painful beyond endurance. The severity of the episodes, the potential impact of a future episode on an individual's functioning, the attitude of the patient toward taking medication for long periods, and many other factors determine whether and for how long a patient continues on treatment. In one study of lithium compliance it was found that 50% of the patients who were on it stopped taking the drug against medical advice. They missed the euphoric feelings and sense of well-being experienced during mild manic states.

Precautions are necessary while on lithium because, according to the National Institute of Mental Health (NIMH), lithium can be poisonous if taken in excessive doses. Care must be taken not to exceed the prescribed dosage because there is a narrow range between the therapeutic and toxic levels.

Because lithium is excreted from the body almost entirely by the kidneys, any injury or weakening of the kidneys that brings on an inability to get rid of the proper amount of lithium may allow lithium to accumulate to dangerous levels in the body. Consequently lithium should not be taken by patients with severely impaired kidney function.

The excretion of lithium in the kidneys is closely linked to that of sodium (table salt is sodium chloride). The less sodium in the body, the less lithium is excreted. Thus there is a greater chance of lithium build-up and possible lithium toxicity. Because of the way too little sodium is implicated in lithium build-up low-sodium diets can be especially harmful to the patient taking lithium. Diuretics can also be harmful since they cause the kidneys to excrete sodium. As a result, lithium levels rise.

Patients with heart disease and others who have a significant change in sodium in their diet or periodic episodes of heavy sweating should be especially careful to have their lithium blood levels monitored regularly. Lithium should not be used in the first three months of pregnancy. Women should not breastfeed when they are taking lithium, except in rare circumstances when, in the view of the physician, the potential benefits to the mother outweigh possible hazards to the child.

Other effects of lithium include nausea, lethargy, moderate thirst, hand tremors, greatly increased urination, possible weight gain, memory deficits and the slowing of mental processes. Toxic doses can cause vomiting, diarrhea, extreme thirst, weight loss, muscle twitching, abnormal muscle movement, slurred speech, blurred vision, dizziness, stupor or pulse irregularities.

With careful adherence to the instructions for taking this medication, regular blood level checks and observations for any of the above signs, these problems can almost always be avoided. (See also DRUG THERAPY; LITHIUM PROPHYLACTIC TREATMENT.)

Kolata, Gina, "Experts Say Treatments Affect Recall," *The New York Times*, October 19, 1988.

lithium prophylactic treatment   Lithium's greatest value is its effectiveness in preventing or reducing the occurrence of future episodes in manic-depressive illness. It has not been shown to be highly effective in treating an ongoing depressive episode.

The use of lithium is often referred to as "lithium prophylaxis" or "lithium prophylactic treatment." The prophylactic value of lithium in unipolar illness is not certain at this time, although several major studies indicate that lithium treatment usually hastens the disappearance of recurring depressions or reduces their severity.

Lithium is not a cure for recurrent manic or depressive illnesses. When fully effective—and if it's kept up—it will prevent the illness for the rest of one's life. It can be prescribed by a psychiatrist and is administered to patients as a white powder taken orally in capsule or tablet form. It should not be discontinued without consulting the physician.

In lithium prophylactic treatment, lithium is administered after the patient has recovered from a manic or depressive episode to prevent or dampen future attacks. Some patients respond quickly to treatment and have no further episodes of mania or depression. Others respond more slowly and continue to have moderate mood swings even months after therapy is started. These highs or lows usually become progressively less severe with this treatment and often disappear completely. With some patients, lithium may not prevent all future manic and depressive episodes, but it may reduce or lessen their severity. In some cases, there are patients who are not helped at all by lithium and who continue to have episodes at the same frequency and severity as before lithium therapy. A physician cannot predict with any certainty how lithium will work in an individual case. This can be determined only by actual use of the medication.

In general, lithium is not the treatment choice for ongoing depression but may be effective in cases that do not respond to other treatments.

A CHECKLIST FOR PATIENTS TAKING LITHIUM

1. Take the medication on a regular basis as prescribed by the physician.
2. Obtain regular blood tests for lithium levels.
3. Have the physician take blood tests for lithium levels 12 hours after the last dose.
4. Inform the physician if other medications are being taken, since they can change lithium levels.
5. Notify the physician whenever there is a change in diet, since it may cause the lithium level in the body to change.
6. Advise the physician about any changes in frequency of urination, voiding of fluids (e.g., diarrhea, vomiting, excessive sweating) or illness, since adjustment of dosage or further testing may be required.
7. If planning to become pregnant, advise the physician.
8. Since it takes time for mood swings to be completely controlled by lithium, do not get discouraged, but continue taking the medicine until advised otherwise by the physician.

living with a depressed person See ROLE OF FAMILY AND FRIENDS.

Logan, Joshua A famous stage and screen director (1908–1988), coauthor and producer or coproducer of some of Broadway's most enduring hits, such as *South Pacific* and *Mr. Roberts*. For many years he was a victim of manic depression and rumors abounded about his ups and downs of mood. On two occasions the problem became so great he was hospitalized for extended periods because of his excessive mood swings.

During the early years of Logan's illness it was not common knowledge that manic depression could be treated and controlled by lithium. But when Logan learned of this treatment in 1969 he began taking lithium as a preventive. Subsequently he gained a reputation for his frankness in talking about manic depression.

In his obituary in *The New York Times* he was quoted as writing in his book, *Movie Stars, Real People, and Me:* "I had been ignorant all my life about such things. At least I could tell others so they would never be as ignorant as I was." As part of his candor about his illness Logan took part in medical seminars, appeared on television and talked extensively about depression. But he also made it clear that he felt its manic phase contributed to his creativity. The *Times* obituary went on to quote him as saying "Without my illness, active or dormant, I'm sure I would have lived only half of the life I've lived and that would be as unexciting as a safe and sane Fourth of July. I would have missed the sharpest, the rarest and, yes, the sweetest moments of my existence."

New York Times, "Joshua Logan, Stage and Screen Director, Dies at 79," *The New York Times,* July 13, 1988.

loss The primary losses that can cause depression and GRIEF are losses by death. But there are other life happenings that provoke a sense of loss, too. Among the most usual are: separation (such as divorce or the end of a relationship); loss of a pet; disability from loss of an arm, leg, eyesight, hearing or other bodily function; illness and accidents; alienation of friends and family; loss of a job, home, money and material things; and situational changes such as retirement, geographical uprootings, departure of children from home. Other losses researchers pinpoint are lost opportunities and expectations and lost self-esteem, status, reputation, faith and hope.

While researching loss by death Dr. Michele M. Van Eerdewegh, assistant professor of psychiatry at Washington University School of Medicine in St. Louis, conducted two studies on the effects of parental death on young to adolescent children, and found that children cope better with the loss than the widow or widower. Although children are saddened by the loss, Van Eerdewegh noted that the intensity of the reaction is a lot less for the children than for the surviving parents because the children do not have to shoulder the responsibility of both parents. Difficulties for the child occur when the surviving parent makes extraordinary demands or is seriously depressed.

In her studies Van Eerdewegh and her associates observed that the immediate reaction of a child to the death of a parent is usually mild and short-lived. The children might suffer from a mild sadness lasting a month or two, with some lingering symptoms for up to one year, and there may be some regret and guilt. For example, very young children may fear that their behavior was the reason for the death while an older child may feel guilt about not having been a better son or daughter.

Other responses (that are normal grief reactions and should diminish as the child works through the loss) might include increased anger, irritability, difficulty in sleeping or a change in appetite. Many children could become withdrawn.

Van Eerdewegh's studies showed a problem with bedwetting by girls between six and 12 who had lost a parent. In a bereaved group, 17% had difficulty with it, compared with none in a control group. "Perhaps the most significant response to a parent's death is a noticeable drop in school performance," stated Van Eerdewegh. "What's going on in school is a very good barometer of what's going on inside the children."

Among the 105 bereaved children in Van Eerdewegh's initial study, only six suffered from severe depression, and most were adolescents. That's similar to the control group, where four were depressed. What interested Van Eerdewegh, however, was that the surviving parent (the mother) of five of the six bereaved, depressed children suffered from depression. That led Van Eerdewegh to think that even if the death triggered onset of depression in some children, there were other intervening factors—some probably biological or genetic, and others of a more reactive nature in response to the mother's own mental state.

"Children probably have differential responses according to their developmental age," reported Van Eerdewegh. "The older the child is, the more likely he or she is to show a reaction similar to an adult reaction."

As a result of her observations, Van Eerdewegh stressed that the surviving parent should not require too much from the child who has lost a parent. "An overly demanding parent could cause the child to become overly responsible or, to the other extreme, totally irresponsible later in life," she warned. "The child could also rebel or just give up ever trying to accomplish anything."

A surviving father is more likely to demand too much from his daughter than he would his son, stated Van Eerdewegh, citing housework and child care as examples. The same holds true for surviving mothers and sons. Troubles also can arise when a boy has lost his father, or a girl, her mother. These children have a high risk factor for the development of mental disorders later in life. Since the child who has experienced a loss needs a person of his or her own sex to show the normal roles expected of that sex, Van Eerdewegh recommended that the surviving parent try to find a substitute for the child, such as a member of the child's extended family—say, an uncle, if the bereaved child is a boy. And if the child needs professional counseling Van Eerdewegh suggested finding a therapist who is the same sex as the child.

Researchers have found that children who lose a sibling in childhood often find it difficult to mourn the loss through normal grieving. As a result the loss can remain bottled up and become unfinished psychological business that can leave the surviving sibling vaguely depressed for years. In fact, problems associated with this difficulty often do not emerge until adulthood.

In an article "When A Young Sibling Dies" Mary Amoroso reports on a study on sibling loss, conducted by psychologist Dr. Helen Rosen while Rosen was a professor at Rutgers University. Now a professor at Bryn Mawr, Rosen said: "In general I found that people who'd lost a sibling in childhood found their loss was treated as a very minor thing. The feeling was 'You're young; you'll get over it.' Also, they had felt a tremendous need to protect and take care of their parents. This took precedence over their need to grieve. They didn't want to do anything that would cause their parents more pain. And some children tried to be a replacement child to make up to their parents for the lost child. Some had actually changed career plans to take up where the deceased child had left off."

Amoroso also reported on the work of Rob Stevenson, a New Jersey certified counselor in death education who counsels children and adolescents who have lost siblings. "The grief process takes about a year for a lot of people," advised Stevenson. "With younger people, they have school, they are more resilient, and they have a strong energy source, all of which they can use to postpone grieving for a year, two years, even five years."

According to Amoroso, the experts offer the following advice on what families and teachers can do to make sure that surviving siblings who suffer a loss aren't overlooked:

1. Keep the lines of communication open. If a parent has trouble expressing his feelings, let the child know that. Saying nothing can make a child feel confused and alone.

2. Acknowledge the child's loss. Too often, the parents receive all the condolences, and the child's grief is all but forgotten.

3. Try to make sure there are others around to whom a child can talk—aunts, uncles, a school counselor, or a support group.

4. Try to avoid idealizing the deceased child since it's hard for surviving siblings when they have to compete.

5. Make sure the child's school is notified about the death in the family. Teachers and counselors should be sensitized to the need to offer condolences and to listen to the child, but by the same token the death should not be brought up constantly. Sometimes children need the normality and the neutrality of school to help them escape the tension of a grieving household.

6. Understand that children act out their grief in different ways. A child's grades may drop, his behavior may become rocky, he may seem distant or he may seem oblivious to the family's pain. Helping him to verbalize his loss and to say goodbye to his sibling will aid him in resolving the pain.

In *The Seasons of Grief* Donna A Gaffney, a family therapist, also emphasizes the need to encourage children to keep talking about the death and loss of someone close to them. Similarly, Alicia Carmona, a psychiatrist who specializes in the treatment of children in her private practice and at the Institute of Living in Hartford, stresses the importance of allowing children to express their feelings both negative and positive. "Often adults are afraid to hear negative feelings about the dead from children, but the more they can express their feelings, the better it is," she stated in an article, "A Therapist's Guide to Explaining Death to Children."

Carmona pointed out that explanations have to be age-appropriate. She advised that with young children you can talk about the cycles of life as relating to seasons, bugs and animals while being careful not to give the children a false understanding of death, such as "sleep" or "gone away." Children ages 7 to 11 are better equipped to understand death, but they need to be reassured that they will not be abandoned, that other people will take care of them. Teenagers may feel guilty and think that in some way they might have prevented the death, so they need the kind of reassurance that helps them understand they must not feel responsible.

Whatever the reaction is, both adults and children must be able to express their feelings about loss and death for as long as it is helpful to them. In the final analysis, most researchers agree that emotional recovery from loss (especially loss by death) is longer and more difficult than has often been assumed in the past. They conclude that failure to achieve the resolution of a loss after a significant amount of time following the traumatic loss of a loved one is not a sign of an inability to cope or to free oneself from the emotional bond to a deceased loved one but rather a common response to the situation. (See also BEREAVEMENT; GRIEF, CAUSES AND EFFECTS OF; GRIEF THERAPY/TREATMENT; MOURNING; STAGES OF GRIEF; Appendix 6.)

Amoroso, Mary, "When A Young Sibling Dies," *The* [Hackensack, N.J.] *Record,* March 19, 1989.

Gaffney, Donna A., *The Seasons of Grief* (New York: New American Library, 1988).

Kochakian, Mary Jo, "A Therapist's Guide to Explaining Death to Children," *The* [Hackensack, N.J.] *Record* (Special from *The Hartford Courant*), July 8, 1988.

loss of a parent (effect on children)
See LOSS.

loss of a sibling   See LOSS.

L-tryptophan   L-tryptophan, an essential amino acid, is one of the dietary building blocks that body tissues use to manufacture proteins. Because our bodies cannot manufacture their own L-tryptophan, it must be ingested in the food we eat—for example, through eggs, milk, meat, turkey, beans and wheat.

L-tryptophan is the only dietary substance scientists have consistently linked to depression. This is because L-tryptophan is used by the brain to manufacture SEROTONIN, one of the amine transmitters. When there is an inadequate amount of L-tryptophan in the diet, brain serotonin levels fall, which may contribute to depression. At the Massachusetts Institute of Technology, for instance, scientists have found that the level of serotonin in the brain is directly influenced by the amount of L-tryptophan in the diet. As yet, all of the answers concerning L-tryptophan as a solution to depression are not in, but for some patients it has been moderately effective. For others its effectiveness as a treatment for depression has been inconsistent and only partially beneficial.

In recent years millions of Americans have come to rely on L-tryptophan in tablet, capsule and powder form as a relaxant and sleep aid. A doctor's prescription has not been needed to obtain it, since the Food and Drug Administration classifies L-tryptophan as a food additive, not as a drug. It has been available through health food stores or chemical-supply companies.

In November 1989, however, the FDA asked manufacturers and retailers to voluntarily remove products with L-tryptophan from shelves immediately. The FDA said it had found an "unequivocal link" between consumption of L-tryptophan supplements and a sudden outbreak of a rare blood disorder called eosinophilia-myalgia syndrome. This syndrome is marked by extremely high fever, muscle aches, joint pain, and swelling of the legs or arms. The illness results in elevated white blood cell counts. Rashes and impaired breathing may also occur.

Despite the federal recall, some stores have continued to sell dietary supplements with L-tryptophan. But until scientists are able to pinpoint the cause of the outbreak of illness, it is advisable to adhere to the FDA recall and refrain from taking products containing L-tryptophan.

Doherty, Matthew J., "L-tryptrophan Is Still Around Despite Recall," *The* [Hackensack, N.J.] *Record,* December 1, 1989.

lymphocytes Mobile white blood cells found in the blood and the lymphoid tissue; known to play a key role in mobilizing the body's defense mechanisms against disease.

M

Madopar The trade name for benserazide/LEVODOPA, now under clinical investigation for the treatment for PARKINSON'S DISEASE.

magnetic resonance imaging (MRI) A diagnostic system that uses radio waves rather than radiation to create images of the human anatomy and provide clear anatomical pictures. It produces images similar to X rays but without the hazard of radiation. As it allows researchers and clinicians to take three-dimensional pictures of the body and its organs, the pictures produced by it are unlike anything available from other devices that rely on either X rays or sound waves.

Because of MRI scans clinicians are able to examine parts of the body that X rays are unable to contact and are more readily able to identify crucial changes in brain activity and body biochemistry. Among other things, MRI is used to diagnose brain and nervous system disorders; bone, joint and muscle dis-

orders; tumors; heart and blood vessel problems; and several types of cancer. It also shows diagnostic potential for evaluating such neural diseases as Alzheimer's and Parkinson's disease. All of this can be done without subjecting patients to invasive procedures.

For an MRI scan a patient is placed inside a long cylindrical magnet with a magnetic field thousands of times stronger than the Earth's. Though the patient doesn't feel it, the magnetic force pulls the nuclei or atoms within the body into alignment. Then the MRI machine sends out a radio signal, forcing the displaced nuclei out of line. When the radio waves stop, the magnet draws them back into alignment. As the nuclei return to their original position, they emit a faint radio frequency signal, a phenomenon called nuclear magnetic resonance. The signals from these nuclei differ, and these differences are processed by a computer. An image is projected on a video monitor, showing not only soft tissue in the body, but also the biochemical processes within them. Like other imaging techniques, MRI scans show "slices" of the body.

Because MRI technology is considered non-invasive, it offers fewer risks than some diagnostic alternatives. In some instances, it may reduce the need for lengthy hospital stays, thereby holding down healthcare costs. The average cost for an MRI scan is approximately $700 to $800, though in some cases it can be higher.

University of Texas Health Science Center at San Antonio, "Images For Research," *The Mission,* 16:3(Summer 1989).

major depression A term that is used to indicate a clinical depression that meets specific diagnostic criteria as to duration, functional impairment and involvement of a cluster of both psychological and physiological systems. It is a term that overlaps with CLINICAL, UNIPOLAR or ENDOGENOUS DEPRESSION.

male postpartum depression Although this type of depression is usually associated with women who have recently given birth it is common for some husbands to go through it to some degree. Those who experience it may feel an unconscious or disguised jealousy at their new lifestyle of sharing their wife's love with the newcomer in the family. As they feel left out when a wife appears to be preoccupied with the care of a baby, they react temporarily by doing such things as making their own demands for her attention or complaining of headaches and other small ills. Male postpartum depression is not a long-lasting situation and often passes after a one or two week duration.

manic-depressive A person suffering from a psychotic form of depression that includes mania as well as depression. A manic-depressive illness (also called BIPOLAR DEPRESSION) is characterized by alternating cycles of mania and depression—or inappropriate highs and terrible lows. Though not nearly as prevalent as other forms of depressive disorders, millions of people experience this emotional roller coaster in which the mood switches are sometimes dramatic and rapid, but most often gradual.

When in the depressed cycle, people can have any or all of the symptoms of a depressive disorder (see COMMON SIGNS AND SYMPTOMS). Manic episodes typically are characterized by elation, poor judgment, embarrassing social behavior, overtalkativeness, increased sexual activity, hyperactivity and tremendous energy, decreased need for sleep, grandiose notions, a feeling of being capable of carrying out any undertaking and a tendency to overlook painful and harmful consequences. In extreme cases, manic-depressives may suffer from thought disorder and jump from one idea to another with no apparent connection, sometimes to the point of delusions and hallucinations.

On the average, manic attacks persist from one to three months, while the depression cycle lasts from two to four months. There is no timetable as to how often or when manic or depressive episodes will occur. In manic-depressive illness, there may be several episodes of mania and only one of depression, or just the opposite. Research suggests that the interval between episodes tends to shorten with each subsequent attack. (See also DRUG THERAPY; PSYCHOTHERAPY; TREATMENT OF DEPRESSION.)

marital distress Dr. Ian H. Gotlib of the Department of Psychology, University of Western Ontario, and his colleagues have done extensive research and studies on depression and marital distress. The results of their studies thus far clearly demonstrate that all is not well within the marital relationships of depressed persons. In this situation the depressed persons' interactions are characterized by poor communication, friction, tension, overt and covert hostility, and a tendency for positive verbal messages to be delivered with negative nonverbal effect. Moreover, disturbed marital relationships have been found not only to precede the onset of depressive episodes, but also to be associated with the course of the depression and, in some cases, to persist following symptomatic recovery.

"There is also evidence that depressed individuals interact more politely and positively with strangers than they do with their spouses, suggesting that their communication deficits may be particularly exacerbated when interacting with intimates," wrote Dr. Gotlib and Jill M. Hooley of Harvard University in "Depression and Marital Distress: Current Status and Future Directions." "Finally, there is evidence to suggest that while individual therapy may be effective in reducing levels of depressive symptomatology, it tends not to ameliorate difficulties in interpersonal functioning; therapies that include a focus on the marriages of depressed persons may be necessary to achieve both symptom relief and a reduction in the high level of marital discord.

"Although there is a consistent association between depression and marital distress," the researchers continued, "we have seen that the nature of the link is complex. Available data suggest that a number of causal pathways are likely to be operating, all of which deserve scrutiny in future investigations."

The researchers conclude that although a considerable amount of work has been done on the link between depression and marital functioning the study of marriage and depression is still in its infancy and much remains to be learned. They believe, however, that the study of the relationship between depression and marital distress holds great promise to contribute significantly to the understanding of the etiology and maintenance of depression and to the empirically based development of programs designed for the treatment and, ultimately, the prevention of this disorder.

Gotlib, Ian H. and Hooley, Jill M., "Depression and Marital Distress: Current Status and Future Directions," in S.W. Duck (ed.), *Handbook of Personal Relationships* (New York: John Wiley, 1988).

Marsilid See IPRONIAZID.

masked depression A condition in which depression is hidden behind a facade. Victims appear to be living normally (see COREY, RICHARD), but it is common for them to lack an awareness of what they are really going through. They are only in touch with the feelings, thoughts and ideas that they can experience without coming into contact with their depressive illness. While inner turmoil and turbulence suck away at them beneath their false exterior, they outwardly do what is expected of them in a superficial way. But inside they close off more and more of their selves to escape the depression. As part of their facade their faces are generally fixed and immobile and show little or no emotion.

According to Dr. Stanley Lesse, a New York neurologist and psychiatrist who has studied masked depression extensively, this form of depression appears to be increasing in frequency. It is also referred to as "depression sine depression," "depressive equivalents," "affective equivalents," "hidden depression" and "missed depression." Many patients considered as having "borderline syndrome" properly should be labeled "masked depression."

In a 17-year clinical study of 1,465 patients who had severe masked depression Dr. Lesse found that this syndrome is most commonly seen in middle-aged women and that masked depressions are most commonly hidden behind hypochondriacal complaints, psychosomatic disorders and phobias.

He also found that the psychologic aspects of this syndrome usually were not appreciated for a number of years, during which time the patients were exposed to an inordinate number of consultations and testings. Inappropriate medical and surgical treatments were frequent, and they usually resulted in significant iatrogenic overlays. By the time the masked depression syndrome was recognized the underlying depression was usually of severe proportions. Feelings of hopelessness were observed in most of the patients, and suicidal ideas were present in almost half of them.

Lesse, Stanley, "The Masked Depression Syndrome—Results of a Seventeen-Year Clinical Study," *American Journal of Psychotherapy*, 37:4(October 1983).

mastectomy The excision or amputation of the breast. Following a mastectomy the risks of depression are higher than is commonly realized. According to a study by Dr. Robert O. Pasnau of the University of California at Los Angeles Medical School, a quarter of the 63 women in the study reported suicidal thoughts within a year after the operation.

However, Dr. Pasnau pointed out that having reconstructive breast surgery significantly reduced the emotional distress in the women, and the sooner they had the reconstruction, the less distress they suffered. Dr. Pasnau noted that the greatest problem is a feeling of the loss of femininity. Women who had the reconstruction right away never had to mourn that loss.

medical insurance programs for depressive illness See HEALTH INSURANCE PROGRAMS.

melancholia A mental condition characterized by an overriding inability to experience pleasure, even in situations that are normally pleasurable. Melancholic individuals describe their depression (usually worse in the morning) as distinct from the sadness or grief they have felt before—even in connection with the death of a loved one. Along with their depressed mood and loss of pleasure, individuals with melancholia may also experience early awakening, loss of appetite and weight, inappropriate guilt feelings and marked changes in activity levels.

melatonin A hormone secreted by the PINEAL GLAND, a bean-sized part of the brain, for a fixed period every 24 hours during darkness. The period is set by a biological clock, which is light-sensitive. If there are eight hours of darkness, it can produce its quota. If there are only six it falls short.

The role of melatonin is not yet fully understood. Some research groups have tied SEASONAL AFFECTIVE DISORDER (SAD) to melatonin because of the way it is produced in the dark, particularly during winter when the days are shorter and darker.

In "A New Light on the Blues" Glennys Bell wrote: "Melatonin is still a mystery; its role in humans still being discovered, but it has great potential. It could join other brain hormones such as endorphins—the intriguing opiates of the mind—as the big headline makers of the 90s."

Along with being linked to mood disorders, such as SAD, Bell pointed out that melatonin may also be involved in other problems such as carbohydrate craving obesity (CCO) and premenstrual syndrome (PMS).
Bell, Glennys, "A New Light on the Blues," *The Bulletin*, July 25, 1989.

memory loss Although memory loss is associated with ELECTROCONVULSIVE THERAPY (ECT), it now appears that ECT produces less temporary confusion and memory loss than it did in its earlier days. Even under the best conditions, though, researchers who have studied ECT and memory loss say that many patients experience transient memory loss of events surrounding the treatment as well as immediate loss of memory for current and past events. However, the memory loss gradually recedes and after several months patients can remember new events—though some may be left with a gap covering a few weeks before, during and after their treatments and some may also have some spotty memory loss going back months before their treatment.

In discussing the many-faceted phenomenon of memory loss in both therapy and other situations, Robert O'Brien and Dr. Sidney Cohen wrote in *The Encyclopedia of Drug Abuse:*

Neither the mechanisms of memory itself, nor those of memory loss induced by drugs or other factors, are well understood at present, but both continue to be the subject of much scientific study. The memory process includes short-term and long-term storage and retrieval facilities which appear to be centered in the brain's limbic system. Electrical stimulation of this area has enabled some patients to recall long-forgotten events and other information.

Information storage seems related to such chemical structures as proteins and nucleic acids. Pituitary hormones may also contribute to the memory process. Information appears to be filed chronologically and by sense; that is, there is a separate memory "file" for vision, hearing, taste, and so on.

Symptoms of memory loss, regardless of the cause, include inability to concentrate, absent-mindedness, poor sequence retention and general temporal confusion.

O'Brien, Robert and Cohen, Sidney, *The Encyclopedia of Drug Abuse* (New York: Facts On File, 1984).

men See SEX FACTORS.

menopause At one time mental health experts believed that women who experienced depression during change of life were suffering a special kind of depressive disorder referred to as INVOLUTIONAL MELANCHOLIA. This diagnosis is no longer in use, but the belief that women who go through menopause are particularly vulnerable to depression is still common among the public.

However, research has shown that depressive disorders at menopause do not differ from those experienced at other ages and that women most likely to experience change-of-life depression typically have a history of past depressive episodes.

In the 1970s the idea that depression during menopause might be a myth was speculated upon by Dr. George Winokur at the University of Iowa and Dr. Myrna Weissman, then at Yale and now at Columbia College of Physicians and Surgeons. In the 1980s Dr. Robert O. Pasnau of the University of California at Los Angeles Medical School also referred to depression during menopause as a myth and pointed out that systematic studies have shown that women in this age group are no more likely to experience depression than are women of other ages (nor men, as a matter of fact). In still other research, a 1986 British study that found a rise in the rate of depression among women aged 45 to 49 compared with women of other ages also found that the rise in depression was strongest among women who had not yet reached menopause. (See also MID-LIFE.)

Meyer, Adolf A Swiss-born and trained American psychiatrist and professor of psychiatry (1866–1950) at Cornell University and Johns Hopkins University. He was a leading figure in American psychiatry between 1895 and 1940, and in 1904 he suggested that the term "melancholy" gave a stamp of certainty to a vague condition in which there was no positive evidence of disease. He also proposed using the term "depression" to differentiate between melancholy (or severe depression) and the more widespread form that nearly everyone experiences.

MHPG test (3-methoxy-4-hydroxyphenylglycol test) In a chapter in *Inpatient Psychiatry* Dr. A.L.C. Pottash et al. explain the MHPG test as follows:

Some clinicians have found measurement of pretreatment urinary 3-methoxy-4-hydroxyphenylglycol (MHPG) to be of assistance in the prediction of a response to specific antidepressant medications. MHPG is the major metabolite of brain norepinephrine. While there has been some disagreement about the use of urinary MHPG as a diagnostic test for depression and some discussion in the basic science community regarding the relative contribution of the brain and periphery to the MHPG measured, most, but not all, studies support the use of the MHPG test to predict response to medication.

Prior to collection of a 24-hour urine, the patient may be on a regular diet but preferably will have been off psychoactive drugs for at least 1 week. Creatinine clearance and total urinary volume are measured at the same time as MHPG to rule out incomplete collection. In patients who are candidates for treatment with antidepressants, low pretreatment MHPG levels have predicted favorable response to use of antidepressants such as imipramine and maprotiline.

Pottash, A. et al., "The Use of the Clinical Laboratory," ch. 9 in *Inpatient Psychiatry-Diagnosis and Treatment*, 2nd ed., Lloyd I. Sederer (ed.) (Baltimore/Los Angeles: Williams & Wilkins, 1986).

mid-life   Mid-life is a time when some people evaluate the past and succumb to disillusionment, despair and depression (see SEX FACTORS). In *Feeling Good* Dr. David D. Burns writes:

As you review the past you may conclude that your life hasn't really amounted to much in comparison with the starry-eyed expectations of your youth. This is a stage in which you review what you have actually done with your life compared with your hopes and plans. If you cannot resolve this crisis successfully you may experience disappointment and depression. You have not experienced the joy and fulfillment you expected. You have a sense of inadequacy and think of yourself as a failure. You feel you have accomplished nothing worthwhile and that your life is not worth living. You feel that what you have done isn't good enough.

While all of the foregoing is true in certain situations—and while depression can certainly be a factor during a mid-life crisis—a more positive and encouraging view is that today's generation of midlife people have the tools to be more mentally and physically fit than any previous generation *if* they examine and redefine their lives and, according to their personal choice, make the years ahead all those years can be.

In his book *The Seasons of a Man's Life* Yale Professor of Psychology Daniel Levinson said it well when he wrote:

Middle age is usually regarded as a vague interim period, defined primarily in negative terms. One is no longer young and yet not quite old—but what *is* one in a more positive sense? The connotations of youth are vitality, growth, mastery, the heroic; whereas old age connotes vulnerability, withering, ending, the brink of nothingness. Our overly negative imagery of old age adds greatly to the burden of middle age. It is terrifying to go through middle age in the shadow of death, as though one were already very old; and it is a self-defeating illusion to live it in the shadow of youth, as though one were still simply young. Each phase in the life cycle has its own virtue and limitations. To realize its potential value, we must know and accept its terms and create our lives within it accordingly.

Burns, David D., *Feeling Good: The New Mood Therapy* (New York: New American Library, 1980).

Levinson, Daniel J. et al., *The Seasons of a Man's Life* (New York: Alfred A. Knopf, 1978).

Midwest AIDS Biobehavioral Research Center (MABRC)   Located at the University of Michigan Institute for Social Research at Ann Arbor, this organization has the general goal of contributing to the improvement of psychiatric assessment procedures for the treatment of patients with HIV (human immunodeficiency virus) infection. Given documented indications of mild early cognitive manifestations of CENTRAL NERVOUS SYSTEM HIV infection, researchers have been particularly interested in examining relationships between affective illness and organic impairment.

To do this MABRC has explored relationships among self-reported measures of depression and anxiety, somatic symptoms and neuropsychological impairment.

Although MABRC states that the clinical implication of their findings are limited at this time, the findings do suggest that patient symptom self-reports can be used to differentiate among the several possible etiologies of affective and cognitive symptoms in HIV illness. Preliminary observations of response to antidepressant or psychostimulant treatment suggest that clinical improvement may be independent of the underlying etiology.

miscarriage Following a miscarriage (the spontaneous termination of pregnancy between conception and the 20th week of gestation) women can experience the same hormonal involvement that makes for POSTPARTUM DEPRESSION. Many women regard this loss as the death of their child, and the loss they experience can bring on months of depression, grief, soul-searching and agonized hunts for the causes. In an August 15, 1988, article in *Newsweek,* Ingrid Kohn, professional coordinator of the Pregnancy Loss Support Program in New York City, stated: "For a woman a miscarriage is not just the loss of a wanted baby, it's a loss of her self-esteem and an assault on her sense as a competent woman."

Husbands may also feel the loss greatly but they often aren't sure how to show it. Because they feel they must be strong for their wives they often have little room to grieve themselves. Moreover, family and friends may not comprehend the GRIEF and physical trauma a couple experiences. This, in turn, can compound the depression and despair the couple can feel.

Actually, miscarriage is one of the most common phenomena in medicine, and one of the most emotionally devastating. The size of the baby has nothing to do with the degree of grief either. A three-month miscarriage to one couple may be as difficult as a STILL-BORN to another couple.

No one knows for sure how often miscarriages occur. However, in one comprehensive study on pregnancy and reproduction led by Dr. Allen J. Wilcox of the National Institute of Environmental Health Sciences in Research Triangle Park, North Carolina the researchers found that 31% of all conceptions end in miscarriage, usually in the early months of pregnancy. Other estimates reported in the *Newsweek* article indicate that as many as one in every three pregnancies ends in failure. By rough estimates perhaps one out of every four women knows she has had at least one miscarriage. Roughly one in 300 has had three or more.

Scientists continue to probe for cause and effect. Prime suspected causes are a woman's age and chromosomal, hormonal or anatomical abnormalities. In addition there are many theories that attempt to account for other miscarriages, but there is still no reliable data. Most researchers and medical professionals believe that even after several miscarriages the odds are good that a woman will carry a future pregnancy to term. (See also NEWBORN DEATH; STILLBIRTH; Appendix 6.)

Amoroso, Mary, "When A Hope and a Dream Are Stillborn," *The* [Hackensack, N.J.] *Record,* July 21, 1987.

Anon., "A Special Kind of Grief," *University of California, Berkeley Wellness Letter,* August 1988.

Beck, Melinda et al., "Miscarriages," *Newsweek,* August 15, 1988.

Kolata, Gina, "Study Finds 31% Rate of Miscarriage," *The New York Times,* July 27, 1988.

monoamine oxidase (MAO) An enzyme that breaks down NEUROTRANSMITTER molecules into inactive substances. As it destroys BIOGENIC AMINES it stops the message that tells a brain cell to fire. Once the cell has been triggered it then receives a sufficient dose of monoamine oxidase to erase the triggering message.

monoamine oxidase (MAO) inhibitors The main type of MAO inhibitors are isocarboxazid (Marplan); phenelzine sulfate (Nardil); and tranylcypromine sulfate (Parnate). Some years ago they were the first ANTIDEPRESSANTS to receive widespread use for patients who were classified as victims of an atypical depression, characterized by phobias and high levels of anxiety, chronic anger, hypochondriacal complaints or impulsive self-destructive behavior. Later they fell into relative disuse when the newer and somewhat safer TRICYCLIC COMPOUNDS were developed. In recent years the MAO inhibitors have experienced a resurgence of popularity.

According to Dr. Ira Lipton who has continued Dr. Nathan Kline's Manhattan practice, the MAO inhibitors are increasing in clinical use today because some research has confirmed that certain groups of atypical patients respond better to the second-generation MAOs (those that followed MARSILID) than to other drugs.

"Up until the last few years doctors were still reticent about prescribing MAO's because of the original Marsilid problem and the side effects of dietary problems in which certain foods will produce a hypertensive nerve reaction and a serious blood pressure rise," stated Lipton. "For some patients MAO's still tend not to be the first line of treatment because there are people who— even though they have symptoms that are consistent with the atypical picture—respond to tricyclic drugs, so we're better off trying them. They're safer and there are less side effects."

Some of the research that has confirmed that certain groups of atypical patients respond better to MAOs than to other drugs was done by Dr. Frederic M. Quitkin of the New York State Psychiatric Institute and Columbia's College of Physicians and Surgeons. Dr. Quitkin and his group found the MAO inhibitors particularly useful for the above-mentioned atypical patients. Most depression patients lose weight and have trouble sleeping, but atypical patients eat more and sleep excessively and—while the illness is episodic in many people—these cases tend to be chronic. In the past patients of this type were classified as neurotic and not considered candidates for drug treatment. But in the Quitkin study of almost 200 such patients, the team found a MAO inhibitor significantly more effective than one of the standard tricyclics.

Other research has documented that MAO inhibitors are often remarkably effective for patients with recurrent obsessive thoughts and compulsive ritualistic habits, and for patients who do not respond to tricyclics, especially those who have experienced so many years of depression that the illness has become an unwelcome life-style.

Persons taking MAO inhibitors require careful medical management and close supervision and teamwork with a physician because these drugs are extremely potent, and adverse reactions are frequent and can be severe.

All patients should avoid certain drugs— tricyclic antidepressants, cold tablets, decongestants, hay fever medicine, asthma inhalers, allergy pills, stimulants such as amphetamines, anticonvulsants and narcotics— because when MAOs are used in combination with many other types of drugs such an intense additive effect can be produced that even death may result.

Individuals on MAOs should also refrain from eating certain foods because the combination of some foods with MAO inhibitors can trigger very high blood pressure, rapid pulse, headaches, vision problems and, sometimes, paralyzing or fatal strokes. Specific foods to avoid are chocolate, cheese, yogurt, pickled fish, soy sauce, pods of broad beans, canned figs, bananas, avocados, raisins, liver, yeast, meats prepared with tenderizer, sour cream, wine, beer, ale and alcohol. Caffeine should be used in moderation. MAOs require two to three weeks to become effective. (See also DRUG THERAPY.)

mononamines Complex chemicals produced by the central nervous system and crucially involved in the functioning of the brain, e.g., dopamine, norepinephrine, serotonin.

mourning Today more and more researchers are coming to a sharper understanding of mourning (a period in which people deal with the effects of LOSS). In fact, Dr. Mardi Horowitz, professor of psychiatry at the University of California in San Francisco, who has long been a leader in research on mourning, has found in his studies that the issue of mourning and GRIEF is a pressing one.

As research on the subject spawns a variety of findings, certain new studies now: (1) challenge some of the most common clinical beliefs about mourning: (2) say that some of the widespread beliefs are largely myth; and (3) conclude that the normal range of reactions to loss is far wider that once thought. Later in this entry we will discuss this research. But first we will examine the most common clinical findings and research.

Some of the most usual signs of mourning are: a flatness of feeling; an inability to work or to finish projects; a powerlessness in starting new relationships; and an incapacity to be caring or creative, or even to experience pleasant feelings. Generally such feelings fade as time passes, but when people have trouble mourning, those emotions can persist for months or years.

Researchers who have followed what has been thought to be the "normal" path of grieving say that signs that the mourning is ongoing and in a stage where the mourners might have become frozen can include recurring nightmares (or night terrors) so real that dreamers may wake up screaming. The bereaved may also continue to be plagued by anxiety, fear, depression, despair, rage, shame or guilt.

Even though the primary loss that causes mourning, depression and grief is a loss by the death of a loved one, there are other types of losses that bring about strong emotional reactions and periods of mourning. Specifically, these other losses can be separation (such as divorce or the end of a relationship); loss of a pet; disability from the loss of an arm, leg, eyesight, hearing or other bodily function; illness and accidents; alienation of friends and family; loss of a job, home, money and material things; and situational changes such as retirement, geographical uprootings and departure of children from home. Mourning can also result from disappointments, lost opportunities and the inability to live up to one's expectations—all of which can bring a loss of self-esteem, faith and hope and a feeling that individuals have lost status and reputation in other people's eyes.

In his studies on the type of mourning that involves death Horowitz has seen that the course of mourning can begin even before death. Most deaths come slowly through illness, allowing time for emotional preparation. At this point, though, some of those close to the dying person may be unable to acknowledge that death is near. These people can feel confused or inexplicably angry. In extreme cases, such people avoid the dying person, which can lead to intense remorse after the death. If the approach of death is acknowledged, however, it can present an opportunity to go over the events of life and reconcile any grievances. Even with the best preparation, however, news of the death generally comes as a shock.

After death and before the mourner has begun to grasp the loss, the emotional turmoil often revolves around a wish to do something to protect or please the dead person. This desire might be served by having the kind of funeral he would have wanted. It's common for mourners in this period to feel numb to all emotions. This is a necessary prelude in which they generally regain a sense of equilibrium that will allow them to confront the loss, observed Horowitz. He has found that at this phase some mourners make extreme efforts to put the death out of mind. Sometimes they abuse drugs or alcohol or throw themselves into a frenzy of work, athletics or sexual activity.

Ultimately mourners reach a point where they go through a mental review of their life with the deceased. Vivid memories begin to flow, and the feelings that memories arouse alternate between intrusive thoughts of the deceased or intense sadness that make it hard for the mourner to concentrate on anything else, or putting the death out of mind so that mourning proceeds in manageable doses. Horowitz said that many irrational thoughts come up during mourning, such as "If I'd been a better person they never would have died." Normally, people let go of these ideas, but some get stuck in them, especially if they felt a strong ambivalence or anger toward the dead person.

Once the mental review of life with the deceased is completed, persons involved in the normal course of mourning can experience an intense yearning for the company of the dead person. Ordinarily this signifies a last-ditch effort to deny the death, but gradually yields to an emotional acceptance of it. Dr. George Pollock, a psychiatrist and director of the Chicago Institute for Psychoanalysis, has found that a child's death is difficult to mourn and that for most parents whose child has died, mourning is never completed. Pollock believes it is much easier to mourn the death of a parent than a child, because to a child, the parent is the past, while to the parent the child is the future.

With the completion of mourning, people once again feel a sense of mastery of life and, though some grief persists, mourners decide that life can continue without the dead person. According to Horowitz, they're ready, for instance, to take on the risks of a new relationship.

Some researchers find that failure to mourn can result in the highly intense and out-of-control experience of pathological grief. As Horowitz puts it, this failure may be associated with a continuing impairment in work, creativity or intimacy that can go on distorting a person's character for years. Consequently, a person suffering from the resulting reactive depression may be unable to feel emotion and to experience some types of positive stages. There may be anxious, depressed, enraged, shame-filled or guilty moods, or psychopathological syndromes.

As an example, Horowitz cites the case of a patient whose mother had died when he was 13 and who had never mourned her. At age 27 the patient had problems involving phobic withdrawal from love and work and avoidance of developing career-related skills. Dur-

ing the course of psychoanalysis it gradually became apparent that he had never mourned his mother. In his paper "A Model of Mourning: Change in Schemas of Self and Others," Horowitz describes the case as follows:

During the first two years of treatment he remained indifferent to the analyst's vacations or work-related trips. Weekends apart meant nothing. Then he threatened to leave analysis on a variety of pretexts, citing the analyst's inadequacy. With each challenge, he observed the analyst's reactions carefully. Because the analyst did not appear anxious and did not act firmly to urge him to stay in treatment, he decided—unconsciously, I believe—that the analyst could tolerate his own fear of losing the patient. The patient identified with the analyst's ability to tolerate sadness and anxiety at impending separation and loss. For the first time he began to feel the analyst's departure on vacations as painful. He mourned each weekend as a loss. Earlier childhood fears of abandonment surfaced in conscious memories. Missing the analyst, and being pleased at reunions, then awakened more positive memories of his mother. Only then, gradually, did he begin to grieve. He entered an intrusive phase with sobbing, over vivid visual memories of his mother's funeral. He spent an extended period of working through these reactions.

Granted, the above example of pathological mourning is far removed from "normal" by either older or newer studies on what is (or isn't) normal. But findings from the latest studies—studies that reportedly have monitored the course of grief more closely than ever before—continue to indicate there is a far wider range of normal reactions to a grave loss than what some earlier research had supposed. The studies also find that mourning can take many forms.

Dr. Camille Wortman, a psychologist at the University of Michigan who has researched mourning extensively, emphasizes that the studies show we need to expand our notions of what is a normal reaction to loss. She points out that, primarily, the large body of clinical wisdom about grief is based on studies of people who have sought therapy for their problems. Until the last five years or so there have been few carefully designed studies that systematically tracked for several years the emotional course of ordinary people who have suffered a loss. To Dr. Wortman it is not inevitable that severe distress or depression must follow a loss. Nor is the absence of such a response necessarily pathological.

Other researchers also refute the notion that everyone who is mentally healthy will undergo a period of distress after experiencing a loss. A 1986 study of Mormons who had recently lost a spouse showed that only about one in five was seriously depressed in the months that followed. To counteract the fact that some people may regard such survivors as unfeeling and unloving, Dr. Wortman stressed that those survivors may be exhibiting a psychological strength and a resilience that permit them to handle their grief in a relatively unshaken manner. Even though they are going through a period of sorrow and separation they are able to go on with their lives without becoming deeply depressed.

At the same time, however, Dr. Wortman acknowledges that a failure to be severely distressed can be a result of emotional numbness or an unhealthy denial of the reality of the loss, both of which can lead to a painful situation later. Still, she believes her research indicates that if people are not greatly distressed at first after a loss they probably never will be, and many persons who are most upset immediately after a loss tend to be among the most upset a year or two later.

Because of today's new research Dr. Wortman also questions the widespread belief that people should recover from a loss within a certain time frame, after which they reach a final stage of acceptance. A great deal of research, past and present, has stated

that a failure to reach this stage is an indication of pathological mourning and a need for therapy. But Dr. Wortman does not agree that people who may benefit from therapy to help them deal with their depression and anxiety are experiencing abnormal or pathological grief, since the new research continues to show that the normal range of reactions to loss is far wider that once thought.

Still another belief that is being questioned in light of the new research is the view that ultimately people should discover some meaning in their loss in order to come to terms with and end their mourning. But in a 1983 HARVARD STUDY of widows and widowers and in a study by Dr. Wortman of parents whose infants died suddenly, about 40% of those who mourned were still asking why the loss had occurred for as long as four years later. More than half who had lost a loved one in an auto accident failed to find any meaning in it four to seven years later.

As studies on mourning continue researchers reemphasize that we are just beginning to realize the full range of normal grief. Studies also show that, apart from the differences between mourners, the kind of death can make a great deal of difference. Untimely or sudden deaths are generally harder to get over. (See also BEREAVEMENT; GRIEF, CAUSES AND EFFECTS OF; GRIEF THERAPY/ TREATMENT; LENGTH OF GRIEVING PROCESS.)

Horowitz, Mardi J., "A Model of Mourning: Change in Schemas of Self and Others," *The Journal of the Psychoanalytic Association*, 1988.

Goleman, Daniel, "New Studies Find Many Myths About Mourning," *The New York Times*, August 8, 1989.

———, "Study of Normal Mourning Process Illuminates Grief Gone Awry," *The New York Times*, March 28, 1988.

mourning, from death by suicide   Researchers report that some kinds of death are more difficult than others to mourn. Some of the research focuses on suicide, which experts say is one of the most difficult deaths to mourn. "In addition to suicide being a loss the survivor suffers, he also experiences it as an accusation of sorts—that his love was not good enough to keep the loved one alive, or that their relationship was not important enough to stay alive for, for instance," said Henry Seiden, a psychologist and coauthor of *Silent Grief: Living in the Wake of Suicide.*

The typical response of the survivors of a suicide is—out of shame—to be silent about the fact the death was a suicide, Dr. Seiden explains. That interferes with the normal course of mourning. The best thing is to talk about it, because when mourners are quiet about loss by suicide each feels he or she is alone. Survivors can thus be stuck in feelings of guilt, anger or shame for years. Seiden points out in his book that suicide survivors suffer and mourn in three ways: first, because they are grieving for a dead person; second, because they are suffering from a traumatic experience called post-traumatic stress disorder; and third, because they don't talk about it.

Depression, in the case of suicide survivors, is often long-lasting and deep, explains Seiden. "It paralyzes people," he wrote. "They lose weight or overeat; they can't form new relationships because their self-esteem is so low; if one person rejects them so will everyone else. Some can't get jobs, some are too depressed to ask for a raise."

Part of the relief from the depression (and from the confusion, anger and guilt) mourners feel lies in learning how to talk about the suicide—and that cannot be stressed or repeated enough. A mourning period that results in a return to a normal life and adjustment to the death is also essential.

As in other types of losses and subsequent mourning, failed or faulty mourning can result in the highly intense and out-of-control experience of pathological grief, and this failure may be associated with a continuing impairment in work, creativity or intimacy that can go on distorting a person's character for years. For people who stay in their grief and mourning some form of outside help is necessary.

Seiden, Henry and Lukas, Christopher, *Silent Grief: Living in the Wake of Suicide* (New York: Scribner, 1988).

mourning, from death of a child See MOURNING.

mourning therapy See GRIEF THERAPY/TREATMENT.

N

Nathan S. Kline Institute (NKI) The Nathan S. Kline Institute for Psychiatric Research, an agency of the New York State Office of Mental Health, is a multi-disciplinary organization dedicated to the study of the etiology, treatment and prevention of mental illness. Originally called the Research Center of Rockland State Hospital and, later, the Rockland Research Institute, the Nathan S. Kline Institute was renamed in 1983 for its noted founder who, as a leading force in modern psychiatry, was its director for 30 years. He contributed significantly to the use of psychoactive drugs for treating mental illness, which, in turn, revolutionized psychiatric medicine. This included important breakthroughs in treating affective disorders and depression.

NKI is located on the campus of the Rockland Psychiatric Center (RPC) in Orangeburg, New York about 20 miles from New York City. The two facilities collaborate closely in patient care. NKI's director, Robert Cancro, M.D., is the chairman of the department of psychiatry at NYU School of Medicine, and many NKI researchers are faculty members of NYU. The institute is also affiliated with the Albert Einstein College of Medicine. (See also KLINE, NATHAN S.)

National Alliance for Research on Schizophrenia and Depression (NARSAD) A Chicago-based organization that is privately funded to raise and distribute funds for scientific research into the causes, cures, treatments and prevention of severe mental illnesses, primarily the schizophrenias and the depressions.

Since its formation in 1986 it has become a significant factor in the scientific community. It complements rather than duplicates the federal funding efforts of the National Institute of Mental Health (NIMH). One of the purposes of its founding was to establish an award process that would identify the most promising research and enable investigators to receive the necessary funding to initiate research quickly. To achieve this, the organization assembled a group of distinguished psychiatric researchers who agreed to become its Scientific Council. The council's review committees solicit and evaluate research proposals and respond to grant requests. For information contact: National Alliance for Research on Schizophrenia and Depression, 208 S. LaSalle St., Suite 1438, Chicago, IL 60604. Phone: 312-641-1666.

National Center for Health Statistics A primary agency within the U.S. Department of Health and Human Services that is responsible for gathering and disseminating data and statistics on major health issues in the United States. As part of its functions it provides information to researchers and other professionals who are concerned with the delivery and quality of health services in the country. For information: 3700 East-West Highway, Room 1-57, Hyattsville, MD 20782. Phone: 301-436-8500.

National Depressive and Manic Depressive Association (NDMDA) A national association that recognizes the biochemical nature of bipolar and unipolar affective disorders and the disruptive psychological impact of the illnesses on patients and families. Its purpose is to provide personal

support and direct service to persons with major depression or manic-depression and their families; to educate the public concerning the nature and management of these disorders; and to promote related research. It is a rapidly growing organization with local chapters throughout the United States and Canada. For further information contact: NDMDA, Merchandise Mart, Box 3395, Chicago, IL 60654. Phone: 312-446-9009. (See also BIPOLAR DEPRESSION; UNIPOLAR DEPRESSION.)

National Foundation for Depressive Illness A group of professional and lay people whose goal is to advance private and public education in the area of depression and its treatment. The organization has an 800 number (1-800-248-4344), which gives a recorded message detailing the symptoms of depression and offering to send a list of local referrals and literature to persons who write for them. There is a charge to cover postage and handling. Address: National Foundation for Depressive Illness, Inc., P.O. Box 2257, New York, NY 10116. Phone: 212-620-7637. Donald F. Klein, M.D., is the current president.

National Institute of Alcohol Abuse and Alcoholism (NIAAA) A federal agency that predates the Alcohol, Drug Abuse and Mental Health Administration (ADAMHA). Organized in 1971 its function is to provide leadership, policies and goals for the government's work in the prevention, control and treatment of alcohol abuse and alcoholism and the rehabilitation of affected individuals. It also publishes periodic reports to the U.S. Congress on alcohol and health. Address: P.O. Box 2345, Rockville, MD 20852.

National Institute of Mental Health (NIMH) A U.S. government agency that supports and conducts research to improve the diagnosis, treatment and prevention of mental illness. NIMH-supported studies alleviate suffering and bring hope to people who have a mental disorder, to those who are at risk of developing one, and to their families, friends and coworkers. Thus, this agency's mental health research benefits millions of Americans and reduces the burden that mental disorders impose on society as a whole. NIMH is a part of the Alcohol, Drug Abuse and Mental Health Administration, a component of the U.S. Department of Health and Human Services.

One of its most important programs is D/ART (see DEPRESSION/AWARENESS, RECOGNITION, AND TREATMENT PROJECT), a national project to educate the public, primary care physicians and mental health specialists about the symptoms and treatments of depressive disorders. Through D/ART it has set in motion the development of written and audiovisual materials for the public; training programs for mental health specialists; clinical training grants for universities and medical schools to develop short-term educational programs for mental health specialists and primary care physicans; and media kits and training programs for community volunteers. The ultimate goal of this NIMH campaign is to alleviate suffering due to depressive disorders. Address for D/ART: Depression, 5600 Fishers Lane, Room 15C-05, Rockville, MD 20857. Phone: 301-443-4140.

National Institute of Mental Health Epidemiologic Catchment Area (ECA) Program   This program is a series of epidemiologic research studies performed by independent research teams in collaboration with the staff of the Division of Biometry and Epidemiology of the NATIONAL INSTITUTE OF MENTAL HEALTH (NIMH).

The program is a landmark in psychiatric epidemiology and psychiatric research in the United States. The basic goals of the program are to estimate rates of prevalence and incidence of specific mental disorders, to estimate rates of health and mental health services use, to study factors influencing the development and continuance of disorders and to study factors influencing use of services. Studies have been conducted in major sites within the United States. (See also EPIDEMIOLOGIC CATCHMENT AREA STUDY.)

Freedman, Daniel, "Psychiatric Epidemiology Counts," *Archives of General Psychiatry,* 41(October, 1984).

Regier, D.A. et al., "The NIMH Epidemiologic Catchment Area Program," *Archives of General Psychiatry,* 41(October 1984).

Eaton, W.W. et al., "The Design of the Epidemiologic Catchment Area Surveys," *Archives of General Psychiatry,* 41(October 1984).

National Institute of Mental Health Treatment of Depression Collaborative Research Program (TDCRP). The first multi-site coordinated study initiated by the National Institute of Mental Health (NIMH) in the field of psychotherapy research. This study investigated the effectiveness of specific forms of brief (16-week) psychotherapy for the treatment of non-bipolar, non-psychotic depressed outpatients.

The two forms of psychotherapy studied were INTERPERSONAL PSYCHOTHERAPY (IPT), as described by Gerald Klerman, Myrna Weissman and their colleagues in Boston and New Haven, and COGNITIVE BEHAVIOR THERAPY (CBT) (see COGNITIVE THERAPY), as described by Aaron T. Beck and his colleagues in Philadelphia. These therapies were compared with the antidepressant drug, imipramine. A pill-placebo control group was also included, and the two pharmacotherapy conditions, combined with a clinical management component, were administered double-blind.

The study was carried out at three institutions: the University of Pittsburgh, with Dr. Stanley Imber and Dr. Paul Pilkonis; George Washington University, with Dr. Stuart Sotsky and Dr. David Glass; and the University of Oklahoma, with Dr. John Watkins and Dr. William Leber. The study was coordinated by the NIMH, with Dr. Irene Elkin and Dr.

Tracie Shea as coordinator and associate co-ordinator.

Initial results indicated that both anti-depressant drug treatment and the specific psychotherapies can be helpful in reducing depressed symptoms. This does not mean, however, that both are equally effective for all patients. Work continues (in this study and others) to try to understand for which patient each of these treatments may be particularly beneficial. It is also likely that some patients may benefit most from a combination of antidepressant drugs and some form of therapy, although the TDCRP study did not address that issue.

Subjects of the study were outpatients with major UNIPOLAR DEPRESSION. The study excluded patients who were psychotically depressed as well as those with bipolar or manic depression. (See also BIPOLAR DEPRESSION; MANIC-DEPRESSIVE.)

National Institute on Drug Abuse Established in 1973 this agency is a constituent part of the Alcohol, Drug Abuse and Mental Health Administration (ADAMHA). Like NIAAA (see NATIONAL INSTITUTE OF ALCOHOL ABUSE AND ALCOHOLISM) its function is to provide leadership, policies and goals for the government's work in the prevention, control and treatment of narcotic addiction and drug abuse. It is also involved in the rehabilitation of affected individuals. Address: 5600 Fishers Lane, Rockville, MD 20857.

National Mental Health Association A nationwide, voluntary, non-governmental organization dedicated to the promotion of mental health, the prevention of mental illnesses, and the improved care and treatment of people with mental illnesses. Its 650 chapters and divisions and more than one million citizen volunteers work toward these goals through a wide range of activities in social action, education, advocacy and information. For information: National Mental Health Association, 1021 Prince St., Alexandria, VA 22314-2971. Phone: 703–684-7722.

National Self-Help Clearinghouse A clearinghouse founded in 1976 to facilitate access to self-help groups and increase the awareness of the importance of mutual support. It: (1) encourages and conducts training activities (including the training of professionals) about self-help and ways to work with mutual aid groups; (2) carries out research activities, including research about the effects of self help, the character of the self-help process, and relationships with the formal caregiving systems; (3) maintains a data bank and "switchboard" to provide information about and referral to self-help groups and regional self-help clearinghouses; and (4) addresses professional and public policy audiences about self-help group activities, links between self-help and professional providers, and self-help's relevance to public policy issues. It also publishes the following manuals and newsletters: *Self-Help Reporter*, published quarterly, $10; *How to Organize a Self-Help Group*, $6; *Organizing a Self-Help Clearinghouse*, $5; *New Dimensions in Self-Help*, $5. For information contact: National Self-Help Clearinghouse, Graduate School and University Center of the City University of New York, Room 620, 25 West 43rd St., New York, NY 10036. Phone: 212–642-2944. (See also SELF-HELP/SUPPORT ORGANIZATIONS.)

National Sudden Infant Death Syndrome (SIDS) Foundation An organization founded in 1962 to provide emotional support to grieving families of SIDS victims through local chapters. It supports research and educates the public through newsletters, a telephone support network and chapter development guidelines. Address: 8200 Professional Place, Suite 104, Landover, MD 20785. Phone: 800–221-SIDS.

Native Americans Extensive depression is a problem in the Native American community for the following reasons:

1.   The disruptions and dislocations of the established order of tribes and pueblos, combined with a steady disinte-

gration of both nuclear and extended families.

2. The change of traditional ways of earning a living and the ensuing high unemployment rate among adults on many reservations.

3. The poverty, hopelessness and loss of status and self-esteem caused by the first two reasons.

4. The differing values of Anglo and Indian societies and the sociocultural stress that follows.

5. Alcoholism and the much publicized fetal alcohol syndrome, which occurs when pregnant mothers drink.

6. The consequent high incidence of developmentally disabled infants and small children who will become adolescents and adults with psychological problems and behavior disorders.

Together these reasons contribute to serious depression and prompt ongoing research on both depression and suicide. According to Dr. Irving Berlin of the University of New Mexico, who has done considerable research on Native Americans, one aspect of research receiving great emphasis involves children who are victims of mothers too depressed to take care of them. When these children learn to distrust adults the result can be severe depression and withdrawal from others. Berlin points out that studies of third-grade children have indicated very depressed children can be identified in this age group.

The Bureau of Indian Affairs Boarding Schools (which are a part of the Indian education system) can contribute to children's depression, too. Many children are sent to these boarding schools because their parents are not available as caretakers when they reach school age. Large numbers of these children were brought up without opportunities to learn their tribe's traditions and values, and researchers have found out that many are withdrawn and depressed. Researchers also say that many boarding-school-educated adults have become what is described as the "lost generation," without strong tribal ties. And, because of interper-sonal problems, depression and alcoholism, these adults are unable to relate to either their parents or their children in traditionally supportive ways.

Berlin reports that among Indian adolescents suicide has increased about 200% in two decades and suicide attempts have increased about 500%. Most suicides are attributed to chronic depression related to early parental loss. Several different kinds of intervention for depression and its related problems are being tried. Among them are efforts that recognize depression in grade school as an indicator of later depression and possible suicide attempts.

As this work with depression continues, some of the intervention efforts have shown that as adolescents begin to work together on the practical learning of trades and art skills, their self-esteem increases, they appear less depressed, and they are able to work more easily with other people in a variety of tribal projects.

Berlin, Irving N., "Psychopathology and Its Antecedents among American Indian Adolescents," in Benjamin B. Lahey and Alan E. Kazdin (eds.), *Advances in Clinical Child Psychology*, vol. 9 (New York: Plenum, 1986).

———, "Effects of Changing Native American Cultures on Child Development," *Journal of Community Psychology*, 15(July 1987).

———, "Prevention of Adolescent Suicide Among Some Native American Tribes," *Adolescent Psychiatry*, 12(1985).

———, "Suicide among American Indian Adolescents: An Overview," *Suicide and Life Threatening Behavior*, 17(Fall 1987).

Nebuchadnezzar A Babylonian king (605–562 B.C.) who presided over a huge and powerful empire and who was known as an important monarch and great builder and doer. However, he was also known for his erratic moods, and the Book of Daniel in the Bible depicts him as a conceited and domineering king and tells of his going mad and eating grass. He suffered greatly from peaks of intense activity that were interspersed with what appears in retrospect to be extreme and deep depression.

Historically Nebuchadnezzar is familiar in Judeo-Christian lore as the man who cast Shadrach, Meshach and Abednego into the fiery furnace. But despite his problems with deviant moods and behavior he had a long and successful regime in which the Babylonian Empire reached its zenith.

neurohormones   See HORMONE.

neurotic depression   In "Neurotic Depression: a Diagnosis Based on Preexisting Characteristics" Dr. George Winokur of the University of Iowa College of Medicine and his colleagues wrote:

An ordinary dictionary definition of a neurotic is an emotionally unstable individual. A definition of neurotic-reactive depression would include those patients who suffer from a depression in the context of chronic gross personality problems and a history of a stormy lifestyle, with or without the presence of precipitating factors. The terms neurotic depression and reactive depression have often been used synonymously, but the fact is that depressions reactive to life stresses may be entirely different from those depressions that occur in the context of an unstable personality and a stormy lifestyle. A person suffering from a neurotic depression may have little in common with a person who suffers a depression as a reaction to a life stress.

In general, in a depression that is referred to as neurotic—with its accompanying personality problems—people feel self-pity, impatience, anxiety, fear and anger at the world. They regard themselves as victims of their own suffering.

In depressions caused by severe or prolonged stress and a failure to adapt to life stresses, unresolved conflicts and a feeling of great inadequacy in personal striving take over.

The onset of neurotic/reactive depressions (which can fluctuate from mild to severe) can be gradual and build up slowly over several weeks. The duration varies and throughout the depression the victim's mood is unpredictable.

Winokur, George et al., "Neurotic Depression: A Diagnosis Based on Preexisting Characteristics," *European Archives of Psychiatry and Neurological Sciences,* 236(1987), 343–348.

neurotransmitters   Chemicals produced by the CENTRAL NERVOUS SYSTEM that transmit electrochemical signals from one nerve cell in the brain to another. As "messengers" they set in motion an endless number of functions, including the regulation of pain, learning, thoughts, memory and the desire to eat, drink and sleep. They also affect moods, feelings and behavior. Approximately 40 neurotransmitters have been identified, but according to Dr. Candice Pert, National Institute of Mental Health (NIMH) and a codiscoverer of the endorphin neurotransmitters, there could be 100 to 200 different kinds.

Although many neurochemicals can play roles in depression, three neurotransmitters—DOPAMINE, SEROTONIN and NOREPINEPHRINE—have been implicated as culprits in depressive illnesses. Research suggests that a depletion or abundance, or problems in regulating them as they journey through the brain, may account for and be related to the symptoms and episodes of depression and mania.

new age of melancholy   A phrase used to describe the prevalence of depression at the end of the 20th century. Some people believe that current high rates of depression are simply a reflection of a society that is increasingly "psychologically minded." But when we look back at history—with or without statistics—men and women from the beginning of time have experienced bouts of depression in varying degrees.

In *From Sad To Glad*, Dr. NATHAN S. KLINE wrote:

When we turn to the past we find this illness running like a dark thread through the whole fabric of man's recorded experience. A brief historical scan of depression is instructive for more than mere academic reasons. It clearly demonstrates that this is a natural illness, something inherent in the human condition and not just a by-product of the anxieties created by modern times. A view of the past is useful also in providing some perspective on how man has tried to explain and cope with this common problem through the ages.

In reviewing the history of depression social historians note that there have been particular times when the incidence appeared to rise to epidemic proportions. In turn, they theorize that periods of great social change are times when individual depressions flourish. For instance, the last half of the 16th century, the Elizabethan Age (1558–1603), was known as the great age of melancholy (see ELIZABETHAN ENGLAND).

Everyone seems to have a rationale for our new age of melancholy. The most common reasons include societal issues and social changes; decline in moral values; erosion of the family; unhealthy and unnatural contemporary life styles; drug and alcohol abuse; economic factors; overpopulation; and the fear of nuclear war. Some researchers also blame the rise of individualism, the emphasis on self, the baby boom, elevated self-expectations and even the cult of female thinness.

In "Why Is There So Much Depression Today?" given as part of the G. Stanley Hall Lecture Series in Washington, D.C. in 1988, Dr. Martin E.P. Seligman, a psychologist at the University of Pennsylvania, said: "Something has happened, roughly since World War II, in America so that depression is about ten times as common as it used to be. Large scale studies show that the lifetime prevalence of depression in young people now exceeds by roughly a factor of ten the

prevalence in young people fifty years ago. There seems to be something about modern life that creates fertile soil for depression." (See also AGE OF DEPRESSION.)

Kline, Nathan S., *From Sad to Glad* (New York: Putnam, 1974).

Seligman, M.E.P., "Why Is There So Much Depression Today?" G. Stanley Hall Lecture Series (Washington, D.C. 1988).

newborn death   In the past, when newborn death and infant mortality were much more frequent than they are today, babies sometimes were not even named at birth. Before investing them with the badge of personhood people waited to see whether they survived. If they didn't, no formal period of mourning nor established customs or conventions, such as funerals, allowed the parents an outlet for their GRIEF.

Today, however, medical professionals and psychologists believe that the grief that follows a newborn's death must be acknowledged if a person is to recover from the magnitude of a loss for which they are unprepared—and a loss that often brings with it slights from well-intentioned but tongue-tied family members and friends who avoid the bereaved parents completely or act as though nothing happened. This silent refusal of others to discuss the loss (or their cheerful determination not to mention it) can intensify the parents' grief rather than relieve it, since it's reasonable to want to discuss this special kind of grief and ask loved ones for support.

Sometimes the grieving process can take a year or two as people go through the normal psychological passages of BEREAVEMENT. During this period every parent grieves in his or her own way and in his or her own time. Often a husband and wife may grieve at different intervals and go through different stages of grieving at different times. It helps to have a sympathetic physician who'll encourage parents to talk to him and to each other.

Medical professionals also suggest that parents be encouraged to hold and photograph their lifeless infant, name the child and plan its funeral arrangements. In addition, they say parents should get mementos of the child—a photo, footprints, the receiving blanket or a lock of hair. According to studies published in the *Medical Journal of Australia* and reported in the *University of California, Berkley Wellness Letter*, this physical contact can be beneficial and lead to a better resolution of grief. (See also STILLBIRTH, Appendix 6.)

Amoroso, Mary, "When A Hope and a Dream Are Stillborn," *The* [Hackensack, N.J.] *Record*, July 21, 1987.

Anon., "A Special Kind of Grief," *University of California, Berkley Wellness Letter*, August 1988.

Beck, Melinda et al., "Miscarriages," *Newsweek*, August 15, 1988.

Kolata, Gina, "Study Finds 31% Rate of Miscarriage," *The New York Times*, July 27, 1988.

New Jersey Self-Help Clearinghouse
The *first* statewide and computerized operation of its type in the nation, this clearinghouse—a project of St. Clares-Riverside Medical Center in Denville—provides information and referral, free consultation, and training services for persons interested in finding or forming self-help groups throughout New Jersey. It maintains and continually updates a data base of information on over 3,500 group meetings within the state, over 500 national headquarters and demonstration models, and over 200 helplines/hotlines. An important component of this organization's work is the development of new groups as needs arise. For example, if a caller inquires about a support group for manic depression and the computer search yields nothing in the caller's area, the Clearinghouse would invite the person to start a group, offering technical assistance, linkage with other existing groups and resource organizations and a free listing in its computer. In that way, future callers could be referred to that individual as a contact person interested in starting such a group.

The Clearinghouse publishes *Helping Ourselves-Helping Others: A Guide to Starting Mutual Aid Self-Help Groups for Depression and Manic Depression* ($9, postpaid) and *The Self-Help Sourcebook: Finding and Forming Mutual Aid Self-Help Groups*. The latter is a 138-page national guide ($8, book-rate postage or $9, first class postage). For information write: Self-Help Clearinghouse, St. Clares-Riverside Medical Center, Pocono Road, Denville, NJ 07834. The Clearinghouse welcomes phone requests for information and referral on Mondays through Fridays, 9:00 A.M. to 5:00 P.M. At other times it utilizes an answering machine to take calls, which it returns on the next work day. In New Jersey phone: 1-800-367-6274; outside of New Jersey: 201-625-9565. (See also SELF-HELP/SUPPORT ORGANIZATIONS.)

nihilism   A pessimistic doctrine that believes traditional values and beliefs are unfounded; that there is no truth or meaning to anything; that existence is senseless and useless; that all of life involves suffering and agony. Nihilists believe the world and the people and objects within it offer only evil and distress.

In his book *Up From Depression* Dr. Leonard Cammer stated that nihilism may be partial or total in a depressed person's denial of existence. "He or she believes that everything is dead and gone," he wrote. "It's useless and dried up." According to Cammer, the depressed individual will see you and talk with you but will contend that neither you nor he is there and that the surroundings are not there either. To him, everything is vapor and shadows, a complete nullity. Such delusions rarely contain mental pain, and suicidal thoughts are usually absent. But the conviction of nothingness breeds an inability to function in terms of reality and logic.

Cammer, Leonard, *Up From Depression* (New York: Pocket Books, 1969).

nomifensine (Merital)   A drug that acts on the neurotransmitter, dopamine. Because it had serious side effects (see DRUG THER-

APY, SIDE EFFECTS), it was taken off the market in 1986.

norepinephrine   One of the chemical compounds (a biogenic amine) identified as a NEUROTRANSMITTER, which, as a key chemical required by certain nerve cells in the brain, transmits electrochemical signals or impulses from one brain cell to another. As a neurotransmitter, an amine activates the "on" switches in the nerve cells of the brain.

Norepinephrine is released by nerve cells when a person takes amphetamines and gets "high." Under normal conditions, it is involved in the maintenance of arousal, alertness and euphoria. For some time it has been implicated as a culprit in depressive illnesses, since research has suggested that a depletion, abundance or problems in regulating transmitters as they journey through the brain may account for and be related to the symptoms and episodes of depression and mania. About 20 years ago researchers hypothesized that too little of the transmitted norepinephrine caused depression, and too much caused mania. More recent research, however, has shown that depression often involves disturbances in several transmitters, not just a simple high or low level in one.

Researchers believe that norepinephrine has a many-faceted role in depression. Both unipolar and bipolar research subjects react with a similar exaggerated release of it when clinically stressed, even though the "resting" levels of the transmitter are quite different in the two groups. Moreover, all the antidepressants eventually affect the norepinephrine system, even those designed to affect SEROTONIN. In discussing norepinephrine's role in depression, Dr. William Potter, chief of clinical pharmacology at the National Institute of Mental Health (NIMH), stated: "Norepinephrine is a device for focusing in on stimuli from the environment. The depressed person suffers from characteristic distortions—for example, seeing criticism where there is none—because he is unable to take in and process information correctly."

(See also BIPOLAR DEPRESSION; UNIPOLAR DEPRESSION.)

normal depression   In its normal state the occasional depression that afflicts everyone during difficult times is usually transient and a temporary reaction to life's circumstances. It is not as severe or lasting as clinical depression, nor is it manifested by dramatic behavioral change. Although it is often combined with feelings of anger, conflict, disappointment, discouragement and sadness, most people continue to function until it passes and they emerge from it by themselves without requiring treatment.

normal grief   See GRIEF.

nutrition   See DIET.

O

obsessive-compulsive disorder   In obsessive-compulsive disorders some people suffer from obsessions (recurrent, intrusive thoughts). Others are overwhelmed by compulsions (actions they feel they must perform). And in some cases persons experience a combination of the two.

A study on obsessive-compulsive disorder published in the December 1988 issue of the *Archives of General Psychiatry* estimated that from 1.9% to 3.3% of Americans will have this disorder during their lives. The estimate comes from part of a national survey of 18,572 men and women conducted door-to-door in New Haven, Baltimore, St. Louis, the Piedmont region of North Carolina, and Los Angeles.

Previous estimates have put the prevalence of obsessive-compulsive disorder at about one person in every 2,000. But researchers now say the disorder has been vastly underreported. In actuality it may afflict one in 40 Americans at some point in their lives.

Some of the characteristics victims exhibit, in varying degrees, are

- fluffing up pillows on sofas as soon as people get up, so the pillows are always just so;
- emptying ash trays the minute someone puts out a cirgarette;
- being unable to sleep unless shoes are lined up evenly;
- feeling they need to buy an even dozen of any item;
- returning to their parked cars several times to be sure the emergency brake is on;
- checking and rechecking whether every door is locked and every appliance is turned off before they leave their homes;
- washing their hands excessively;
- fearing they may harm someone they love.

Although obsessive-compulsive disorder has long been regarded by psychotherapists as one of the most difficult problems to treat, new techniques using medication or behavior therapy have proven highly effective in recent years. The most promising new drug treatments for obsessive-compulsive disorder are three drugs developed as antidepressants: clomipramine, fluoxetine and fluvoxamine. (See also NEUROTIC DEPRESSION.)

Cammer, Leonard, *Up From Depression* (New York: Pocket Books, 1969).

Goleman, Daniel, "Obsessive Disorder: Secret Toll Is Found," *The New York Times,* December 13, 1988.

Old Order Amish study A study that focused on the genetic aspects of bipolar (see BIPOLAR DEPRESSION), or MANIC-DEPRESSIVE, disorder among the Old Order Amish community, a group of over 12,000 people living in relative isolation in Lancaster, Pennsylvania. When a report on the study was published in 1987 a close comparison of the affected and the well family members revealed a genetic marker, which was mapped to the tip of the short arm of chromosome 11. At the time the research indicated that at least some cases of manic depression are caused by a dominant gene on the tip of the short arm of chromosome 11, and the researchers believed that there was a genetic transmission of the illness within families and that the research marked the initial proof of a link to a specific region of a chromosome. (The chromosomes in our body cells carry the blueprint of our inheritance as well as our physical and behavioral traits.) The study was the first evidence for a gene linked to a predisposition to manic-depressive illness.

Scientists working on this project used the most modern techniques of molecular biology to determine the chromosomal location of the gene that appeared to convey a strong risk of developing the illness. However, in "Manic-Depression Gene Tied to Chromosome 11" in *Science*, Gina Kolata pointed out that since a large percentage of persons with the gene never get the disease it does not necessarily follow that there is a genetic transmission of the illness within families.

Although the Old Order Amish study was hailed as a significant advance in understanding an important illness and as a step toward better diagnosis and treatment, by late 1989 new evidence from a National Institute of Mental Health (NIMH) study cast serious doubt on the faulty gene's role in manic-depressive illness and said the new data drastically reduced the probability that such a gene was at the location suspected.

"It means we are sort of back to square one," said Dr. Kenneth K. Kidd of Yale University, a contributor to both the original and later studies. Kidd pointed out that the new evidence does not mean that the original was in error. But what was once considered powerful evidence has now diminished to merely suggestive.

Much of the earlier evidence was reported by Dr. Janice A. Egeland, a professor of psychiatry at the University of Miami School of Medicine, who for more than a dozen years has documented genetic research into manic-depressive illness among this Old Order Amish population. As a graduate student at Johns Hopkins University pursuing genetic studies and completing her dissertation, Egeland established a working relationship with the Old Order Amish community and has continued to work with this group for more than two decades.

There are several reasons for studying the Amish. First, this is a closed population with a limited gene pool. Second, the Amish have large extended families with many relatives, both well and affected, for comparison of possible genetic markers linked to the illness. Third, finding cases and diagnosing manic-depression was easier in a culture where there are clearly defined behaviors and where there was an absence of alcohol, drug abuse and aggressive behaviors, which can mask the illness. The large extended families, with clear cases of manic depression, provided a natural resource for study, which could not be found in an academic or hospital setting. In fact, when a member of the Old Amish community is deeply depressed the Amish explain the behavior by saying "Siss im blut" (it is in the blood).

An additional advantage of studying manic depression in the Amish is that they tend to keep good genealogical records and few Amish enter or leave the community. The entire population is descended from 50 or fewer couples who emigrated from Germany between 1720 and 1750.

In the Old Order Amish study, Egeland, along with other researchers from the University of Miami School of Medicine, Massachusetts Institute of Technology and Yale University School of Medicine, found the previously-mentioned genetic marker—a piece of DNA so near the manic-depression gene that it is inherited along with the disease-causing gene. Although the group of researchers did not yet know what the manic-depression gene is, they were intrigued by the fact that at least one gene in this region of chromosome 11 might be involved in the

synthesis of the NEUROTRANSMITTER DOPAMINE. Dopamine is thought to be involved in the genesis of manic depression.

Since the Old Order Amish study reports were published in 1987 other groups have begun looking for the chromosome 11 linkage in families in whom manic depression appears to be inherited through a dominant gene. One study focused on non-Amish North American Caucasians and another on Icelandic families. Those research groups have reported no linkage to genes at the tip of chromosome 11, which means, say the researchers, that more than one gene may cause manic depression. Dr. Egeland agrees that other genes are expected to be important for manic-depressive illness and that it is also expected that more than one gene will be identified for the disorder.

In the Amish study later evidence on the suspected faulty gene suggested that it might lie near the gene for the enzyme tyrosine hydroxylase. That enzyme is vital to the brain's production of catecholamines, messenger chemicals that transmit signals from brain cell to brain cell.

Dr. John R. Kelsoe (formerly at NIMH and now at the University of California at San Diego) and Dr. Edward I. Ginns of NIMH cloned the gene for the enzyme tyrosine hydroxylase. They initially thought a faulty version of the gene might be a factor in the depression. But new research by Dr. Ginns and Dr. Karen O'Malley of Washington University in St. Louis showed that the gene in the enzyme could not be involved because its location is quite distant from the suspected gene. That work led the scientists to an exhaustive re-analysis of the original data and to new information coming out of the continuing study of Amish families.

"It was a very sobering realization," said Dr. Egeland, although she added that she still believes the Amish population is a valuable resource for studying the disorder.

As work continues to determine whether more than one gene plays a role or whether there is a single faulty gene at a different location, the significance of the Amish find-ings is that it opened up new research areas. Scientists hope these findings will ultimately prove valuable in diagnosing the condition and predicting who may develop it. They also stress that in spite of setbacks they are confident in their objectives and in the power of their techniques for probing gene chemis-try.

National Depressive and Manic Depressive Association, *Q & A: The Amish Study Findings* (Chicago: National Depressive and Manic Depressive Association, March 1987).

Kolata, Gina, "Manic-Depression Gene Tied to Chromosome 11," *Science*, March 6, 1987.

Egeland, J.A. et al., "Bipolar Affective Dis-orders Linked to DNA Markers on Chro-mosome 11," *Nature*, 325(February 1987).

Schmeck, Harold M., Jr., "Scientists Now Doubt They Found Faulty Gene Linked to Mental Illness," *The New York Times*, November 7, 1989.

organic brain symptom   See ELDERLY.

over-the-counter medications (OTC) OTC drugs are those that can be purchased without a prescription. Some are subject to abuse, particularly those that contain seda-tive or stimulant ingredients. Among the most abused are sleeping aids and appetite depressants.

Persons experiencing even a mild form of depression should not medicate themselves with these drugs. Consistent use of depres-sants that affect the CENTRAL NERVOUS SYSTEM can result in a real psychological depression, and an overdose of depressants can affect areas of the cerebral cortex and stop the respiratory system.

Sleeping aids can be easily abused be-cause, after only a few days of regular use, they begin to lose their effectiveness and increased doses may be required to induce sleep. When this happens depressives can develop a dangerous pattern of dependency and addiction. As they feel the need to use sleeping aids more and more, they find it increasingly difficult to stop using them. Thus the sleeping problem becomes worse, and depressives are apt to conclude there is no way they can give up the pills. The National Institute of Mental Health (NIMH) advises that sleeping pills should not be taken alone for depression.

P

Pakistan   An Asian country formed from parts of the former British India. Many peo-ple within the country (even if severely de-pressed) deny a diagnosis of depression and substitute instead such somatic symptoms as "I cannot sleep because of a headache" or "I cannot go to work because of a weakness" (the latter to save themselves from the humil-iation of being labeled "lazy" or "good for nothing").

"Depression is an elicited symptom rather than an offered complaint," explained Dr. S. Haroon Ahmed, professor and head of the Department of Neuropsychiatry at the Jinnah Post Graduate Medical Centre in Karachi. "It may be because we do not have a popular word for depression in Urdu. Secondly, in our culture physical illness attracts more at-tention than psychological, hence depression transforms into somatic experiences and ex-pression."

Since the pattern of depressive symptoms differs from culture to culture and depends upon the socioeconomic status, Dr. Ahmed who has done considerable research on cul-ture and symptomatology in depression con-ducted a study to record the socioeconomic variables and symptoms of 100 depressed patients from the outpatient Department of Neuropsychiatry at Jinnah Postgraduate Medical Centre. The hundred cases were se-lected from a total of 6,152 patients attending the center, of whom 1,801 had a hospital diagnosis of depression where anxiety, obsession and schizophrenia were also included.

The results of the study showed that depression was more common among females than males and more common in married people than in single persons. The mean age of the 100 patients was 39.5 years. More than half of the depressives had migrated from India and belonged to a lower socioeconomic group with an average income of less than one thousand rupees per month. Also, more than half were illiterate and living in housing that was shared by two or more families.

The somatic symptoms offered were giddiness, palpitation, headache, general weakness, frequent and/or burning urination, and gastrointestinal problems. Biological symptoms were anorexia, sleep disturbance, menstrual disorders and impotence. Psychic anxiety, suicidal tendency, phobia and psychomotor retardation were major psychological symptoms. Obsession and delusion were minimal.

The summary of these results indicates that in this study depressions in Pakistan were presented principally as depressed mood, somatic symptoms, anxiety, motor retardation and suicidal ideas. Guilt feeling was expressed by only a few of the subjects.

Ahmed, S. Haroon and Arif, M., "Culture and Symptomatology in Depression," *Pakistan Journal of Medical Research*, 21(April-June 1982).

Ahmed, S. Haroon, "Treatment Response and the Clinical Continuum of Illness," in *Mental Disorders, Alcohol-and-Drug-Related Problems* (Amsterdam: Excerpta Medica, 1985).

Pan American Health Organization (PAHO)

The world's oldest international health agency. Since its founding in 1902, it has served the countries of the Western Hemisphere in seeking to prevent and control disease and to promote health. PAHO is also the coordinating agency for health of the Inter-American system and the regional office for the Americas of the World Health Organization (WHO) and thus a part of the U.N. family. Its headquarters are in Washington, D.C. where its regional experts cover the spectrum of issues affecting health in the Americas.

panic attacks   The DIAGNOSTIC AND STATISTICAL MANUAL OF MENTAL DISORDERS (DSM-III-R) defines panic attacks as periods of intense fear or discomfort, with at least four of the following symptoms: (1) shortness of breath or smothering sensations; (2) dizziness, unsteady feelings or faintness; (3) palpitations or accelerated heart rate; (4) trembling or shaking; (5) sweating; (6) choking; (7) nausea or abdominal distress; (8) depersonalization or derealization; (9) numbness or tingling sensations; (10) flushes or chills; (11) chest pain or discomfort; (12) fear of dying; (13) fear of going crazy or of doing something uncontrolled.

One study of depressed women with panic attacks, conducted by Dr. Charles VanValkenburg of the University of Minnesota Hospital and his colleagues, involved a group of 288 depressed female inpatients, admitted to the University of Iowa Psychiatric Hospital. Forty-three of the women (15%) had secondary panic attacks. Compared to other depressives, the subgroup with panic attacks had significantly higher frequencies of anorexia, weight loss, gastrointestinal disturbances, hypochondriasis and psychomotor agitation and significantly lower frequencies of melancholic symptoms, including loss of interest in usual activities, guilt feelings, delusional thinking, psychomotor retardation and orientation or memory impairment. Patients with panic attacks were less likely to have a depressed parent and were more likely to be described as having been nervous, worrisome, sensitive and sexually dysfunctional before the onset of depression.

According to the DSM-III-R description, panic attacks usually last minutes or, more rarely, hours. The attacks, at least initially, are unexpected and are not triggered by situations in which the person is the focus of others' attention. The "unexpected" aspect of the panic attacks is the essential feature of the disorder, although later in the course of the disturbance certain situations (e.g., driving a car or being in a crowded place) may become associated with having a panic attack. Panic attacks typically begin with the sudden onset of intense apprehension, fear or terror. Often there is a feeling of impending doom. In the great majority of cases of panic attack seen in clinical settings, the person has developed some symptoms of agoraphobia—the fear of being in places or situations from which escape might be difficult or in which help might not be available in the event of a panic attack. (See also ANXIETY.)

VanValkenburg, Charles et al., "Depressed Women: With Panic Attacks," *Journal of Clinical Psychiatry*, 45:9(September 1984).

paranoia A term used loosely in ancient Greece in the sense that a 20th-century person might use "crazy" or "out of his mind." It emerged as a medical term in the 18th century, being used by R.A. Vogel in 1772 as a general term equivalent to madness. The term was used in 1863 by KARL L. KAHLBAUM (1828–1899), a German psychiatrist, to designate various persecutory and grandiose states. As a chronic functional psychosis of insidious development, paranoia is characterized by persistent delusions of persecution and grandeur, usually without hallucinations.

In the persecution state there is an excessive or irrational suspiciousness and distrustfulness of others, and the paranoiac may wish to do violence to the imaginary persecutor. Persons affected by paranoia cannot be convinced that someone—or some thing—is not out to harm them. As a result of their twisted and distorted thinking they may refuse medication because they believe it is poison and that people giving it to them want to kill them. They may also refuse to eat because of a similar fear.

In the grandiose state people may see themselves as exalted persons with a mission of great importance to accomplish. Paranoid states can occur with the use of amphetamines.

paresthesia A numbness or tingling sensation.

Parkinson's disease (PD) A chronic, slowly progressive neurological disorder that affects the part of the brain that controls voluntary movement. The onset is gradual, usually beginning as a slight tremor in the hands, when at rest, and an involuntary nodding of the head. As the disease advances tremor, stiffness and slowness are characteristic features. Speech may be slow. Movement may be difficult to initiate. Late in the course of the disease some patients may develop DEMENTIA.

In patients with PD, depression is the most common mental disturbance, according to Dr. Richard Mayeux of the Departments of Neurology, Psychiatry and Rehabilitation Medicine, College of Physicians and Surgeons, Columbia University, and one of the world's leading authorities on depression in Parkinson's. As a result of studies they have conducted he and his colleagues hypothesize that depression in PD is associated with a reduction in brain serotonin. Other researchers disagree and consider depression to be related to the degree of disability and the severity of illness in PD because its prevalence is similar to that in patients with chronic illnesses, such as arthritis.

In *The Relationship of Serotonin to Depression in Parkinson's Disease* Dr. Mayeux wrote: "We have observed a relationship between depression and reduced cerebrospinal fluid (CSF) levels of the metabolite of serotonin, 5-hydroxyindoleacetic acid (5-HIAA), during a dopamine agonist withdrawal period. While this does not imply that depression is endogenous, it suggests that depression in patients with PD may be related to alterations in biogenic amines. A relationship between depression and serotonin has also been found in some depressed patients without PD. This relationship between depression and reduced CSF 5-HIAA in PD suggests that reduced serotonin in the brain may be related to the cause of depression."

To clarify their initial studies and their hypothesis that depression in PD is associated with a reduction in brain serotonin, Dr. Mayeux and his colleagues conducted further studies based upon previous work. Of the 41 new subjects, there were 27 men and 14 women. Their mean age was 66.3 years (range 48 to 83 years), mean years of education was 14.2 (range 5 to 19 years) and mean duration of illness was 7.6 years (range 2 to 30 years). Seven met criteria for major depression, 15 met criteria for primary degenerative dementia, and three met criteria for both. The remaining 16 patients were free of dementia or depression. This further work on the relationship of serotonin to depression in Parkinson's disease added additional evidence to the researchers' hypothesis that depression in patients with PD is related to a reduction in brain serotonin. The relationship may be present in demented patients with PD who are also depressed.

In summing up the studies Dr. Mayeux wrote: "While interesting, this observation needs to be confirmed by others. Our study does not distinguish between a reactive or primary depression in PD. Nevertheless, there is clearly a biochemical correlate that may allow for the development of a rational treatment for this behavioral problem."

There is some indication that individuals with Parkinson's Disease lack the substance DOPAMINE, which is involved in control of muscle activity by the nervous sytem. Because of this association some Parkinson's patients are given a substance that is converted into dopamine in the brain (see LEVO-DOPA). This drug can relieve the symptoms for a while. Some of the researchers indicate that it takes two to three years from diagnosis until patients need levodopa, abbreviated as L-dopa.

The therapeutic effects of L-dopa (also referred to as SINEMET) in the treatment of Parkinson's were demonstrated 20 years ago in initial large scale clinical trials and considered a historic advance in the treatment of the disease. During this earlier period the peripheral side effects seen in the early course of high-dose levodopa treatment were reduced with the subsequent introduction of dopa decarboxylase inhibitors (carbidopa and benserazide). Since then the combination of levodopa and a dopa decarboxylase inhibitor rapidly became, and remains, the most widely used treatment of idiopathic Parkinson's disease.

With most patients, though, the initial response to levodopa diminishes with prolonged use. A common side effect is fluctuating motor performance, which can take about three to five years from the time patients first need L-dopa to when their balance is impaired and they are unable to work. This is so common that researchers have found that approximately 50% of patients treated with levodopa for five or more years develop fluctuations in motor response. In these patients the length of therapeutic benefit derived from each dose is diminished.

Traditionally the approach employed to control this is to reduce individual doses of levodopa and increase dosing frequency. However, the effectiveness of this approach is limited, so the challenge to researchers is to develop controlled-release and longer-acting preparations of levodopa.

To achieve this, researchers have been studying other agents and, according to Dr. Thomas Hutton of Texas Tech University, Parkinson's disease patients may soon benefit from an improved form of L-dopa, which is released in the body over time. SINEMET CR, developed by Dr. Hutton, is at this writing being evaluated by the Food and Drug Administration for licensing.

In 1989 other researchers announced that they had found a new drug, Deprenyl. This drug, with the chemical name selegiline, slows Parkinson's pace and delays the symptoms. This finding is the first time that any drug has been shown to delay the symptoms of any neurological disease, since existing treatments have focused on relieving symptoms. Based on studies of animals, researchers think the new drug actually prevents the death of brain cells. However, the researchers who tested the drug cautioned that the study was small and that it was not possible to prove, short of autopsy, that the drug prevented the death of brain cells in Parkinson's patients.

The researchers, Dr. James W. Tetrud and Dr. J. William Langston of the California Parkinson's Foundation in San Jose, found that Deprenyl significantly delayed the onset of symptoms requiring treatment with L-dopa. The study involved 54 patients in early stages of the disease.

The 27 patients who took Deprenyl went for an average of 549 days after entering the study before they needed L-dopa. The 27 patients who took a placebo needed L-dopa after an average of 312 days. The drug also slowed the worsening of the disease as measured by five scales by 40% to 83% a year. Deprenyl, which was approved by the Food and Drug Administration in June 1988, did not produce any notable side effects, the researchers said.

In an article in *The New York Times* Gina Kolata quoted Dr. Christopher G. Goetz, a neurologist and Parkinson's disease expert at Rush-Presbyterian-St. Luke's Medical Center in Chicago, who said: "The concept that you can prevent the natural progression of a neurological disease is revolutionary." However, researchers cautioned that their findings should be regarded as preliminary and in need of confirmation. They said a much larger, federally sponsored study involving 800 patients, scheduled to be released in 1991, was under way and should provide definitive evidence. (See also MADOPAR.)

Kolata, Gina, "Researchers Find New Drug Slows Parkinson's Pace," *The New York Times*, August 4, 1989.

Mayeux, Richard et al., "The Relationship of Serotonin to Depression in Parkinson's Disease," *Movement Disorders* 3:3(1988).

———, "Altered Serotonin Metabolism in Depression Patients with Parkinson's Disease," *Neurology*, 34(1984), 642-6.

———, "Clinical and Biochemical Features of Depression in Parkinson's Disease," *American Journal of Psychiatry*, 143(1986), 756-9.

Hutton, J.T. and Morris, J.L., "Long Acting Levodopa Preparations," *Neurology* Supplement, October 1989.

pathogenesis The origin and development of a disease.

pathological grief See GRIEF.

Perls, Frederick S. Known as Fritz Perls (1894–1970), this 20th-century innovator in the field of humanistic psychology was a developer and main proponent of GESTALT THERAPY. His workshops and demonstrations have been considered the most famous and dramatic presentations of Gestalt therapy.

PET scan (positron emitting tomography) A scan used to look into the living, functioning human brain that allows clinicians and researchers to diagnose disorders by watching the brain as it functions. As PET provides a computer-constructed image in any plane, it enables the clinicians and researchers to look at any cross section, transsection or visual slice of the brain.

Though researchers still are testing PET's accuracy in diagnosing brain disorders, positron emission tomography shows great promise in testing various hypotheses about NEUROTRANSMITTERS that allow nerve cells to talk to each other.

Stamm, Karen, "Images For Research," *The Mission*, 16:3(Summer 1989). Published by the University of Texas Health Science Center at San Antonio.

pharmaceuticals   Pills, capsules, liquids and other preparations that have a medical use.

pharmacotherapy   See DRUG THERAPY.

phobia   An overwhelming apprehension or excessive or unreasonable fear that can provoke intense anxiety or lead to anxiety attacks. Sometimes anxiolytics or anti-anxiety drugs are used as a temporary therapy for simple phobias.

phototherapy   See LIGHT THERAPY.

physiological changes   Besides chemical disturbances, certain physiological changes are associated with depression, though not all are found in every case. Muscle tension and heart and respiration rates may increase. Cells may retain more salt than usual, bringing about an imbalance in the electrical charges within the nervous system. At times blood pressure may decrease, which in turn may produce some feelings of dizziness or weakness.

Along with generalized aches and pains, other physiological side effects may be chest pains, backaches, stomach cramps or aches, headaches and odd feelings of pressure in the head, ears or neck. There may be coldness of the extremities and numbness or tingling of the hands and feet.

In addition, there can be changes in sexual activity, bowel habits, weight, appetite and sleep patterns. Still other physiological effects may be fatigue, sweating, nausea and dryness of the mouth.

pineal gland   A pea-sized endocrine organ. It is located in the brain at the entrance to an important canal for the circulation of spinal fluid and has a role in controlling the flow of cerebrospinal fluid.

It secretes the hormone MELATONIN for a fixed period every 24 hours, during darkness. The period is set by a biological clock that is light-sensitive. If there are eight hours of darkness, it can produce its quota. If there are only six it falls short. Some researchers have tied SEASONAL AFFECTIVE DISORDER to melatonin because of the way the hormone is produced in the dark, particularly during winter.

Since we do not yet fully understand everything relating to the pineal gland's functions, research groups continue to investigate its role. In "A New Light on the Blues" Glennys Bell wrote: "The pineal gland is only slowly giving up its secrets . . . As organs go, the pineal gland has not had an illustrious history, despite its good beginning when Aristotle nominated it as the 'site of the soul.' Early Greek anatomists knew of it and Herophilus suggested in the 4th century B.C. that it was ' the sphincter of thought,' the mind's valve."
Bell, Glennys, "A New Light on the Blues," *The Bulletin*, July 25, 1989.

Plath, Sylvia   An American poet and novelist (1932–1963) who wrote *The Bell Jar,* a classic description of the progression of depressive illness in an intelligent young woman. The novel was first published pseudonymously in England in 1962, and Dr. Nancy Andreasen of the University of Iowa School of Medicine has indicated that medical readers can learn more about depression from reading it than from reading many psychiatric texts.

Throughout Plath's life, she was inwardly depressed while attempting to maintain an outward appearance of cheerfulness and efficiency, so Andreasen believes Plath seems to have suffered from recurrent ENDOGENOUS DEPRESSIONS. In "Ariel's Flight: The Death of Sylvia Plath," Andreasen describes the two major episodes of depression Plath experienced.

The first occurred between her junior and senior years at Smith College when she began to have feelings of decreased energy and interest, nagging self-doubt, hopelessness about the future and inexplicable outbursts of tears while serving as a guest managing editor at *Mademoiselle* magazine during the summer. When she returned home the symptoms worsened markedly and Plath suffered from profound apathy, severe insomnia and a progressively stronger suicidal urge. Her symptoms finally culminated in a serious and nearly successful suicide attempt. During her hospitalization she was first treated with insulin, unsuccessfully, and then with electrotherapy, to which she responded well.

Subsequently Plath was able to return to Smith and function well enough to graduate summa cum laude. Then, after a brief teaching stint at Smith, marriage to English poet Ted Hughes and the birth of her two children, Plath and her family moved to England. She apparently remained well until 10 years later, when she again experienced depressive symptoms.

Andreasen suggests that writing *The Bell Jar*, a semiautobiographical work about a woman caught up in rebellion against the constricting forces of society and her emotional and psychological conflicts and crises resulting from family tensions, may have caused Plath to relive the old feelings of hopelessness and despair. It may also have reawakened conflicts about men since her marriage to Hughes had ended. The book's final pages contain the prophetic statement that the symbolic "bell jar" with its stifling distortions may again descend, perhaps somewhere in Europe. This suggests, wrote Andreasen, that Plath could have been struggling with early depressive symptoms as much as a year before her death.

Plath's severe depression during the weeks prior to her death by suicide in London in 1963 was characterized by the same insomnia and hopelessness she had experienced during the final stages of her first episode.

Andreasen, Nancy, "Ariel's Flight: The Death of Sylvia Plath," *Journal of the American Medical Association*, 228:5 (April 29, 1974).

positron emitting tomography See PET SCAN.

postpartum depression The transient "baby blues" many women experience in the early weeks following childbirth.

When a new or first-time mother gets overwhelmed with the care of an infant her symptoms generally include crying, anxiety and a feeling of being caught in a gloomy and hopeless situation. Some women are unable to sleep. Others have no appetite.

One of the causes may be hormonal because, as a woman's body returns to a nonpregnant condition after childbirth, it undergoes a tremendous hormonal upheaval. The biological mechanism that would explain the hormonal involvement, however, has yet to be discovered. Whatever the mechanism is, though, it occurs at the same time that the new mother may be experiencing radical and stressful social changes in her life.

Another contributing factor can be lack of an extended family, which adds to the isolation that many new mothers feel. In an extended family, a relative sometimes sees that a new mother needs a break and helps out with moral support as well as with physical care of the baby. All new mothers do not have extended families, however, so in some parts of the country services such as Mothertime (with national headquarters at 140 Christie St., Leonia, NJ 07605; phone: 201-585-0846) are springing up to help mothers during the early weeks at home with a new baby. The services provide trained *doulas*—a Greek word meaning "mother's mother"—to go into homes a few hours each day for several weeks to provide postpartum home care, help with housework, care for older children and offer confidence-building information and encouragement.

Although a period of "the blues" is common among women in the first week or two after birth and typically begins after the elation of giving birth fades, new research findings from Europe contradict the risks of depression for women after childbirth. Dr. Robert O. Pasnau of the University of California at Los Angeles Medical School, who reviewed the European findings in the November 1989 issue of *The American Journal of Psychiatry*, stated that some of the findings have been corroborated by American studies and that depression associated with childbirth is exaggerated. Earlier studies estimated the risk of such depression after birth at between 8% and 15%. But those studies did not compare new mothers with women of similar age who had not gone through childbirth. However, a 1988 British study that included a comparison group found there was no higher rate of moderate depression among new mothers. Moreover, a series of British studies in the 1980s found that depression within a year of giving birth was more strongly related to marital conflicts and other setbacks, like the death of a loved one, than to motherhood.

Dr. Pasnau found that the most alarming finding in the survey of new studies related to women who become psychotic after childbirth, with symptoms like hallucinations and delusions. For example, in 1985 researchers at the University of Edinburgh Medical School in Scotland reported visiting 82 women 15 years after they had been hospitalized for psychosis. Of the 82, two had killed their infants, one was suspected of having done so and a fourth had tried to.

According to a study by Dr. Robert Kendell, a psychiatrist at the Edinburgh Medical School, about half the women who become psychotic after childbirth are extremely depressed, while about a quarter become psychotic during a manic episode. Studies have found that women who have had postpartum depression or psychosis have a heightened risk of a later episode. A 1985 Scandinavian study found that postpartum depression recurred after one-third of subsequent childbirths; a 1987 British study found that 20% to 25% of women who became psychotic after childbirth had a repeat episode after the birth

of another child. (See also POSTPARTUM PSYCHOSIS.)

Goleman, Daniel, "Wide Beliefs on Depression in Women Contradicted," *The New York Times*, January 9, 1990.

postpartum psychosis   When POSTPARTUM DEPRESSION expands from a mild depression and "baby blues" to a full-blown psychosis with severe thought disorder and complete dissociation, some victims of postpartum psychosis are vulnerable to suicide. In other situations, infanticide may—and has—resulted, as apparently normal new mothers suddenly snap and kill their new babies.

According to a report in *Time* magazine, about 8% to 12% of women who give birth suffer a blacker torment than the emotional letdown and "baby blues" experienced by 50% to 80% of new mothers. As the former group become seriously depressed for months, the mothers undergo mercurial mood swings, lose their appetites, go sleepless for nights on end and become plagued by thoughts of suicide or fantasies of killing their baby by dropping it down the stairs, burying it in the backyard or cutting it up with a kitchen knife. "These are invasive, terrifying ideas that can drive them crazy," psychiatrist Ricardo Fernandez of Princeton, New Jersey said in the article. "A lot of women have a tremendous amount of guilt and shame because of these thoughts." Fortunately, most new mothers never act on these impulses, but a few become sufficiently psychotic to resort to infanticide.

No one is completely sure what causes either postpartum depression or postpartum psychosis but both physical and psychological causes have been suggested. One of the physical causes may be a hormonal involvement, but not every aspect of that involvement has yet been discovered.

The article in *Time* reported that medical treatment for postpartum disorders has become quite effective. It may include medication, hospitalization, electroconvulsive ther- apy and counseling. Some women, including those who have experienced problem preg- nancies or who have a family history of men- tal illness, are thought to be at higher risk of developing postpartum trouble. Preventive injections of progesterone immediately after birth may be suggested for women who have suffered from depression after a previous birth.

The legal defense of temporary insanity as a result of postpartum psychosis has been used in court hearings on infanticide cases. The defense has sometimes been successful. In October 1988 in the first successful use in New York of the insanity defense in the case of a postpartum psychosis, a former pediatric nurse who admitted killing two of her new- born children (and was accused of trying to suffocate a third child) was cleared of murder charges by jurors who found her "not re- sponsible" for a crime because she suffered from postpartum depression. The judge or- dered her to undergo psychiatric testing. The insanity defense is expected to be used again in other cases, though there is controversy about it and not all attorneys agree that women suffering from this depression are always out of their minds and unaware of what they are doing.

Within the past few years women who have experienced postpartum distress have started support groups such as the Pennsylva- nia-based Depression After Delivery, with chapters around the country. These groups are one excellent source for obtaining sympa- thetic and ongoing help.

Toufexis, A. et al., "Why Mothers Kill Their Babies," *Time*, June 20, 1988.

Clark, Patrick and Marques, Stuart, "Birth Blues Clear Baby-Killer Mom," *New York Daily News*, October 1, 1988.

premature death from grief See GRIEF, CAUSES AND EFFECTS OF.

premenstrual depression Menstrual cycles have been associated with depressed feelings, irritability and other behavioral and physical changes in some women for many years, but in the past the role of menstruation in depression has been neglected as a re- search subject. Now, however, scientists are researching the premenstrual syndrome (PMS) and applying their expertise to contro- versies about its causes, implications and re- lation to depressive disorders. In "Depres- sion: Is There a Quick Fix For This Danger- ous Disease?" Carol Duchow Gurin and Joel Gurin report on the findings of psychiatrist Barbara Parry, who has done research on the subject at the National Institute of Mental Health (NIMH). PMS is a cyclic problem and Parry notes that PMS and SEASONAL AFFEC- TIVE DISORDER (SAD), also a cyclic problem and much more common among women than men, may be biologically linked. She has also stated that there may be something about reproductive endocrinology and the cyclic physiology of women that predisposes them to these forms of depression.

Parry points out that the symptoms of PMS and SAD are very similar. In both cases, women feel lethargic, oversleep and overeat, and especially crave carbohydrates. She has also found that several women had "seasonal premenstrual syndrome." They have pre- menstrual symptoms primarily during the winter, and during the winter months they're only depressed when they're premenstrual. According to Parry, the LIGHT THERAPY that works for SAD may also turn out to work for PMS. PMS sufferers may also be helped by another technique for resetting the body's clocks—sleep deprivation. Researchers have found that missing an occasional night's sleep, or shifting sleep patterns a few nights in a row, can temporarily alleviate depression in some people. Though this treatment is still experimental, Parry has found that it may help many PMS sufferers as well.

Gurin, Carol Duchow (with Gurin, Joel), "Depression: Is There a Quick Fix For This Dangerous Disease?" *Ms*, December 1987.

primary depression A depression in which the mood is not related to a preexisting mental disorder or to a known organic fact, such as a physical condition, substance abuse disorder or a medication.

In a coauthored article on depression Dr. David A. Lewis and Dr. George Winokur of the University of Iowa College of Medicine explain that primary depressive disorders occur in individuals with no previous history of any other psychiatric illness and can be divided into UNIPOLAR and BIPOLAR DEPRESSIONS. Some patients with primary affective disorder complain of a dysphoric mood described as feeling depressed, sad, blue, low, gloomy or "down in the dumps." However, other patients may complain primarily of feeling hopeless, irritable, fearful or anxious.

Additional psychological symptoms include loss of interest in normal activities, diminished pleasurable experiences or anhedonia, interpersonal withdrawal, feelings of helplessness, and recurrent thoughts of death or suicide.

Although the most frequent symptoms are psychological in nature, it is not uncommon for persons with primary depression to initially mention somatic symptoms such as headache, diffuse pains, fatigue, palpitations, gastrointestinal disturbances and weight loss. These physical complaints may sometimes be of hypochondriacal proportions, although they frequently appear valid.

Lewis, David A. and Winokur, George, "Depression," *Medical Grand Rounds*, 3:4(1984).

prodromal period The time in which symptoms appear before the actual onset of depression. The main features are anxiety, tension and difficulty in making decisions. The prodromal period varies in length and may not be obvious in someone with an ACUTE ONSET.

Prozac See FLUOXETINE.

psychodynamic therapies Psychodynamic therapies are based on the assumption that internal conflicts, such as conflicted feelings (e.g., wanting independence and dependence, hating and loving the same person) are at the heart of a depressive's disorder. Such unresolved conflicts are often rooted in early childhood, and many evolve from child-parent relationships. Resolving them is essential to successful TREATMENT, so short-term versions of psychodynamic therapies are used to treat clinical depression. A key aspect of the treatment involves bringing the conflict into a therapeutic situation where it can be dealt with and resolved.

Some researchers studying psychodynamic therapies give this form of therapy mixed reviews for its effectiveness in treating depression. Others applaud its efficacy for patients who cannot or do not wish to take drugs for various reasons. More research remains to be done on this subject before definite answers are available. But the first steps have been taken to analyze information on the relationship of specific patient characteristics to specific treatment outcomes, and of significant importance to researchers are the clues that are beginning to emerge about which patients do best on which treatments. (See also COGNITIVE THERAPY; INTERPERSONAL PSYCHOTHERAPY; PSYCHOTHERAPY; COUNSELING.)

psychological drug dependence A craving or compulsion to continue the use of a drug because it gives a feeling of well-being and satisfaction. The syndrome is also known as behavioral, psychic or emotional dependence.

Psychic dependence can vary in intensity from a mild preference for a drug to a strong craving for it. The World Health Organization defines psychic dependence as "a feeling of satisfaction and a psychic drive that requires periodic or continuous administration of a drug to produce a desired effect or to avoid discomfort." An individual can be psychologically dependent on a drug and not physically dependent, and the reverse is also true.

psychoneuroimmunology A branch of science that deals with the role played by mental-emotional stress in disturbing immune processes in such a way as to precipitate disease.

psychosis A medical term for deep depression and other severe mental disorders that interfere with a person's capacity to meet the ordinary demands of life. A psychotic episode can bring about such symptoms as hallucinations, delusions, extreme confusion, disorientation, aggressive behavior and loss of contact with reality. It affects a person's ability to think, respond emotionally, remember, communicate, interpret and behave appropriately.

Schizophrenic and manic-depressive psychoses are examples of what has been called functional psychosis. In toxic psychosis, psychotic-like behavior results from impairment of brain cell function.

With treatment, many people (though not everyone) recover from a psychotic episode, regardless of how distressing the actual episode seems to be while the person is experiencing it.

psychosomatic A term that applies to the relationship of mind and body. It is used to describe disorders in which psychological factors have played a crucial role in leading to physical disease. Both mental and physical symptoms are likely to be present. In psychosomatic medicine, the treatment of both body and emotions is emphasized.

psychotherapy Psychotherapy comes in many variations and is offered for groups, families, couples and individuals. There are "talking therapies" during which problems are discussed and resolved through the emotional support, insights and understanding gained from the verbal give-and-take. Depression "talking therapy" is an examination of the emotional and intellectual experience of depression and how best to deal with it. For patients who are not too severely depressed this can often help as much as drugs.

Other therapies concentrate on behaviors: Patients are taught to be more effective in obtaining rewards and satisfaction through their own actions. Some therapies examine the past, seeking resolution of present problems by shedding light on earlier experiences. Others focus strictly on current conflicts and interpersonal problems.

Although people are sometimes counseled to avoid rushing into therapy too rapidly, many mental health experts suggest seeking help if the symptoms of depression persist for more than two weeks and/or they cause a noticeable impairment in ordinary function. A good place to seek initial help or leads is through a physician's office, family service agency or local health or mental health clinic or center. Other possibilities include a general hospital's department of psychiatry or outpatients' psychiatric clinic; a state hospital outpatient clinic; a university or medical school-affiliated program; a family service or social agency; and private clinics or facilities. (See also COUNSELING; TREATMENT OF DEPRESSION.)

R

Rand Corporation-based medical outcomes study (MOS) An $11.5 million project, the largest and most comprehensive quality-of-care research effort to date; conducted by a team of doctors and social scientists from RAND, the New England Medical Center, UCLA, the University of California, San Francisco, Dartmouth Medical School and the University of Washington.

The California-based RAND is a private, nonprofit institution engaged in research and analysis of problems affecting the nation's security and domestic welfare. In one of the most striking of MOS's initial findings researchers found that the impact of depression on patients' day-to-day functioning has not only been underestimated but is also comparable to that of a serious heart condition and greater than for many other major, chronic medical diseases.

According to the study, patients with depression spent more days in bed and had more bodily pain than patients with back, lung or gastrointestinal problems, angina, hypertension or diabetes. Only arthritis proved more painful and only serious heart conditions produced more bed days. Some 22,462 patients and 523 physicians took part at sites in Boston, Chicago and Los Angeles. The patients were all English-speaking adults who visited participating clinicians between February and October 1986. The physicians and their practices represented a variety of specialties and structures.

One research team analyzed an 11,252-patient cross section of the MOS sample, comparing questionnaire responses from patients with depression, patients with chronic medical problems and patients who were ill but had no chronic condition. Some of the 2,467 depression patients were also interviewed by telephone.

In an article in the *Journal of the American Medical Association* that reported on this study, researchers found that:

1. In routine activities such as climbing stairs, walking, dressing, going to work and visiting friends, patients with depression are at least as impaired as those with chronic medical conditions, and often more so.

2. Day-to-day functioning is especially poor when patients suffer from both depression and a chronic medical condition. Those with coronary artery disease and depressive symptoms, for example, encountered twice as much trouble with social relationships as for either condition alone.

3. Patients who exhibited merely the symptoms of depression functioned nearly as poorly as those formally diagnosed as having depressive disorder. Moreover, many were receiving care from general medical clinicians rather than mental health specialists.

"Our results suggest that depression may be more like major medical conditions in its disabling effects than has previously been appreciated," said Dr. Kenneth B. Wells, a member of the RAND staff and professor of psychiatry at the UCLA Neuropsychiatric Institute. "They also underscore the importance of accurate diagnosis and proper care, even for patients who are not necessarily complaining of the condition."

Wells, Kenneth B. et al., "The Functioning and Well-being of Depressed Patients," *Journal of the American Medical Association*, 262:7(August 18, 1989).

rapid eye movement (REM) One of the various stages of sleep, and the stage in which a person dreams. Since all of the orders of the sleep cycle are biologically essential, a person deprived of REM may become hostile, irritable and anxious.

Normally REM sleep periods, which last from 10 to 60 minutes, are spaced about 1.5 hours apart, with the longest periods toward the end of sleep, near dawn. In depression the normal pattern reverses, with REM sleep occurring early in sleep, and the first REM period may be the longest. A few studies suggest the other extreme is true for manic patients—with the first REM period occurring later than normal and with waking occurring earlier. (See also SLEEP AND SLEEP DISORDERS.)

Corfman, Eunice, *Depression, Manic-Depressive Illness, and Biological Rhythms* (Rockville, Maryland: Alcohol, Drug Abuse and Mental Health Administration, 1982; DHHS #82-889).

rational-emotive psychotherapy (RET)
A holistic approach to emotional growth that

stresses action, encourages the discovery and expression of emotions and emphasizes the interrelationship of thinking, emotions and behavior. RET's followers believe that RET helps people develop their power to: (1) overcome emotional stress and interpersonal problems; (2) channel their energy more creatively; and (3) become happier, more successful and more fulfilled persons in every area of their lives.

Dr. ALBERT ELLIS introduced rational-emotive therapy in 1955 and founded the Manhattan-based Institute for Rational-Emotive Therapy—a not-for-profit educational organization—in 1968. RET and other cognitive behavioral techniques are now practiced by over 10,000 mental health and educational professionals worldwide. One emphasis of the Institute for Rational-Emotive Therapy is counseling depressives and teaching depressed individuals that by learning to alter their dysfunctional beliefs, they can develop greater capacities for dealing with their current problems and living freer and more emotionally satisfying lives.

Rauwolfia serpentina (reserpine) A plant with a root that bears a striking resemblance to a snake—hence, *serpentina*. It grows wild in the hill country of India and many other parts of the world. It is the root that provides the active pharmacological ingredients. Its medicinal powers are chronicled in ancient Sanskrit and Hindu manuscripts, and long before the 20th century, healers used its medicinal powers to treat a long list of ills, including snake bite, fever, stomach ulcers, high blood pressure and complications of pregnancy. It was also noted for its soothing effects as a sleeping potion. Because of its calming powers it became a standard treatment for the insane.

It was ignored by Western medicine except for scattered accounts detailing its use as an antidote to some highly agitated forms of behavior for patients with mental disorders. In fact, no one thought to test the properties of the remedy until 1931 when two physicians, Dr. G. Sen and Dr. K.C. Bose, published a medical paper claiming the successful Rauwolfia treatment of several violently disturbed patients.

The following 20 years brought a trickle of other accounts, and by the early 1950s some obscure medical journals published literature attesting to the promise of Rauwolfia (or reserpine, as the drug is known) for patients suffering from a variety of psychiatric disorders.

In 1953 Dr. NATHAN S. KLINE played a pioneer role in the modern development of reserpine when he agreed to experiment with Rauwolfia (or the reserpine extract) on patients suffering from schizophrenia and other mental disorders. In his position as a mental hospital research director he was chiefly concerned with schizophrenia. In testing reserpine on both schizophrenics and manic-depressives he found that in some cases reserpine did affect behavior patterns.

As Kline experimented he found that the drug was clearly a sedative, while at the same time it made some patients more active. The theory was that the sedation was confined to particular centers in the nervous system, damping down anxiety reaction without impairing other responses.

Though Kline found that reserpine is not a drug for depressives, as it may push them into deeper withdrawal, reserpine proved to be an enormously important drug in itself. Its discovery was significant because it stimulated a massive search for psychotropic drugs. Moreover, as a tranquilizing medication it replaced locked cells and straitjackets and helped point the way to a chemical approach to mental illness. Although it was also found useful in the treatment of high blood pressure, its tendency to cause depression soon prompted considerable caution in its use.

Kline, Nathan S., *From Sad to Glad* (New York: Putnam, 1974).

recurrent episodes "Recurrent" refers to a new episode of depression that follows a recovery. The episode reappears at different intervals, with normal periods, called remissions, appearing in between. Often referred to as the "recurrent nature of affective disorders," the phenomenon was first noticed in Europe. Later, in the United States, the introduction of psychoactive drugs (and the need this brought to study psychiatric histories) put clinicians into the position of needing to do in-depth studies of recurrences, count episodes and estimate cycles.

Research has now shown that persons with bipolar disorders (see BIPOLAR DEPRESSION) are particularly likely to suffer recurrences since most patients who have a manic episode go on to have a course marked by multiple recurrences of major depressive and manic episodes.

According to a consensus statement from the 1984 Consensus Development Conference on Mood Disorders: Pharmacologic Prevention of Recurrences (convened by the National Institutes of Health in conjunction with the National Institute of Mental Health) studies have suggested that as many as 50% of patients with recurrent unipolar disorders who recover from a given episode have a recurrence within the first two years after recovery. The likelihood of recurrence is greatest in the four to six months following initial symptomatic recovery. This risk levels off markedly between six and 12 months and is still lower after the patient has been well for 18 months. Some evidence suggests that the length of well intervals between episodes decreases for the first few episodes and then remains steady, while the duration of episodes remains fairly constant. ELECTROCONVULSIVE THERAPY is used for some unremitting or suicidal depressions.

Many of the answers to the causes of recurrent episodes and how to prevent them are still elusive, and researchers are investigating: (1) why some patients develop severe recurrent illnesses while others do not; (2) why some patients respond well to preventive treatment while others do not; and (3) why some patients lose benefits after an initial response to treatment.

re-grief therapy A method used by Dr. Vamik Volkan, a psychiatrist at the University of Virginia Medical school, to help persons suffering from pathological GRIEF to recognize the actuality of the death and get the normal mourning process moving ahead. His approach makes use of a common phenomenon in those with mourning problems: the possession of a special object that links them to the dead person, such as a piece of jewelry. These links are more than just treasured keepsakes. They are jealously guarded and hold an eerie fascination for the mourner. As these objects become symbolic tokens jointly "owned" by both the mourner and the deceased person, they are a way of keeping the dead person alive.

Because people with this kind of grief are in a chronic state of hope that the dead person will return, Dr. Volkan asks mourners to bring in the linking object and explore its symbolic meaning. This typically allows mourners to face the fact of the death and activate the mourning they haven't completed.

Goleman, Daniel, "Study of Normal Mourning Process Illuminates Grief Gone Awry," *The New York Times*, March 29, 1988.

research diagnostic criteria (RDC) A diagnostic tool that specifies 10 depressive symptoms that are used to diagnose endogenous depression. Four symptoms are in group A (distinct quality of mood, lack of reactivity to pleasurable environmental stimuli, mood worse in morning, pervasive anhedonia) and six are in group B (guilt or self-reproach, middle or terminal insomnia, psychomotor agitation or retardation, poor appetite, loss of weight, pervasive or nonpervasive anhedonia). The symptoms are scored as present or absent and all are given equal weight. For a patient's condition to be diagnosed as endogenous at least one symptom must come from group A. Diagnosis is made at three levels of certainty: nonendogenous, probable endogenous and definite endogenous.

reserpine See RAUWOLFIA SERPENTINA.

retirement Some researchers believe retirement (with the boredom and lack of self-esteem that sometimes accompanies it) contributes to depression among older people (and especially men) who see their self-worth in terms of work and productivity. Along with retirement, possible health problems, waning strength and death of friends and loved ones, the awareness of mortality and, often, a sense of uselessness combine to make older persons vulnerable to depression.

re-uptake process A way in which the brain normally regulates the chemical flow of the NEUROTRANSMITTERS (the NOREPINEPHRINE and SEROTONIN systems) by having some cells absorb the excess of this chemical flow. Depressed people apparently need more norepinephrine and serotonin than their brains allow them to use, so drugs are used to block the re-uptake in order to leave more of the chemicals available to work against depression.

reverse-sad (summer depression) In the more common SEASONAL AFFECTIVE DISORDER (SAD) people suffer from fall and winter depressions that alternate with HYPOMANIA or nondepressed periods in spring and summer. In recent years, however, scientists have documented reverse cases in which reverse-SAD people have spring and summer depression and fall and winter hypomania. Those with the reverse-SAD syndrome report that their depression typically starts in the March-June period and ends between August and October. While those with winter depression can be helped by increasing their exposure to real or simulated sunlight, people with summer depression seem to improve when they are exposed to cold.

Three researchers, Dr. Thomas A. Wehr, Dr. David A. Sack and Dr. Norman E. Rosenthal of the National Institute of Mental Health (NIMH), have noted that the first case of summer depression and winter mania was described in France in the 1800s. Other researchers have since told of patients whose seasonal depression switched from winter to summer. Dr. Wehr and his colleagues suggest that summer depression may be more common than is generally realized and may account for the peak in suicides in late spring and summer.

In a study conducted by Dr Wehr and his colleagues the researchers observed 12 patients with reverse-SAD, all of whom had a lifetime diagnosis of BIPOLAR DEPRESSION. Their depressions usually began between March and June and ended between August and October. Manias or hypomanias generally started between September and October and concluded between March and May. The symptoms of depression and hypomania were similar to those found in the winter variety of SAD.

As with the winter SAD patients, several summer SAD patients noted a relationship between latitude or climate and severity of illness. Some patients reported that they did not have symptoms when they lived farther north. Others reported that when they traveled south in the spring, their summer depressions began earlier in the year. Conversely, summer vacations in the north were accompanied by clinical improvements, and in some cases improvement occurred when patients bathed in cold lakes.

The striking resemblance between the clinical picture and environmental sensitivity of summer and winter SAD patients to different environmental stimuli prompted Dr. Wehr and his colleagues to explore the effects of having a single patient with summer SAD stay in an air conditioned apartment for several days during the summer and periodically subject herself to very cold temperatures. After five days the patient showed a marked antidepressant response and she relapsed nine days after this treatment was discontinued.

Researchers have yet to identify the fundamental cause of seasonal affective disorders, and they now feel that at this time they are in the same situation with reverse-SAD as they were with winter SAD some years ago. Future controlled studies are required to explore the clinical usefulness of temperature modification in reverse-SAD patients.

rituals   See FUNERALS.

role of family and friends   An initial concern for family and friends living with a depressive may be that the person seems to be irritable much of the time. Next, the depressive may start to withdraw, turn down social activities and suffer delusions, though in the beginning delusions are so subtle they hardly seem abnormal. Later the depressive will exhibit helplessness, lose all energy and have no interest in doing much. Personal hygiene may be neglected.

It is difficult and exhausting to live with this, so while trying to pull the depressive out of the severe blue mood persons living with him or her may start to feel angry, hostile, irritated, frustrated and impatient. These feelings are normal, however, so the family and friends of depressives do not need to feel guilty about feeling this way. What they *do* need to do is to realize that the depressed person is in pain and needs help. They should encourage the depressed person to get appropriate treatment from a mental health professional, when symptoms linger beyond a reasonable time, or if there seems to be no apparent reason for the individual's persistent feelings of unhappiness and gloom. But since the very nature of depression can keep a depressive from seeking help, he or she may be reluctant to see a doctor. Consequently those close to the person may have to work hard to effect this. On occasion, this may require making the appointment and accompanying the depressed person to the appointment. But the earlier the depressed person receives help, the sooner the symptoms will be alleviated and the speedier the recovery will be. With treatment most depressed people eventually do get better. Keep that in

mind and keep reassuring depressed persons that with time and help, they *will* feel better.

Though a depression may appear relatively mild, it does not exclude the possibility of suicide, because sometimes seemingly mild depression has much deeper roots. It is not true, as many people believe, that a person who talks about suicide will not attempt it. Those who attempt it often appeal first for help by threatening suicide. Therefore, this potential must always be considered by family and friends and if a depressive mentions suicide, report the remarks to the doctor.

To make sure the depressive gets the right treatment, the first step is the family doctor or a clinic. Next, psychiatrists, psychologists, therapists or social workers can engage the patient in PSYCHOTHERAPY (or the "talking treatment"). But only psychiatrists can prescribe drugs. After treatment is obtained, family and friends may need to encourage a depressed individual to stay with the treatment until symptoms begin to abate (several weeks) or to seek different treatment. They may also need to monitor whether the depressed person is taking the prescribed medication.

Another thing family and friends can do is to provide emotional support. This involves showing encouragement, understanding, patience, and love, even when this gets hard. This helps far more than blame and argument.

Never compound the feeling of guilt that depression brings by implying that a depressed person is lazy or weak, and refrain from accusing the person of faking illness and saying he or she can "snap out of it."

The National Institute of Mental Health (NIMH) recommends applying the following "Dos" and "Don'ts":

DO

- maintain as normal a relationship as possible
- point out distorted negative thinking without being critical or disapproving

- acknowledge that the person is suffering and in pain
- smile and encourage honest effort
- offer kind words and pay compliments
- express affection
- show that you care, respect and value the depressed person

DON'T

- blame the depressed person for his or her condition
- criticize, pick on, "put down" or voice disapproval until the depressed person is feeling better
- say or do anything to acerbate his or her poor self-image

SAD See SEASONAL AFFECTIVE DISORDER.

Schedule for Affective Disorders and Schizophrenia (SADS)

Developed by Robert Spitzer, Jean Endicott and their associates. Designed for recording information regarding a person's functioning and symptoms. Involves a 78-page protocol that presents a detailed interview schedule containing many highly structured and specific questions. Has been widely used for clinical and research purposes.

Schedule for Standardized Assessment of Depressive Disorders (WHO/SADD)

An instrument used in the World Health Organization (WHO) Collaborative Study on Standardized Assessment of Depressive Disorders; it was designed to be easy to master and to be adaptable to a variety of interviewing styles. The schedule is composed of three parts. Part 1 covers basic data necessary for the identification of the patient, such as age, sex, residence, marital status, education and occupation. Part 2 consists of a series of rating scales for the assessment of the clinical condition of the patient and questions covering his or her psychiatric history. Part 3 covers the diagnosis and the classification of the diagnosis.

schizoaffective disorder A diagnosis made by the presence of typical schizophrenic and affective symptoms during the same episode. This category of illness presents particular problems in classification, however.

According to Dr. George Winokur of the University of Iowa College of Medicine, the term has historically implied a mixture of schizophrenic and affective symptoms. But where schizoaffective disorder fits in relationship to these separate categories of illness is uncertain. Does schizoaffective disorder fall within the schizophrenic realm, the affective realm or neither? At present, states Winokur, clinical data are inadequate to determine the question of etiology. The presence of schizophrenic symptoms mixed with affective symptoms generally predicts a poorer prognosis, but this is not always the case.

Some researchers have concluded that in schizoaffective patients with demographic features more characteristic of schizophrenia, a relatively poor prognosis can be anticipated. Among the features that have been cited for a poor prognosis are early onset, insidious onset, family history negative for clear affective disorder or positive for clear schizophrenia, chronic course, and prodromal traits such as social isolation, peculiar behavior or long-standing role impairment. The converse of these features has implied a good prognosis. (See also SCHIZOPHRENIC DEPRESSION.)

Winokur, George, "The Schizoaffective Continuum: Euclid's Second Axiom," *Annals of Clinical Psychiatry*, 1(1989), 19–24.

Cook, B.L. and Winokur, G., "Nosology of Affective Disorders," in John G. Howells (ed.), *Perspectives in the Psychiatry of the Affective Disorders* (New York: Brunner Mazel, 1989).

schizophrenia A mental disorder and psychotic illness. Researchers pinpoint the main types as catatonic, disorganized, paranoid and undifferentiated. The illness is characterized by withdrawal from reality and the environment and by a disentegration of personality expressed as distorted behavior, private fantasies and disordered emotions and thoughts.

It was formerly called dementia praecox when, in 1896, EMIL KRAEPELIN grouped what were previously considered unrelated mental diseases (simple, hebephrenic, catatonic and paranoid) under the heading of dementia praecox, a condition of diminished mentality that he theorized was incurable. Later in 1911 Paul Eugen Bleuler, a Swiss psychiatrist and neurologist (1857–1939), concluded that the disease was not one of dementia but rather a disharmonious state of mind in which contradictory tendencies exist together, splitting the harmony of the mind. Based on this conclusion, he introduced the term schizophrenia to mean "splitting of the mind," a relevant term for our current definitions of the disorder.

In *The Encyclopedia of Suicide* Glen Evans and Norman L. Farberow point out that through the years the search for the underlying causes of schizophrenia has centered on both functional and organic factors. Because antipsychotic drugs have a marked effect on reducing the symptoms of the disorder, many authorities now believe that further research in the biochemistry of the brain is promising. Investigators have searched for products in schizophrenics' blood that are not found in normals and have tried to analyze disorders in the neurotransmitter substances in the brain.

At Washington University School of Medicine in St. Louis researchers have proposed a new scientific model that attributes schizophrenia to an abnormality in the left hemisphere of the brain in an area that controls attention.

The model links the disease to an impairment in the brain's limbic system, where certain structures band together in circuits that orchestrate attention, along with other emotional and behavioral processes. It is one of the few to connect the debilitating psychotic symptoms of schizophrenia to anatomical abnormalities in the brain.

The Washington University researchers also suggest that schizophrenics may have a deficiency—rather than an excess—of DOPAMINE, a neurotransmitter long implicated in the disease.

"The model offers possible explanations for many aspects of schizophrenia, and attempts to link cognitive function to the anatomy of the disorder," explained Dr. Terrence Early, assistant professor of psychiatry at Washington University. "It's defined precisely enough that it can be tested fairly well, and it suggests a number of avenues of study.

"We are proposing a disruption in left hemispheric function and specifically that an impairment in the anatomical circuit containing key structures within the brain's limbic system is fundamental to the disorder. Though prevailing neurochemical theories stress a dopamine excess, we are speculating that patients with schizophrenia have something like reduced dopamine input to the ventral striatum in the left hemisphere."

Although researchers have found medications that help schizophrenia they still do not know the causes. A better understanding of the illness depends on the results of ongoing research.

The main symptoms of schizophrenia are hallucinations; delusions; stupor, incoherence and faulty thought processes; negativism; progressive deterioration; impulsive acts and bizarre behavior; withdrawal and tendency to live in an inner world; and an incapacity to maintain normal interpersonal relationships.

Schizophrenia commonly strikes its victims during late adolescence or early adulthood and at first may be hardly noticeable. However, as the disorder progresses in severity, schizophrenics may develop significant impairments.

Evans, Glen and Farberow, Norman L., *The Encyclopedia of Suicide* (New York: Facts On File, 1988).

schizophrenic depression   A term used when SCHIZOPHRENIA and depression interweave as one illness. Schizophrenia and depression combined affect about 14.5 million Americans. According to the NATIONAL ALLIANCE FOR RESEARCH ON SCHIZOPHRENIA AND DEPRESSION, $36 billion is spent each year on medical and social services for victims of schizophrenia and depression. The indirect costs total $67.4 billion.

Many researchers believe that schizophrenia, and its break with reality, is the primary illness. Others contend that SECONDARY DEPRESSION and minor depressive illness often occur in medical illness and in non-affective psychiatric illness such as schizophrenia. They suggest the following mixtures or classifications: (1) patients are truly schizophrenic and the affective symptoms are matters of relative insignificance; (2) the patients' disorders are affective in nature and the schizophrenic symptoms are simply inconsequential; (3) the SCHIZOAFFECTIVE DISORDER may possibly be an autonomous illness in itself—that is, a third psychosis. All agree, however, that this psychotic disorder, mixed with depression, can lead to complex mixes of beliefs and fantasies.

In a study at the University of Pennsylvania conducted by Dr. AARON BECK and Dr. David Braff and reported in *Feeling Good: The New Mood Therapy* by Dr. David Burns, depressed individuals were compared with schizophrenic patients and with non-depressed persons in their ability to interpret the meaning of a number of proverbs, such as ''a stitch in time saves nine.'' Both the schizophrenic and depressed patients made many logical errors and had difficulty in extracting the meaning of the proverbs. They were overly concrete and couldn't make accurate generalizations.

Although the severity of the defect was obviously less profound and bizarre in the depressed patients than in the schizophrenic group, the depressed individuals were clearly abnormal as compared with the normal subjects.

In practical terms, the study indicated that during periods of depression people lose some of their capacity for clear thinking.

Negative events grow in importance until these events dominate people's perspective and reality to the point that they can't really tell that what is happening is distorted.

When symptoms of depression appear in schizophrenics it is imperative the depression be given immediate attention because schizophrenic depressions account for a large number of suicides.

Burns, David B., *Feeling Good: The New Mood Therapy* (New York: New American Library, 1980).

Winokur, George, ''The Schizoaffective Continuum: Euclid's Second Axiom,'' *Annals of Clinical Psychiatry*, 1(1989), 19–24.

Schumann, Robert   A German composer (1810–1856) who was forced by a hand injury to abandon a career as a pianist and become a composer. Both as a composer and a critic he was a leader of the romantic movement, but throughout his life he suffered from depression and other mental problems.

In *Outlook*, a newsletter of the Department of Psychiatry of the New York Hospital-Cornell Medical Center, Dr. William A. Frosch, vice chairman and professor of psychiatry at Cornell University Medical College and medical director of the Payne Whitney Clinic, writes of Schumann:

Robert Schumann, who was born in 1810, actually had a manic-depressive illness. His father was said to have had a nervous breakdown from which he never entirely recovered. His mother had a chronic depressive disorder. His eldest sister, described as having a ''quiet madness'' became ill at age 17 and drowned herself at 29. One of Robert Schumann's own eight children showed signs of mental illness by the age of 20, was considered incurable two years later and died in a mental hospital at age 51. Early in Schumann's adolescence he experienced repeated attacks of melancholy. At age 20 he wrote of his ''longing to throw myself in the Rhine.''

In 1854 he did throw himself into the Rhine, but was rescued. He then admitted himself to a mental hospital where he died in 1856 at the age of 46.

The ebb and flow of Schumann's moods can be seen by analyzing his productivity. In 1840 and 1849, in a consistently elevated mood, he produced 24 and 27 works respectively. In 1844, a year when he was in low spirits, he produced no music. Despite increasing mental difficulties from 1850 to his death he was relatively free from depression and hypochondria and was correspondingly productive, composing six to 16 pieces each year.

Frosch, William A., "Moods, Madness, and Music," *Outlook*, Fall 1988.

SCID See STRUCTURED CLINICAL INTERVIEW FOR DSM-III-R.

seasonal affective disorder (SAD) A form of depression that occurs only in the winter and fall, when daylight hours are the shortest. Sometimes it is also referred to as "seasonal affective disorder syndrome" (or SADS).

Statistics vary on the number of Americans afflicted by it, and researchers cite different figures. But some put the number of sufferers in the millions and say that more psychiatric complaints are reported during the winter months than at any other time of the year.

Symptoms of this illness have been recognized for centuries. But by the early 1980s the disorder began to receive widespread attention, and in 1987 the American Psychiatric Association labeled SAD as a distinctive psychiatric disorder. Incidence is more common in higher latitudes, diminishing with proximity to the equator. Victims of SAD may start noticing the disorder in their early 20s, and SAD affects three times as many women as men.

In discussing SAD, two researchers—Dr. Patricia L. McGuire and Dr. Robert Moreines—from New Jersey's Fair Oaks Hospital, a psychiatric, diagnostic, therapeutic and clinical research facility with specialty programs in depression research and treatment, explain: "As cold weather sets in and the days grow shorter most people feel a little 'blue.' Just as the seasons are cyclical, the human body has its own internal cycles. We become more vulnerable to stress and depression in the winter. As the season drags on, these feelings intensify. This is often incorrectly dismissed as merely mid-winter blues or cabin fever. For many people, especially women, the mid-winter blues actually encompass a wide range of seasonal psychiatric, biological and socio/cultural problems."

In "Winter Blues Officially an Illness," Dr. Martin B. Keller, director of outpatient research in psychiatry at Massachusetts General Hospital, was quoted as stating that in the fall he gets many calls from people who feel this depression coming on and, like McGuire and Moreines, Keller stresses that this seasonal depression is more than just a passing of the blues. "In this state people appear more energetic, bright-eyed, more enthusiastic," he said. "But if you're trained in this field or if you know the person, you notice they [sic] don't appear quite right. The euphoric, happy state can quickly turn into a temper outburst and a blue mood."

Keller who served on a 12-member panel that studied a series of psychiatric disorders recommended establishing a clinical outline for SAD. He suggested people diagnosed with SAD must have:

Experienced episodes of depression within the same 60-day fall or winter period in three different years, two of them consecutive.

Endured at least three times as many instances of depression within that two-month time period as during other times of the year.

Recovered from the depressive states during another 60-day period occurring at the same time during each of the years in question.

The exact cause of SAD is not known but it is believed that the absence of bright daylight causes chemical changes in the brain. This affects the production of hormones in the body, with changes in intensity leading to imbalances. MELATONIN, a hormone that helps regulate the body's biological clock (and one that is involved in the production of other hormones), is thought to be a key in the disorder.

Melatonin is secreted by the PINEAL GLAND, a bean-sized gland located at the base of the brain. Dr. Norman Rosenthal of the National Institute of Mental Health (NIMH) has theorized that the problem causing SAD originates in this pineal gland. The gland is active only at night, and during the longer nights of winter, it is more active. As a result it throws off the internal body clock in some susceptible individuals.

During the winter, victims of SAD experience depression, fatigue and a low energy level. They generally require more sleep than usual, but never feel as though they have rested enough. They withdraw from friends and family and experience changes in eating patterns, food preferences and weight. Seventy percent of SAD sufferers gain weight during the winter months. These patients are especially prone to carbohydrate binges. Other symptoms that are linked to SAD are anxiety, irritability and decreased sexual drives. In extreme cases people may even become suicidal.

The condition is treatable, but researchers point out that a plane ticket to the Bahamas is not a particularly logical remedy. "That's a very appealing thing to do, but I don't think it's necessarily good medical practice," stated Keller. Instead, Keller said he would approach the ailment like any other psychological disorder: by determining whether counseling or medication would help. In some instances counselors have advised patients to try to get outdoors more during the winter.

Several research centers are studying LIGHT THERAPY. This theory came about when Dr. Rosenthal speculated that an artificially extended day might help. To test the theory he conducted several experiments in which SAD patients sat in front of special high intensity lamps for up to six hours a day. The vast majority of Rosenthal's test group reported that their depression lifted within two to four days. Dr. Rosenthal recommends, however, that light therapy be tried only under the supervision of a qualified therapist.

Dr. Patricia McGuire points out that unless victims of SAD obtain treatment there is a very good chance they will suffer a downward cycle of depression, anxiety and nervousness six months out of the year. It is the hope of all researchers that future studies will lead to a growing understanding of SAD and expand the understanding of who gets the disorder and why. (See also REVERSE-SAD.)

Cool, Lisa Collier, "Fatigue: Are You Fighting an Internal Clock?" *McCall's*, December 1987.

Diamond, John, "Winter Blues Officially an Illness," *The* [Hackensack, N.J.] *Record*, November 30, 1987.

Ubel, Earl, "You Can Fight Depression," *Parade Magazine*, May 8, 1988.

secondary depression Secondary depression is a depression occurring in a person who has a preexisting nonaffective psychiatric disorder or a serious or life-threatening medical illness that precedes and parallels the symptoms of depression. In "Diagnosis of Depression in the 1980s," Dr. Mark S. Gold, director of research at Fair Oaks Hospital in Summit, New Jersey explains it this way: "Secondary depression and minor depressive illness occur in medical illness and in non-affective psychiatric illness such as obsessive-compulsive neurosis, personality disorders, schizophrenia, drug and alcohol dependence, and sexual dysfunction." Although depression that is secondary to other psychiatric illnesses has been studied to some extent, depression in medically ill patients is less well studied.

The concept of secondary depression was developed at Washington University in St. Louis during the 1960s. Its etiology is not known, and though its symptoms are almost indistinguishable from those of PRIMARY DEPRESSION, secondary depressives have different demographic features and family histories. For example, in "Treatment and Outcome in Secondary Depression: A Naturalistic Study of 1,087 Patients," Dr. Donald W. Black, at the Psychiatric Hospital at the University of Iowa and his colleagues reported that secondary depressives are more likely than primary depressives to be young and male, to have a family history of alcoholism and to have normal suppression to DEXAMETHASONE.

In a study conducted to compare depressions secondary to medical and psychiatric illnesses, Dr. George Winokur of the University of Iowa College of Medicine and his colleagues studied 401 patients with depressions secondary to psychiatric illnesses or depressions secondary to medical illnesses.

In their research they found that the patients with depressions secondary to psychiatric illnesses had an earlier age at onset, were more likely to have suicidal thoughts or to have made suicide attempts, were less likely to have memory problems, were less improved with treatment and more likely to relapse or follow up, and had more alcoholism in their families than patients with depressions secondary to medical illnesses. As a result of this study they concluded that depressions secondary to medical illnesses seem to fit the category of reactive depression, and depressions secondary to psychiatric illnesses fit the definition of neurotic depression.

In the aforementioned study by Dr. Black of 1,087 patients admitted to the University of Iowa Psychiatric Hospital (763 individuals with nonbipolar primary depression and 324 patients with secondary depression), the patients were divided into 4 groups based on the primary mode of therapy received during their hospitalization: (1) ECT, (2) adequate antidepressants, (3) inadequate antidepressants, and (4) patients who received no treatment or therapy. Primary depressives were more likely to have received ECT, and secondary depressives were more likely to have received inadequate antidepressants or no treatment or therapy. A total of 436 primary depressives received adequate therapy, but only 113 secondary depressives did. Overall, primary depressives responded better to treatment (both ECT and antidepressants) than did secondary depressives. A total of 470 primary depressives but only 140 secondary depressives were recovered at discharge. The researchers' conclusion was that secondary depressives are more likely to receive inadequate treatment and are less likely to respond to adequate treatment than are primary depressives.

Speaking generally, however, the effective treatment of secondary depression has not been clearly determined nor has the response to specific treatment, such as ECT and antidepressants, been fully evaluated.

Winokur, George et al., "Depressions Secondary to Other Psychiatric Disorders and Medical Illnesses," *American Journal of Psychiatry*, 145:2(February 1988).

Black, Donald W. et al., "Treatment and Outcome in Secondary Depression: A Naturalistic Study of 1,087 Patients," *Journal of Clinical Psychiatry*, 48:11(1987)

Gold, Mark S., "Diagnosis of Depression in the 1980s," *Journal of the American Medical Association*, 245:15(April 17, 1981).

second (or new) generation of antidepressants   See DRUG THERAPY.

sedative   A drug that tends to calm, moderate or tranquilize a person's state of mind and lessen excessive nervous system activity. (See also TRANQUILIZERS.)

selegiline (Deprenyl)   A drug that slows the progress of PARKINSON'S DISEASE. It is the first drug that has been shown to delay the symptoms of any neurological disease. It does not produce any noticeable side effects. It was approved by the Federal Drug Administration and released in 1989. A federal government-sponsored study on Deprenyl involving 800 patients is underway and is scheduled to be completed in 1991.

self-help   Since the negative thoughts and feelings of depressive disorders—exhaustion, worthlessness, helplessness and hopelessness—make victims feel like giving up, it is important to realize that these negative views are part of the depression and typically do not accurately reflect one's situation. Negative thinking fades as treatment begins to take effect. In the meantime the National Institute of Mental Health (NIMH) recommends the following.

1.   Do not set yourself difficult goals or take on a great deal of responsibility.
2.   Break large tasks into small ones, set some priorities and do what you can as you can.
3.   Do not expect too much from yourself. This will only increase feelings of failure.
4.   Try to be with other people. This is usually better than being alone.
5.   Participate in activities that may make you feel better. You might try mild exercise, going to a movie, a ballgame, or participating in religious or social activities. Don't overdo it or get upset if your mood is not greatly improved right away. Feeling better takes time.
6.   Do not make major life decisions, such as changing jobs, getting married or divorced, without consulting others who know you well and who have a more objective view of your situation. In any case, it is advisable to postpone important decisions until your depression has lifted.
7.   Do not expect to snap out of your depression. People rarely do. Help yourself as much as you can, and do not blame yourself for not being up to par.
8.   Remember, do not accept your negative thinking. It is part of the depression and will disappear as your depression responds to treatment.

self-help/support organizations   The idea of self-help and mutual aid groups for people who face a common concern or condition has become a worldwide phenomenon. In North America alone, an estimated 15 million people attend them, and, according to the New York-based NATIONAL SELF-HELP CLEARINGHOUSE, there are approximately 500,000 groups nationwide.

As more and more mutual aid self-help groups receive increased recognition for social support, practical education and volunteer services, some people believe these groups have become something of an extended family and religion of our times. The groups are not meant to replace needed professional services, however. Rather, they complement and supplement these services, as professionals who have become increasingly aware of their value often refer patients and clients to them. In fact, many victims of depression feel that, along with their medication, it is essential to have community support and a chance to express their feelings and tell their stories of depression and grief to other people who understand and care.

Basically, self-help groups are consumer-oriented, peer-oriented, problem-centered groups in which the member is both the helper and the one to be helped. The groups are important because of their basic theme: "You are not alone." This realization that one is not alone is a great comfort and, through the mutual support the groups offer, all members benefit from the helping process.

Since self-help groups build on the strength of their members, various kinds have arisen to help people through the whole range of life crises and situations. Many bereaved parents, for example, depressed and grief stricken over the loss of a child, are comforted by talking with others who have been through the experience. For them there are such groups as UNITE based in Philadelphia and COMPASSIONATE FRIENDS based in Oak Brook, Illinois. Many self-help/support groups have chapters throughout the country.

Often self-help support groups have HOT LINES that provide people with instant and encouraging help as well as a healing way to gradually enter the mainstream of life again. Across the United States these hotlines cover a wide range of mental health problems, and the numbers that can be called for information and help are often toll-free. Generally they operate on a 24-hour basis. The front pages of county and city telephone directories provide, for easy reference, a list (with phone numbers) of some of the available hot lines.

Names and addresses of support groups can be obtained from self-help clearinghouses such as National Self-Help Clearinghouse; also see Appendix 6. (See also COMMUNITY MENTAL HEALTH SERVICE; GRIEF THERAPY/TREATMENT; TREATMENT OF DEPRESSION.)

senility (organic brain syndrome) See ELDERLY.

serotonin A biogenic amine that assists in the transmission of electrochemical impulses from one nerve cell to another in the brain and activates the "on" switches in the nerve cells of the brain. As one of the NEUROTRANSMITTERS and key chemicals, it is instrumental, along with other brain chemicals, in regulating certain brain activities, including emotion. While studying depression, some researchers have determined that there is also a link between serotonin deficiency and suicide, since researchers have identified a deficiency of this neurotransmitter in the brains of some people who are prone to take their own lives. Thus, their understanding is that serotonin deficiency occurs in people

more prone to impulsive violence and that, when they become depressed, these individuals are then more likely to commit suicide. As a result, serotonin deficiency and depression together expand the risk of suicide more than either one alone.

sex factors Although the interpretation of statistics may vary the National Institute of Mental Health (NIMH) states that during any six-month period 6.6% of all women and 3.5% of all men suffer from depression. Studies have indicated that depressive symptoms are highest in women under 35, and the greatest rates are found in young poor mothers of small children who are single heads of households. These women, faced with raising children with little if any emotional and financial support, appear particularly vulnerable. According to Dr. Myrna Weissman, who conducted depression research at the Yale School of Medicine, it was found that the profile of the person most likely to be depressed has shifted (since the 1930s) from an impoverished middleaged or elderly woman to a young urban woman, either married or single, usually with small children and a family history of depression. Other research by sociologists George W. Brown and Tirril Harris, reported in *The Female Malady: Women, Madness and English Culture, 1830–1980*, showed that women were more likely to suffer from severe depression if they had three or more children under the age of 14 at home; if they had no one to confide in; or if they had lost their mother before the age of 11. For workingclass women, financial and housing problems also contributed.

All the reasons for the higher incidence among younger women are not clear, but genetic, hormonal and sociological influences are being investigated. Researchers from the National Institute of Mental Health (NIMH) point out that the factors contributing to the situation that might be faced by families headed by young single women include inadequate finances, lack of child support payments, and a woman's inability to earn income sufficient to make ends meet. Too often these young women have left school prematurely and lack the educational skills required to gain access to higher paying jobs. Also, unless they can arrange affordable child care, they may not be able to work at all.

The stresses facing women today might seem to contribute to their high rates of depression. Yet some experts argue that women are not more vulnerable to depression than men, but just deal with their symptoms differently. Women, they say, are more apt to admit feelings of depression and seek professional assistance, whereas men may be socially conditioned to repress such feelings.

On the other hand, social conditioning also has been cited as contributing to the higher incidence of depression among women. One theory suggests that young girls are taught to be helpless and therefore are vulnerable to depression when faced with the problems and decisions of adulthood. According to the "learned helplessness" theory, female children are either ignored or punished for taking control of situations. By implication, girls learn that take-charge behaviors suitable for boys are considered unfeminine or not "nice" for girls. Studies show that individuals discouraged from acting on their own behalf tend to become passive and eventually avoid responsibility. A vicious cycle is set in motion, and passsivity leads to lack of control, which leads to feelings of helplessness and depression. In addition to the psychosocial explanations for higher rates of depression among women, hormonal functioning is considered a possible influencing factor, although new research contradicts the risks of depression that women face after childbirth, HYSTERECTOMY and MENOPAUSE. According to these findings, serious depression is far less common after these events than has been believed, while the risks of depression after a MASTECTOMY are higher than is commonly realized.

Between the ages of 45 and 60 depression in women tends to decrease with age. In fact, according to a study by Universtiy of Wisconsin Medical School psychiatry researchers that began as an investigation of risk factors for depression, women aged 50 and older are amazingly resilient to life's stresses. However, in researching depression associated with older women, Marilyn J. Essex, Ph.D., found that a major cause of depression in older women is a lack of intimacy. In her article "Depression Associated with Lack of Intimacy in Older Women" she writes: "Research has consistently shown that intimate or confident relationships are crucial to emotional well-being. As we grow older, however, these relationships are increasingly likely to be lost or negatively affected by other common losses (e.g., retirement, moves, deaths, chronic health problems, financial problems). Because women tend to outlive men, they are even more likely to experience such losses and, thus, are especially at risk for lack of intimacy and consequent depression."

The results of a two-year study on women and depression conducted by a task force of the American Psychological Association and released in 1989 have suggested that forms of psychotherapy lasting as little as 12 to 16 weeks are proving increasingly effective in treating depressed women and that long-term therapy and years of medication may not be necessary for many of the millions of American women who suffer from depression. In reviewing research the task force found that several forms of short-term therapy are well suited for treating women's depression. On their own or in combination with each other or with antidepressant medications, the therapies offer at least temporary relief within three to four months. One of those therapies, known as INTERPERSONAL PSYCHOTHERAPY, focuses narrowly on current "interpersonal problems," such as grief or a dispute over a woman's role in marriage. According to the task force the emphasis on relationships makes the therapy especially appropriate for women who derive much of their identity and sense of well-being from relationships.

The task force also called for wider use of COGNITIVE THERAPY, which aims to correct distorted thinking such as negative and pessimistic views of oneself and the world, and behavioral treatments for depression, which aim to teach social skills, problem-solving, assertiveness and other skills.

Robin Post, a clinical psychologist at the University of Colorado Health Sciences Center and a member of the task force, said that studies indicate those therapies have proven effective in as little as eight to 16 weeks. She said, however, that depression is often cyclical and that some 20% to 45% of women who are helped will experience a recurrence.

The task force made up of nearly two dozen therapists in research and private practice began the study in response to accumulating evidence that depression was increasing, particularly among women. In summing up their findings, the members stated that it was important for women to understand that they can get relief from depression without embarking upon a decade of psychotherapy and years on antidepressant drugs.

Although up until age 65 twice as many women as men are treated for depressive disorders (with the exception of bipolar disorder, which occurs equally in both sexes), depression peaks among men between the ages of 25 and 45 (see MALE POSTPARTUM DEPRESSION). After 65 the depression rates begin to equalize between the sexes.

Some experts attribute the high point of depression among men between the ages of 25 and 45 to failed expectations (see MID-LIFE). Others say there is no overall evidence that depression necessarily arises from failed hopes and plans at this time of life. However, negative events often do begin to occur as people enter their 40s, and in some situations it's probable those events can initiate depression.

Another peak prevalence for depressive symptoms in men tends to appear in the 55 to 70 age range. Some researchers believe RETIREMENT (with the boredom and lack of self-esteem that sometimes accompanies it) contributes to the higher rates of depresssion among older men who are brought up to see their self-worth in terms of work and productivity. Along with retirement, possible health problems, waning strength, death of friends and loved ones, awareness of mortality and, often, a sense of uselessness combine to make older men more vulnerable to depression. (See also AGE FACTORS; MISCARRIAGE; POSTPARTUM DEPRESSION; PREMENSTRUAL DEPRESSION.)

Schmeck, Harold M., Jr. "Depression Studies Bring New Drugs and Insights," *The New York Times*, February 16, 1988.

Showalter, Elaine. *The Female Malady: Women, Madness, and English Culture, 1830–1980* (New York: Pantheon, 1985).

Ubell, Earl, "You Can Fight Depression," *Parade Magazine*, May 8, 1988.

Essex, Marilyn J., "Depression Associated with Lack of Intimacy in Older Women," *Geriatric Medicine Today*, 6:3(March 1987).

Record, The, "Quicker Cures for Depressed Women," *The* [Hackensack, N.J.] *Record* (from *Los Angeles Times News Service*), August 13, 1989.

Goleman, Daniel, "Wide Beliefs on Depression in Women Contradicted," *The New York Times*, January 9, 1990.

shock therapy   See ELECTROCONVULSIVE THERAPY (ECT).

side effects of drugs   See DRUG THERAPY, SIDE EFFECTS.

Sinemet   A currently available drug for the treatment of PARKINSON'S DISEASE. (See also LEVODOPA; SINEMET CR.)

Sinemet CR   A medication for treating PARKINSON'S DISEASE that, at this writing, is under consideration for release by the U.S.

Food and Drug Administration. It has been studied extensively by Dr. Thomas Hutton, professor and director of the Parkinson's Disease Information and Referral Center at Texas Tech University. Other multi-site studies have been done at eight medical centers in the United States. Four different formulations of carbidopa/LEVODOPA, employing a synthetic polymeric matrix to control rates of release of both agents, have been studied in clinical trials. The preparations studied are known by the manufacturer as Sinemet CR, and if Sinemet CR-4 (the last in the series of clinical trials) is approved by the FDA it will be marketed under the name Sinemet CR.

According to Dr. Hutton, Sinemet CR has advantages over currently available SINEMET in the group of advanced Parkinsonian patients that was studied. The number of daily doses required is reduced by about a third, and there is also a significant reduction in the motor fluctuations so characteristic of the illness. The medication is well tolerated, and researchers are now studying whether or not Sinemet CR will stall the onset of motor fluctuations. Although clinical trials have yielded generally promising results, an important consideration is whether the clinical profile of Sinemet CR will continue with long-term administration.

Hutton, J.T. and Morris, J.L., "Long Acting Levodopa Preparations," *Neurology* Supplement, October 1989.

sleeping pills   Short-acting BARBITURATES that are calming and sleep-inducing are commonly known as sleeping pills. The pills act as central nervous system depressants, and their effect lasts about five or six hours. When not abused they produce little or no hangover.

However, sleeping pills can be easily abused because they begin to lose their effectiveness after only a few days of regular use, and increased doses may be required to induce sleep. When this happens depressives can develop a dangerous pattern of dependency and addiction. As they feel the need to use sleeping pills more and more, they find it

increasingly difficult to stop using them. When they try, severe insomnia can be a withdrawal symptom. Thus the sleeping problem becomes worse, and depressives are apt to conclude there is no way they can give up the pills.

Sleeping pills are not antidepressants and the National Institute of Mental Health (NIMH) advises that they should not be taken alone for depression. They are legitimately available only by prescription, but the government estimates that 20% of legally manufactured barbiturates are deflected to the black market and sold illicitly.

sleep and sleep disorders   In the past 30 years scientists have done a great deal of research in sleep laboratories where they study people as they sleep. Information obtained from recording brain activity, heart rate and other body functions is matched with people's own records of their sleep habits. Rhythms relating to sleep are studied by using all-night recordings of electroencephalograms (EECs), which measure brain activity.

Such studies have shown that there are two types of sleep. One, associated with RAPID EYE MOVEMENT, is called REM sleep. The other is called non-REM sleep. Non-REM sleep has four stages. Stage 1 is the lightest sleep, and stage 4 is the deepest.

Sleep problems and disturbances go hand in hand with depression, and studies show that depressed people often miss the most restful stage of sleep. While some tend to sleep all the time, others suffer from insomnia (a disturbance of the biological rhythm of waking and sleeping).

Although research shows insomnia is a common characteristic of depression, it is important to point out that depression alone is not the only cause of insomnia. The latter can also be caused by misinformation about sleep requirements, a preoccupation about getting enough sleep, certain drugs (such as amphetamines) and alcohol.

The various sleep disorders experienced by depressives vary with different types of depression. But studies show that both bipolar and unipolar depressed patients (see BIPO-LAR DEPRESSION; UNIPOLAR DEPRESSION) sleep less, have less deep sleep, take longer to fall asleep, and wake more frequently and earlier in the morning than do normals. Their most common complaints are intense sleepiness in early evening; inability to go back to sleep after awakening during the night; no feeling of rest on waking; and a restless, tired, jittery feeling throughout the day. In mania sleep is further reduced without producing fatigue, a reduction particularly marked, in many cases, the night before the switch into mania, when no sleep at all is common.

In sleep research studies at the National Institute of Mental Health (NIMH) researchers are experimenting with modifying sleep patterns in depressed patients. Keeping patients up for 24 hours, or in some cases the second half of the night, has temporarily alleviated depressive symptoms for a day or two in some people. Dr. Thomas Wehr and a team of scientists are working on the problem of why depriving depressed people of sleep seems to cure the depression—at least until they go back to sleep.

Some depressed people, particularly those whose sleeping patterns have been severely disrupted by depression, are helped by advancing the time period during which they sleep. This treatment is thought to reset the biological clock involved in controlling normal life rhythms, such as eating and sleeping cycles and the production of internal hormones, all of which can be disrupted during a depressive illness.

Hypnotic sedatives that depress the CENTRAL NERVOUS SYSTEM and can be either barbiturates or nonbarbiturates are frequently used to alleviate sleep disorders. But, as previously mentioned, certain drugs and alcohol can actually add to one's sleeping problems. SLEEPING PILLS can be easily abused because, after only a few days of regular use, they begin to lose their effectiveness and increased doses may be required to induce sleep. When this happens, depressives can develop a dangerous pattern of dependency

and addiction. Therefore, the U.S. Department of Health and Human Services advises that sleeping medications should be used only for short-term management of sleep disorders. Initial prescriptions should be limited, and the automatic refilling of prescriptions is not recommended. Some sleeping medications have a prolonged effect and may cause a hangover-like feeling the next day. Alcohol can also disturb the pattern of sleep stages, sometimes promoting sleep, sometimes hindering it.

The amino acid L-TRYPTOPHAN is contained in a number of "health-store" sleep preparations as well as in meat, lettuce and milk. Some claim that L-tryptophan induces sleep "naturally" by stimulating the production of SEROTONIN. This is no longer the prevailing opinion, however, and in November 1989 the Federal Drug Administration asked manufactureres and retailers to voluntarily remove products with L-tryptophan from shelves immediately. The FDA said it had found an "unequivocal link" between consumption of L-tryptophan supplements and a sudden outbreak of a rare blood disorder called eosinophilia-myalgia syndrome. Until scientists are able to pinpoint the cause of the outbreak of illness, it is advisable to adhere to the FDA recall and refrain from taking products containing L-tryptophan.

Patient Care, "Insominia," *Patient Care*, August 15, 1980.

Doherty, Matthew J., "L-tryptophan Is Still Around Despite Recall," *The* [Hackensack, N.J.] *Record,* December 1, 1989.

Social Psychiatry Research Institute A New York-based center that carries on research, evaluation and treatment of depression. Address: 150 E. 69th St., New York, NY 10021. Phone: 212-628-4800. (See also KIEV, ARI.)

sporadic depressive disease (SDD) A term used for the condition of depressives who have no history of psychiatric illness in any first-degree relative.

stages of grief   We know that the course of MOURNING runs through different stages (typically beginning even before the death) as people progress from the onset of GRIEF, through the shock and reality, to functioning as usual. We also know we all react differently to grief. Various researchers have divided grief into different stages. Dr. Elizabeth Kubler-Ross divided it into five stages. Dr. Roberta Temes separates it into three stages (see BEREAVEMENT). Dr. Granger Westberg, a pioneer in the field of religion and health, sums up the varied views on the passages, or stages, of grief in his book *Good Grief*:

1. A state of shock produces overwhelming sorrow and sense of unreality.
2. Emotional release begins as the reality of the loss sets in.
3. A sense of isolation starts and depression is a universal experience.
4. Some people become physically ill because of unresolved grief.
5. Panic sets in when people are unable to concentrate and can think of nothing but the loss.
6. People experience normal guilt or neurotic guilt about a loss.
7. Hostility and resentment can take over and grief-stricken people can become critical of everyone who was related to their loss.
8. There's difficulty in returning to usual activities.
9. Hope breaks through gradually.
10. A struggle to readjust to reality occurs.

(See also GRIEF, CAUSES AND EFFECTS OF; GRIEF THERAPY/TREATMENT; LENGTH OF GRIEVING PROCESS.)

Westberg, Granger, *Good Grief* (Philadelphia: Fortress Press, 1971)

steroids   The term steroid applies to a group of fatlike compounds with similar chemical structure. Basically, steroids are chemical activators and regulators, and they operate most notably in connection with the adrenal cortex and the sex glands. As they are secreted by the glands they are involved in various body functions.

Dr. Nathan S. Kline reported in *From Sad to Glad* that several steroids have been implicated in depressed-patient studies, but the one that showed up most markedly was CORTISOL. Numerous investigations disclosed a sharp rise in cortisol production by depressive patients and a corresponding decrease as recuperation set in. Kline stated that there was also some evidence that the amount of increased cortisol output might be an index to the severity of the case, though views differ on this.

Anabolic steriods (a synthetic compound) have received a great deal of notoriety for their use during athletic training to stimulate muscle development. Physicians and educators fought steroid abuse because of the long-term dangers of athletes taking them orally or by injection. Psychological effects and mood swings are possible side effects.

In the United States anabolic steroids can be obtained legally only by prescription, but there is a large black market. The drugs are legally manufactured by pharmaceutical companies in the United States and overseas and illegally at foreign and domestic underground laboratories.

stillbirth   A stillbirth is the death of a fetus between the 20th week and delivery. It can leave a family unprepared for the grief and depression they feel as they envision the lost baby as a loss of their future and idealized hope. Counselors and obstetrical-gynecological professionals who are close to parents during this time believe the grieving process cannot and should not be denied or minimized. In fact, some feel it can help the process if (when the parents so choose) the full-term or near-full-term stillborn baby, dressed and in a blanket, can be brought to them to see, touch and hold sometime after delivery.

The prime cause of stillbirth seems to be

loss of oxygen to the baby, either because of an umbilical cord accident before or during labor or because of a problem with the placenta. There is no known cause for up to one half of all stillbirths. (See also GRIEF; NEWBORN DEATH; Appendix 6.)

Amoroso, Mary, "When A Hope and a Dream Are Stillborn," *The* [Hackensack, N.J.] *Record,* July 21, 1987.

Anon., "A Special Kind of Grief," *University of California, Berkley Wellness Letter,* August 1988.

stimulants   Drugs that stimulate the CENTRAL NERVOUS SYSTEM and increase the activity of the brain or spinal cord. Amphetamines, cocaine, caffeine and nicotine are classified as stimulants. Since stimulants produce greater energy, increase alertness and create a feeling of euphoria they are often abused. The greatest abuse occurs with amphetamines and cocaine.

stress   Stress is a physical, chemical or emotional factor that causes bodily or mental tension. Though some stress is part of daily life, too much of it on people's minds and bodies can precipitate depression.

In *Depression: How to Recognize It, How to Cure It and How to Grow From it* Wina Sturgeon writes:

There are three aspects of stress which almost always precede a case of depression. First is a period of prolonged stress. This is of course a subjective matter. In one person a three-month stressful period may be considered prolonged. In another, there may be no signs of strain after three years of stress. But eventually the body will react in a negative way. The second aspect—one could almost call these aspects stages, because they come in sequence—is a feeling of being overwhelmed by all the pressures and things to be done. This can result in what could be called "circling" activity, the kind of thing one sees with a mouse caught in a

trap. The circling activity of the person facing a mountain of things-to-be-done may consist of getting on the phone and talking for hours before tackling any of the work. In other words, circling activity is trying to push the mountain out of sight by running all around it picking weeds. The third stage is a feeling of powerlessness. It's a sense of helplessness, a sense that one has no control over one's fate.

Research suggests that brain chemicals can be transformed by stress, particularly when people feel they're not in control, and this can produce depression. Stress also causes certain nutrients to be used by the body at a much faster rate than under normal conditions. As a result, there's a higher need for these nutrients, and usually the need isn't met by diet alone. Furthermore these same nutrients are needed by the central nervous system to manufacture the biogenic amines.

The chemical and behavioral responses of animals to stress are particularly vital to research, because such experiments can't be done on people. In "The Dark Affliction of Mind and Body" Winifred Gallagher reported on experiments done by Jacqueline Crawley, a behavioral neuropharmacologist at the National Institute of Mental Health (NIMH), who found that when a Siberian hamster, one of the few rodents to form enduring partnerships, is taken from its mate, the males in particular show signs of depression, with low serotonin levels, weight fluctuation and inactivity (just as, in humans, widowers show these symptoms and appear to suffer more than widows after a spouse's death). When restored to their mates—or given antidepressants—the animals recover. This sort of reaction to separation, pronounced in primate mothers and babies, underscores the importance of affection and dependency. Simple intimacy seems to offer some protection against depression, which exists at high levels among separated and divorced people.

Researchers also believe massive stress early in life, like the lack of parental love and care, is coded in a girl's memory, creating a sensitivity. Later, divorce reactivates that sensitivity and her first depression results. Subsequently, she may not even require an external stress to become depressed.

According to the Gallagher article, stress experiments have revealed surprising connections between depression and anxiety, and many depressed people are anxious as well. Some anxiety and panic disorders are treated effectively with antidepressants, which implies that the same neurochemicals are involved in both anxiety and depression. Whereas some stresses affect individuals, others affect whole groups, even generations. Because the shift of depression to the younger population has occurred too quickly to have had a genetic origin, epidemiologists think it could be the result of large numbers of vulnerable people being subjected to increasingly common risk factors like divorce and solitary urban life. Just being a baby boomer, competing with a huge number of peers for jobs, housing or a moment in the limelight, might be a risk.

When stress builds up and precipitates or causes depression it is important to obtain help before mental and emotional woes get out of hand. Help and referrals are available through medical professionals, clergy, social workers, psychologists and mental health centers and associations. Tranquilizers can help stress when used as prescribed, but no drugs should be taken except when ordered by a physician.

Gallagher, Winifred, "The Dark Affliction of Mind and Body," *Discover*, 7:5(May 1986).

Sturgeon, Wina, *Depression: How to Recognize It, How to Cure It and How to Grow From It* (Englewood Cliffs, N.J.: Prentice-Hall, 1979).

Structured Clinical Interview for DSM-III-R The Structured Clinical Interview for DSM-III (SCID) is an instrument designed to enable a clinically-trained interviewer to make DSM-III-R diagnoses. The criteria that are included in the SCID are the diagnostic criteria that appear in DSM-III-R. Two standard versions of the instrument are available for diagnosis.

The first version—SCID-P (patient version)—is designed for use with subjects who are identified as psychiatric patients. It contains the following modules, or standards of measurement: mood syndromes; psychotic and associated symptoms; psychotic disorders; mood disorders; psychoactive substance use disorders; anxiety disorders; somatoform disorders; eating disorders; adjustment disorders.

The second version—SCID-NP (nonpatient version)—is for subjects not identified as psychiatric patients. Its diagnostic standards are the same as those of the SCID-P except that it substitutes a psychotic screening module for the more detailed and lengthy psychotic disorder modules that are in the SCID-P. SCID diagnostic materials and further information on SCID can be obtained from Dr. Robert L. Spitzer, Chief, Biometrics Research Department, New York State Psychiatric Institute, 733 West 168 St., Box 74, New York, NY 10032.

Styron, William A prominent American novelist (1926– , *Sophie's Choice, Lie Down in Darkness*) and a victim of clinical depression that affected him so badly he could not read and comprehend a simple newspaper article, let alone write anything.

In 1985 he began suffering from profound depression, which he first thought had been caused by tranquilizers prescribed to ease his withdrawal from alcohol. When the pain from the depression became intolerable he committed himself to the psychiatric ward of Yale-New Haven Hospital in the winter of 1985–86. Although he never attempted suicide during his depression he has said that the possibility was real and the desire great.

In "Styron's Choice" by Philip Caputo, Styron stated that there were probably three causes for his depressive illness. The first was excessive drinking. The second was a genetic link to the problem because both of his parents were depressives. (Along with the genetic link Styron also lost his mother when he was a young boy, and some people believe that persons who have lost a parent early in life are more apt to become victims of depression.) The third reason Styron pinpointed was a problem he was having with a novel he was writing. He knew something was missing in the novel but day after day he could not find the missing element. The more frustrated he became over this the more stress he felt—and the more he drank to relieve the stress the more depressed he grew. Then he drank some more to lift himself out of depression. (After his release from the hospital Styron attended Alcoholics Anonymous.)

Following his release and recovery Styron's doctors assured him he had a 95% chance of never suffering a recurrence of depression. But in summing up his private hell Styron reported in the Caputo article that, along with drugs and psychotherapy, the support of his wife, children and friends was the greatest help in bringing him out of his despair. Said Styron: "I can't imagine anything more horrible than suffering through depression alone."

Caputo, Philip, "Styron's Choice," *Esquire*, December 1986.

substance abuse   A general term used to describe the abuse of drugs.

suicidal warning signs   Many people who commit suicide have given warnings to friends and family. A signal or warning may be a statement such as "I wish I were dead," "I can't take any more—I want out" or "My family and friends would be better off without me." Some people even tell a friend about a plan to kill themselves before they actually take this action. If a friend of yours talks like this, take it seriously immediately and be aware of what your friend has said.

Other warning signs include: disruptive behavior, a high degree of hopelessness, physical illness, excessive substance abuse, changes in eating and sleeping habits, giving away prized possessions, a withdrawal from usual activities and relationships, and reaction to the loss of a spouse, parent, relative or friend.

In *Feeling Good: The New Mood Therapy* Dr. David B. Burns explains that for many people suicide attempts seem to be warm-ups in which they flirt with suicide but have not mastered the particular methods they have selected. The fact that an individual has made this attempt unsuccessfully on several occasions in the past indicates an increased risk of success in the future. It is a dangerous myth that unsuccessful suicide attempts are simply gestures or attention-getting devices and are therefore not to be taken seriously. Burns stresses that current thinking suggests suicidal thoughts or actions are to be taken seriously. It can be highly misleading to view suicidal thoughts and actions as merely a plea for help. Many suicidal people want help least of all because they are 100 percent convinced they are hopeless and beyond help.

To this Glen Evans and Norman L. Farberow add in *The Encyclopedia of Suicide:* "Twelve percent of those who attempt suicide will make a second try and succeed within two years. Four out of five persons who do kill themselves have attempted to do so at least one time previously. Any suicide effort must be taken with greatest seriousness."

Burns, David D., *Feeling Good: The New Mood Therapy* (New York: New American Library, 1980).

Evans, Glen and Farberow, Norman L., *The Encyclopedia of Suicide* (New York: Facts On File, 1988).

suicide   The alarming possibility that severely depressed persons will eventually resort to suicide is one of the greatest complications of depression and grief. In fact, the National Institute of Mental Health (NIMH) has noted that 15% of seriously depressed people will eventually take their own lives.

Sometimes long-lasting feelings of worth-lessness, isolation and pain cause suicidal feelings that remain just thoughts. At other times they lead to actual attempts.

The actual attempts are common among persons hospitalized for depression at some time in their lives, and the greatest risk is during or immediately following hospitalization. Attempts are also common among individuals who experience depression in post-withdrawal states from drugs. The possibility of suicide attempts often increases with advancing age, though in recent years there have been alarming increases in suicide among adolescents and young adults. However, suicide from grief and depression is a potential at any age.

According to the latest statistical data on suicide in the United States released by the National Center for Health Statistics in October 1988 (U.S. Suicide: 1986 Official Final Data), suicide is the 8th-ranking cause of death in the United States. Each year 30,904 people commit suicide. There are 3.6 male completions (24,226) for each female completion (6,678), though there are three female attempts for each male attempt. Firearms are the most common means of suicide among males, while drugs are the most common among females.

In the white population 28,437 take their lives as opposed to 2,467 nonwhites and 1,892 blacks. For elderly people (65+ years) the number of suicides is 6,275. For young people (15–24) the number is 5,120. On the average one old person every hour and 24 minutes commits suicide, and one young person every hour and 43 minutes. On the overall average one person every 17 minutes kills himself. Beyond that, it is estimated that five million living Americans have attempted to commit suicide.

In recent years researchers have identified a deficiency of the neurotransmitter SEROTONIN as one clue to why such a large number of depressed individuals commit suicide. Low serotonin activity has also been linked to aggression and impulsiveness. To support the latter theory, autopsies performed on the brains of suicide victims have indicated that those who committed violent suicide (gunshot and knife wounds) had lower levels of serotonin functioning than those who committed nonviolent suicide (sleeping pills). Some researchers view such suicides as the result of an interaction of depression with a biochemical predisposition to aggression and impulsiveness.

Other views of suicide label it as an act of temporary insanity or a puzzling failure of moral strength. But persons who have suffered severe depression are quick to say that suicide cannot be dissociated from depression and that depression can generate such a strong urge to self-destruction that—when there is no respite from the illness—victims begin to think ceaselessly of oblivion.

In writing about the highly-publicized 1987 suicide of the eminent Italian writer Primo Levi, who was in the depths of clinical depression when he jumped down a stairwell in Turin, novelist WILLIAM STYRON (who battled clinical depression himself) wrote in The New York Times: "Suicide remains a tragic and dreadful act, but its prevention will continue to be hindered, and the age-old stigma against it will remain, unless we can begin to understand that the vast majority of those who do away with themselves—and those who attempt to do so—do not do it because of any frailty and rarely out of impulse but because they are in the grip of an illness that causes almost unimaginable pain."

Many researchers, survivors of depression, and family and friends left behind by suicide victims believe that lives are lost to suicide because of failure to obtain diagnosis and treatment in time. In fact, Styron concluded: "I find it difficult not to believe that if Mr. Levi had been under capable hospital attention, sequestered from the unbearable daily world in a setting where he would have been safe from his self-destructive urge, and where time would have permitted the storm raging in his brain to calm itself and die away, he would be among us now."

Goleman, Daniel, "Study of Normal Mourning Process Illuminates Grief Gone Awry," *The New York Times*, March 29, 1988.

———, "Clues to Suicide: A Brain Chemical Is Implicated," *The New York Times*, October 8, 1985.

Schmeck, Harold M., Jr., "Depression Studies Bring New Drugs and Insights," *The New York Times*, February 16, 1988.

Styron, William, "Why Primo Levi Need Not Have Died," *The New York Times*, December 19, 1988.

Ubell, Earl, "You Can Fight Depression," *Parade Magazine*, May 8, 1988.

suicide prevention centers   The suicide prevention centers around the country are set up to offer—by telephone—immediate help and positive, postponing suggestions to would-be suicides who are still in control of their actions enough to want to talk to someone about their contemplated suicide.

From their side of their cry for help, potential suicides try to communicate their desperation and intent to take their lives. On the other end, the trained person receiving the call will listen, understand, answer and do everything in his or her power to talk the would-be suicide out of his contemplated action. That trained person will listen and talk for as long as the caller wants to pour out his problems and feelings.

In the process the person at the prevention center will use his or her power of persuasion to keep the caller on the line until he or she can obtain a name, address and telephone number from the caller. The goal is to buy time by encouraging the person to at least postpone the act. Once the act is postponed the depressed individual may ultimately feel better and decide to get further help and give life another chance.

For a state-by-state listing of crisis phone numbers and suicide prevention and crisis intervention agencies in the United States

contact: American Association of Suicidology, 2459 S. Ash St. Denver, CO 80222. Phone: 303-692-0985.

suppressed grief   See GRIEF.

supra-additive   Descriptive of an interaction of drugs (synergistic or potentiating) in which the effect of two drugs in combination is greater than it would be if the effects were simply additive. (See also SYNERGY.)

Switzerland   Basel-Stadt was one of the five study areas for the WORLD HEALTH ORGANIZATION (WHO) COLLABORATIVE STUDY ON STANDARDIZED ASSESSMENT OF DEPRESSIVE DISORDERS, designed: (1) to develop and test simple instruments for clinical description of depressive states; (2) to use these instruments to examine series of "average" depressive patients in different cultures; and (3) to set up a network of field research centers. This study area is situated along the Rhine River in the northwest of Switzerland. It borders on the Federal Republic of Germany and France.

Basel-Stadt is almost exclusively an urban canton (a term for one of the states of the Swiss confederation). The catchment area of the University Psychiatric Clinic coincides with the demicanton of Basel-Stadt, which includes the communities of Basel (city), Riehen and Bettingen. This clinic is the only psychiatric institution obliged to admit patients from the catchment area. Most depressive patients are admitted on a voluntary basis, usually on the advice of the family physician or the family.

The selection of patients for the study in the clinic was made in the special ward for depressive patients. Compared with many other areas the population of the Basel catchment area seems to show greater acceptance of psychiatric care. Even patients with mild depression come to the clinic and ask for help. Depressive illnesses of the patients included in the study may therefore be, on the whole, less severe than those of patients admitted to other psychiatric hospitals in the canton or the country. (See also Appendix 1, Tables.)

Sartorius, N. et al., *Depressive Disorders in Different Cultures,* (Geneva: World Health Organization, 1983).

symptoms of grief See GRIEF.

synapse A microscopic gap between the neurons in the chemical network of the brain. Within the brain billions of neurons send and receive electrical messages across these minute gaps by means of specific amounts of neurotransmitters.

synergistic effect See SYNERGY.

synergy The joint action or cooperation of two drugs that, when taken together, are more effective than when used individually.

Because of this phenomenon, an amount of a drug that might normally be safe can have a devastating effect if taken with a drug that acts synergistically. For example, a small amount of alcohol combined with a very small dose of a barbiturate can have a much greater effect than either alcohol or a barbiturate taken alone.

In *The Encyclopedia of Drug Abuse* Robert O'Brien and Sidney Cohen write:

The synergistic process begins in the liver, which metabolizes ingested material. When two drugs are taken together the enzyme system that processes them is overwhelmed because it does not have the capacity to metabolize both at the same time. In the case of alcohol and a barbiturate drug, which compete for the same enzymes, alcohol is always processed first. The barbiturate meanwhile accumulates in the blood where it has an exaggerated effect on the body and the mind. This delayed metabolization of the barbiturate can result in a tripling or quadrupling of its potency when it enters the central nervous system.

The Third Special Report to the U.S. Congress on Alcohol and Health defined an interaction between alcohol or other central nervous system depressants, and a drug as "any alteration in the pharmacologic properties of either due to the presence of the other." The report classified three different types of interactions:

(1) Antagonistic, in which the effects of one or both drugs are blocked or reduced;

(2) Additive, in which the effect is the sum of the effects of each:

(3) Supra-additive (synergistic or potentiating), in which the effect of the two drugs in combination is greater than it would be if the effects were additive.

The SUPRA-ADDITIVE effect is the most dangerous because it can at times prove fatal. Although not quite as dangerous, the antagonistic effect can be hazardous when the therapeutic effects of one drug are reduced by the presence of the other.

Drugs also have a half-life; this is the amount of time it takes for the body to remove half of the drug from the system. For drugs with a half-life of 24 hours or more, such as Valium, half of the first dose may still be in the body when the next is taken. After several days the build up can be fairly large, and when alcohol or another central nervous system depressant is taken the result can be devastating.

O'Brien, Robert and Cohen, Sidney, *The Encyclopedia of Drug Abuse* (New York: Facts On File, 1984).

T

tachycardia Palpitations or an abnormally rapid beating of the heart. It may be the result of emotion, exercise or heart disease.

"talking" treatment See PSYCHOTHERAPY.

tardive dyskinesia (TD) Abnormal movements of the facial and limb muscles seen in some psychiatric patients. It can be a side effect caused by the use of some neuroleptic drugs, and is a distressing condition in which patients make uncontrollable grimaces or jerky movements. Some researchers believe that TD patients have chronically lower levels of DOPAMINE, NOREPINEPHRINE and SEROTONIN in the CENTRAL NERVOUS SYSTEM. Given the precipitant of neuroleptic treatment these patients are more prone to develop TD.

"While the majority of TD cases have been reported in chronic schizophrenics who are the patients most likely to be treated with neuroleptics, the presence of a diagnosis or symptomatology of depression has been implicated as being associated with increased risk for the disorder in several reports," stated Dr. Mary Ann Richardson of the Nathan S. Kline Institute for Psychiatric Research.

In a study conducted by Richardson and her colleagues during a four-month period at a state psychiatric center, male subjects (aged 18 to 44) were screened for study inclusion if they were current inpatients or newly admitted, diagnosed schizophrenics with not less than three years nor more than 20 years since first treatment. Among other findings, the researchers suggest that a schizophrenic patient who has TD is also characterized by a symptom constellation that is affective in quality, but more in the direction of mania than depression.

"That symptoms of mania and TD could be seen together would fit with traditional theoretical mechanisms for both disorders—i.e., that of an increase in amine activity for mania and a supersensitive dopamine receptor for TD," pointed out Richardson in her paper.

In summary, Richardson's paper covers characteristics that discriminate the TD patients from the patients without TD in a population of young male schizophrenics. The characteristics include a longer time since first treatment; symptoms of tension, excite-ment, mannerisms and posturing and hostility; a history of manic symptoms; and a family history of major affective disorder. "The extension of these findings to other psychiatric population (e.g., female schizophrenics) remains for future work, as does a more precise delineation than was attempted in this study of the content and severity of the possible manic symptomatology experienced by patients with TD versus those without the disorder," Richardson concluded.

Richardson, M.A. et al., "Tardive Dyskinesia and Depressive Symptoms in Schizophrenics," *Psychopharmacology Bulletin,* 21(1985).

teenage depression See YOUNG PEOPLES' DEPRESSION.

Tegretol See CARBAMAZEPINE.

thyroid gland Research indicates that this gland, which lies at the base of the neck, may be another biological link to depression, and in the past few years some of the scientific research involving circadian rhythms, the body's natural cycles, has been directed at this gland.

Normally the pituitary gland generates a hormone at night that stimulates the thyroid. But sleep suppresses this procedure. In patients cycling to mania or in depressed patients deprived of sleep, the levels of the thyroid-stimulating hormone fluctuate between highs and lows. Researchers have observed increased levels of thyroid disease in manic-depressive patients, especially those with rapid cycles of the highs and lows.

thyrotropin-releasing hormone test A test sometimes used as an aid in diagnosing depression and assessing thyroid status. Though this test is not as well known as the DEXAMETHASONE SUPPRESSION TEST (DST), clinicians and researchers who feel there are patients who suffer from a subclinical HYPOTHROIDISM consider monitoring for thyroid function an important diagnostic tool. In this test the thyroid-stimulating hormone (TSH) is measured after infusion of protirelin (thyrotropin-releasing hormone, TRH).

In their testing, researchers have discovered that manics seem to have a blunted response compared with that of normal controls. Thus, the thyroid-stimulating hormone (TSH) response to the thyrotropin-releasing hormone infusion (TRH) has indicated that the TRH test can be useful for both diagnosis and treatment planning.

Because of studies that suggest that a significant proportion of patients with depression may have early hypothyroidism, many researchers believe that both depressed inpatients and outpatients (and especially individuals with a poor response to traditional psychiatric treatments) may be appropriate candidates for a comprehensive thyroid evaluation, including the TRH test. This evaluation is especially important if the patient is taking, or being considered for treatment with, lithium carbonate, which is known to cause hypothyroidism in some individuals.

Tofranil   See IMIPRAMINE HYDROCHLORIDE.

touch therapy   Touch is the first sense we use, and today the power of touch to help heal the emotional pain of grief and depression and promote physical and emotional well-being is being investigated by many scientists, including physicians, psychiatrists and biophysicists. Its therapeutic value is considered so promising that Dr. Dolores Krieger, the originator of therapeutic touch, a healing method that involves the laying on of hands, was awarded a government grant to study the act of healing or helping others through touch.

In many ways, however, touch as a tool for healing is as old as mankind. As Sherry Suib Cohen wrote in ''The Amazing Power of Touch'':

What we are now learning about the therapeutic effects of touch, primitive man

may have known instinctively. Pictorial evidence in cave paintings in the Pyrenees shows people using touch to heal as far back as 15,000 years ago. In China, Egypt, and Thailand the traditions of touch healing are demonstrated in early rock carvings and papyrus paintings . . . The many powers of touch were recognized by primitive man and documented in the Bible. And it was Michelangelo, who in his Sistine Chapel masterpiece portrayed God giving life to Adam through the touch of his hand.

toxic   Pertaining to, or due to, a poison. Thus toxicity is the quality of being poisonous and toxicology is the scientific study of poisons, including their action, detection and treatment of conditions caused by them.

tranquilizers   A group of depressant drugs that act selectively on the brain and central nervous system. When used as sedatives they are aimed at reducing the fear, anxiety or anger that are part of depression. They are legally available only on prescription and are manufactured as tablets and capsules in a variety of sizes, shapes and colors—and also as liquids for injection.

Combining tranquilizers with other drugs that act on and slow down the central nervous system (opiates, barbiturates, alcohol and inhalants) is dangerous, since each drug increases the effect of the other. Thus the combined effect is more powerful than the effect of either alone.

O'Brien, Robert and Cohen, Sidney, M.D., *The Encyclopedia of Drug Abuse* (New York: Facts On File, 1984).

trazodone   (Desyrel)   Trazodone is chemically unrelated to either the tricyclics or the MAO inhibitors and represents an entirely different class of antidepressant.

Bristol-Myers, ''Desyrel: A New Generation of Antidepressants,'' *Bristol-Myers Third Quarter Report*, 1982.

treatment of depression   Depression is the most treatable of all the mental illnesses. Individuals no longer have to suffer its debilitating symptoms. With modern treatment methods, even the most serious forms of depressive disorder respond rapidly to treatment. In fact, 80% of people with serious depression can be treated successfully.

Unfortunately, the very nature of a depressive disorder can interfere with a person's ability or wish to get help. Since depression makes a person feel tired, worthless, helpless and hopeless, people with serious depression need encouragement from family and friends to seek the treatments that can ease their pain. Some people need even more help and must be taken for treatment.

When treatment is needed, help is available from physicians, mental health specialists, health maintenance organizations, community mental health centers, hospital departments of psychiatry or outpatient psychiatric clinics, university or medical school-affiliated programs, state hospital outpatient clinics, family service/social agencies and family clinics and facilities. Some hospitals and universities have special research centers that study and treat depression.

The following are the main forms of treatment.

Drugs. Drugs and medication are a common treatment, and some people do very well with them. Some drugs have been in general usage for some time, but newer ones are constantly being tried. Researchers have good reason to be proud of today's drugs, too. Dr. Frederick Goodwin of the National Institute of Mental Health has given a chilling picture of the pre-drug era and patients' lives during that time. According to Goodwin, not counting the suicides, unipolar depressives could expect to spend about a quarter of their adult lives in hospitals, and manic-depressives about half. (See also DRUG THERAPY.)

Electroshock treatment. As an alternative to drugs electroshock treatment is often used for people who are severely ill and who do not respond rapidly enough to drugs. (See also ELECTROCONVULSIVE THERAPY.)

Psychotherapy. A variety of psychotherapies can be used to treat depressive disorders, and PSYCHOTHERAPY is sometimes used in conjunction with drugs. Though people are often counseled to avoid rushing into therapy too rapidly, many mental health experts suggest seeking help if the symptoms of depression persist for more than two weeks—and/or they cause a noticeable impairment in ordinary function.

Counseling. Since people suffering from depression need outlets for expressing their feelings and getting outside of themselves, COUNSELING may be helpful. Both individual and group counseling are available at many community health services. Hot lines and organizations that provide support systems and permit persons suffering from depression to share their experiences with people who have similar experiences also provide encouragement and healing through their meetings and contacts. (See also SELF-HELP/SUPPORT ORGANIZATIONS.)

Combinations of treatments. For some patients, combinations of treatments are most effective, i.e., medications to control symptoms and restore functioning, and psycho-social therapy to address the social and behavioral problems that go with serious disorders. Most clinicians are becoming adept at providing the multiple approaches often needed to help severely depressed people.

In any treatment, if symptoms do not begin to subside after several weeks, the treatment should be reevaluated. People with severe recurrent episodes of depression or mania may need to stay on medication to prevent or alleviate further episodes.

treatment of grief   See GRIEF THERAPY/TREATMENT.

triangularis   The depressor muscles (triangularis) that control the movement of the sides of the mouth. Depression affects the triangularis, and the so-called classic look of a depressed person is a droopy-mouthed person with a slumped posture.

Gallagher, Winifred, "The Dark Affliction of Mind and Body," *Discover*, May 1986.

tricyclic compounds The most widely-used class of the ANTIDEPRESSANT drugs, tricyclics are usually the first treatment for patients with depression. Researchers at the National Institute of Mental Health (NIMH) believe that 80% of patients, on the right dosage of tricyclic drugs, eventually get better.

Some years ago researchers found that the tricyclic compounds had identifiable actions on the NEUROTRANSMITTERS of the brain (the NOREPINEPHRINE system and the SEROTONIN system), which might be involved in depression. One action is preventing brain cells from taking the neurotransmitters out of circulation in a process called RE-UPTAKE.

Depressive symptoms can be alleviated in days or weeks, depending on which tricyclic is used. The symptoms that are alleviated are loss of appetite and weight, decreased capacity to feel pleasure, loss of energy, psychomotor retardation, suicidal thoughts, and thought patterns dominated by hopelessness, helplessness and excessive guilt.

Tricyclics can be extremely toxic in excessive doses, though. Too high a dose, for example, can produce an irregular heartbeat. Other side effects include disturbed vision, sweating, dizziness, decreased or increased sexual desire, constipation and edema.

The tricyclic compounds include: amitriptyline hydrochloride (Elavil, Endep), desipramine hydrochloride (Norpramin, Pertofrane), doxepin hydrochloride (Adapin, Sinequan), imipramine hydrochloride (Janimine, SK-Pramine, Tofranil), nortriptyline hydrochloride (Aventyl, Pamelor), protriptyline hydrochloride (Vivactil) and trimipramine (Surmontil). (See also DRUG THERAPY.)

types of depression Since depression is a complex and many-faceted disorder it comes in various forms and types, as well as a variety of sub-types. Different terms are used to label the various types, and the type or term by which an episode is labeled often depends on whether a person is talking to a clinician, researcher or other mental health specialist. Because of the many terms used to identify the types of depression there are overlapping boundaries and symptoms.

types of grief See GRIEF.

U

unipolar depression A type of depression in which a person may be severely depressed and suffer from MAJOR DEPRESSION but not from MANIC-DEPRESSIVE disorders. It is defined as one depressive episode or a history only of depressive episodes (as opposed to both manic and depressive episodes). Approximately 50% of people who experience a major depression have only one serious episode in their lifetimes. In other cases, the course of unipolar disorder may vary, and episodes may be separated by long intervals, such as years, or they may be closer together. During a "down" episode victims are dispirited and listless and generally find it difficult to go about their work and other activities. Sometimes, however, unipolar depression merely drags a person into a state of the blues without interfering with work. It is a term that overlaps with CLINICAL or ENDOGENOUS DEPRESSION.

Unite, Inc. A support group founded in 1975 for parents who have experienced infant death, miscarriage and stillbirth. There are local group meetings in various areas throughout the country. For information write: Unite, Inc., c/o Jeanes Hospital, 7600 Central Ave., Philadelphia, PA 19111. Phone: 215-728-2082.

V

Valium   See DIAZEPAM (VALIUM).

vitamins   See DIET.

W

weekend depression   A type of depression that is sometimes experienced by people who live alone (often individuals who live within the framework of weekday employment) and who have emotional difficulties when facing solitude. The thought of being alone for a Saturday and Sunday looms as so unbearable they automatically expect to feel wretched and unhappy. Rather than making weekend plans they allow their expectation to fulfill itself. Then they settle for the "blues" while they sleep, lie in bed, watch TV and stare at their four walls.

Wellbutrin   See BUPROPION HYDRO-CHLORIDE (WELLBUTRIN).

Wellness Associates   An educational organization that grew out of the Wellness Resource Center founded by Dr. John W. Travis in 1975. The former center was founded to integrate a wellness program through exploring humanistic and transpersonal psychology, along with nutrition, physical fitness and stress reduction. Reorganized as Wellness Associates in 1980, the organization integrates all the areas of mind, body and spirit that constitute high-level wellness and is based on the premise that each person has his or her own unique path toward wellness. For information contact: Dr. John Travis, Wellness Associates, Box 5433, Mill Valley, CA 94942. Phone: 415-383-3806.

Wertheimer, Max   A German psychologist (1880–1943) whose original research while he was a professor at the universities of Prague and Berlin placed him in the forefront of contemporary psychology and involved him with developing some of the theories of the Gestalt school of psychology. With the advent of Hitler, he came to the United States where he joined the faculty of the New School for Social Research and became a visiting lecturer at Columbia University. He also collaborated with Wolfgang Kohler and Kurt Koffa to introduce a new approach (macroscopic as opposed to microscopic) to the study of psychology. His book *Productive Thinking* was published posthumously in 1945.

WHO   See WORLD HEALTH ORGANIZATION.

WHO/SADD   See SCHEDULE FOR STANDARDIZED ASSESSMENT OF DEPRESSIVE DISORDERS (WHO-SADD).

withdrawal symptoms from drugs   See DRUG ADDICTION; DRUG DEPENDENCY; PSYCHOLOGICAL DRUG DEPENDENCE.

women   See SEX FACTORS.

Woolf, Virginia   An English novelist and essayist (1882–1941) best known for her stream-of-consciousness writing techniques and insightful essays; her *A Room of One's Own* concerned itself with a woman's need for independence and the opportunity to do creative work. She and her husband Leonard Woolf, a critic and writer on economics, established Hogarth Press in 1917.

Despite Woolf's own creativity and literary success she suffered from depression throughout her life. Though she felt her periods of depression eventually enhanced her creativity, she rarely wrote while depressed. During World War I she had a severe mental collapse in which she was unable to function.

Depressed, and fearful that the same kind of mental collapse might return during World War II, she placed heavy stones in her coat pockets, went to a river near her home, and drowned herself in 1941.

workplace, depression in   The National Institute of Mental Health (NIMH) has reported that time lost from work due to depression costs $10 billion annually.

World Health Organization (WHO) An agency of the United Nations that was established in 1948. It is headquartered in Geneva, Switzerland and governed by the World Health Assembly. Its purpose is the "attainment by all peoples of the highest level of health" and it has the primary responsibility for international health matters and public health. Member countries exchange knowledge and experience with the aim of achieving a level of health that permits people to lead socially and economically productive lives. WHO has accomplished notable work, including studies of mental health and the standardization of health statistics, and has worked on other problems of worldwide scope.

World Health Organization (WHO) Collaborative Study on Standardized Assessment of Depressive Disorders In the face of a world total of at least 100 million new cases of clinically recognizable depression each year, this study was designed to develop and test simple instruments for clinical description of depressive states; to examine with these instruments a series of "average" depressive patients in different cultures and to set up a network of field research centers. The five selected study areas—two in JAPAN, one in CANADA, one in IRAN and one in SWITZERLAND—present interesting demographic and cultural differences, as discussed in detail in the WHO publication, *Depressive Disorders in Different Cultures*. A total of 573 patients were selected for detailed assessment using the

WHO/SADD Schedule. Of these 136 were in Basel, Switzerland; 108 in Montreal, Canada; 108 in Nagasaki, Japan; 107 in Teheran, Iran; and 114 in Tokyo, Japan.

Two instruments were developed for the study—a screening form for selecting patients, and a SCHEDULE FOR STANDARDIZED ASSESSMENT OF DEPRESSIVE DISORDERS (WHO/SADD), which was designed to be easy to master and to be adaptable to a variety of interviewing styles.

The WHO Collaborative Study on Standardized Assessment of Depressive Disorders indicated that the patients who seek psychiatric treatment for a depressive illness in the five study areas are strikingly similar to each other in many respects. Although the results support the validity of a distinction between endogenous and psychogenic depressive disorders, there is evidence that the two syndromes should be regarded as two overlapping clusters or extremes of a continuum rather than as two mutually exclusive categories.

In citing the results in *Depressive Disorders in Different Cultures*, the researchers wrote:

The investigators were requested to formulate a diagnosis upon completion of the assessment of every patient and to classify their diagnosis according to two alternative classification systems, one proposed by the Basel group of investigators and the other by the Teheran center.

The Basel system is based on nosological concepts and distinguishes between eight types of depressive condition: periodic (unipolar) depression, involutional (late) depression, circular depression (manic-depressive illness), schizoaffective depressive disorder, exhaustion depression, neurotic depression, reactive depression and other depressive conditions. The Teheran system has five types: endogenous depression, agitated depression, mild endogenous depression, neurotic depression. and reactive depression.

The uneven distribution of the diagnostic subtypes across the centres, with very few or even no cases in some nosological categories in several of the centres, would make difficult the analysis and interpretation of results. Since the investigators agreed that the main dividing line within the continuum of different nosological varieties or syndromes of depression was that separating predominantly endogenous from predominantly psychogenic disorders, a simplified classification of the study patients was obtained by collapsing the diagnostic categories in the following way:

Periodic (unipolar) depression
Involutional (late) depression   } ENDOGENOUS DEPRESSION
Circular (manic-depressive, bipolar) depression

Exhaustion depression
Neurotic depression   } PSYCHOGENIC DEPRESSION
Reactive depression

Schizoaffective depressive disorder
Other depressive disorder   } OTHER DEPRESSION
Unclassified depressive disorder

The investigators found that the most frequent symptoms in all the centers combined were sadness, joylessness, anxiety, tension, lack of energy, loss of interest, loss of ability to concentrate, and ideas of insufficiency, inadequacy and worthlessness. Anxiety and tension appeared to be among the most frequent symptoms in all centers. Suicidal ideas were present in 59% of the patients. Delusions and hypochondriasis were fairly infrequent. Feelings of guilt and self-reproach occurred in varying proportions, and somatic symptoms were present in a considerable proportion of patients. Psychomotor agitation had an average frequency of 42%. (See also Appendix 1, Tables.)

Sartorius, N. et al., *Depressive Disorders in Different Cultures* (Geneva: World Health Organization, 1983).

X

Xanax   See ALPRAZOLAM.

X chromosome   It has long been suspected that some cases of manic-depression might be linked to the X chromosome. Similarly, for some time it was thought some cases might be linked to chromosome 11, as a result of a study published in 1987 that focused on the genetic aspects of bipolar (see BIPOLAR DEPRESSION) or MANIC-DEPRESSIVE disorder among the Old Order Amish community (a group of over 12,000 people living in relative isolation in Lancaster, Pennsylvania). This study revealed a genetic marker, which was mapped to the tip of the short arm of chromosome 11 and appeared to indicate that at least some cases of manic depression might be caused by a dominant gene on the tip of the short arm of that chromosome (see OLD ORDER AMISH STUDY). But by late 1989, new evidence from a National Institute of Mental Health (NIMH) team study cast serious doubt on the conclusions of the Old Order Amish study linking chromosome 11 to manic-depressive illness.

However, both the 1987 and 1989 reports were in agreement that there may be at least two different genes—and possibly more—that predispose people to affective disorder. Dr. Kenneth K. Kidd of Yale University, who contributed to both the earlier and more recent studies linking faulty genes to manic-depressive illness, stated that (in spite of the 1989 NIMH study casting doubt on the conclusions of the Amish study) another study—a large American-Israeli survey using traditional genetic markers—still seems to be unchallenged. That study showed strong links between the mental disorder and a suspected gene on the X chromosome.

One of the hallmarks of X-linked manic depression is the absence of male-to-male transmission. This points to the X chromosome as a possible site of the manic-depression gene. (In a female, the 23rd pair of chromosomes consists of two X chromosomes. A male receives an X chromosome from his mother and a Y from his father.)

In 1987 Dr. Miron Baron, a psychiatrist at the Columbia University College of Physicians & Surgeons and director of the Division of Psychogenetics at New York State Psychiatric Institute, reported finding a genetic culprit underlying bipolar illness—a defective gene on the X chromosome. For the study Baron and his colleagues from Yale University and the Hebrew University-Hadassah Medical School in Jerusalem selected five pedigrees from the patient population of the Jerusalem Mental Health Center.

The Israeli population was especially suited for this type of study owing to the high geographic concentration, the availability of large families in some ethnic groups, and the low rate of alcoholism and drug use, which might complicate the psychiatric diagnosis. The members of one pedigree were Ashkenazi Jews of Polish descent. The others were non-Ashkenazi from Iran, Iraq, Turkey and Yemen. All of the five large families had a high density of manic-depressive illness. Of the 161 study subjects, 47 had bipolar illness or related affective disorders. In four of the families, the illness was strongly linked to one or the other of the two genetic markers being examined—the gene for color blindness and the gene for a deficiency in glucose-6-phosphate dehydrogenase (G6PD). Color blindness and G6PD deficiency (a biochemical defect that can cause anemia) are controlled by genes that are located on the X chromosome. This made this population well suited for genetic studies of disorders thought to be influenced by heredity through the X chromosome. In Baron's study the X chromosome linkage was found only among the non-Ashkenazi groups.

Like Dr. Janice Egeland, principal investigator of manic-depression and chromosome 11 in the Old Order Amish study, the American-Israeli team has not yet identified and zeroed in on the defective gene itself. But since the researchers believe this region lies on the tip of the X chromosome's long arm, it now appears that the gene for one form of manic depression resides in close proximity to the DNA segments that give rise to the inherited traits of color blindness and the biochemical defect, G6PD deficiency. Thus this finding has narrowed the search to a well-circumscribed region of a particular chromosome.

Robinson, Miranda, ''Molecular Genetics of the Mind,'' *Nature*, February 1987.

O'Connor, Joan, ''Probing the Biology of Affective Disorder,'' *Psychiatric News*, November 6, 1987.

Baron, Miron, ''Defective Genes Linked to Manic Depressive Illness,'' *The Psychiatric Times*, December 1987.

Schmeck, Harold M., Jr., ''Scientists Now Doubt They Found Faulty Gene Linked to Mental Illness,'' *The New York Times*. November 7, 1989.

Y

young people's depression   Today depressive illnesses appear to be occurring more commonly among young people. The National Institute of Mental Health (NIMH) reports that approximately 3% to 5% of the teen population experiences clinical depression every year. Among 100 teenagers this means that four could be clinically depressed.

Dr. Gerald R. Klerman, associate chairman for research and professor of psychiatry at New York Hospital-Cornell Medical Center, has noted that the change in age distribution, with the significant rise in the rate of depression among young people, had its start in the 1970s when psychiatric facilities reported that more patients were being diagnosed as depressed and that they were younger than the standard textbook description of depressed patients as middle-aged. This trend very obviously contributes to the dramatic increase in suicide attempts and in death by suicide among adolescents and young adults. Suicide among young people has increased 300% during the past three decades.

Depressed adolescents can experience feelings of emptiness, anxiety, loneliness, helplessness, hopelessness, guilt, loss of confidence and self esteem, and changes in sleeping and eating habits. In addition, they often "act out." That is, they try to "cover" their depression by acting angry, aggressive, running away or becoming delinquent. Manic-depressive disorder in adolescents is often manifested by episodes of impulsivity, irritability and loss of control alternating with periods of withdrawal.

Depression in adolescents can and should be treated, but unfortunately this treatable disorder typically goes unrecognized when it is assumed that such storminess is natural to adolescence. All too often the symptoms are simply chalked up to the "normal adjustments" of adolescence, and as a result depressed young people do not get the help they need. Moreover, young people often don't ask for—or get—the right help because they fail to recognize the symptoms of depression in themselves or in people they care about.

Since adolescents are so noted for their quickly changing moods and behavior, it may take careful watching to see the differences between a depressive disorder and normal behavior. The key to recognizing the depressive disorder is that the change in behavior lasts for weeks or longer.

The National Institute of Mental Health (NIMH) suggests asking and answering the following questions to determine whether young people need treatment for depression:

Do they express feelings of:
   Sadness or "emptiness"?
   Hoplessness, pessimism or guilt?
   Helplessness or worthlessness?
Do they seem:
   Unable to make decisions?
   Unable to concentrate and remember?
   To have lost interest or pleasure in ordinary activities—like sports or band or talking on the phone?
Do they complain of:
   Loss of energy and drive—so they seem "slowed down"?
   Trouble falling asleep, staying asleep or getting up?
   Appetite problems; are they losing or gaining weight?
   Headaches, stomach aches or backaches?
   Chronic aches and pains in joints and muscles?
Has their behavior changed suddenly so that:
   They are restless or more irritable?
   They want to be alone most of the time?
   They've started cutting classes or dropped hobbies and activities?
   You think they may be drinking heavily or taking drugs?
Have they talked about:
   Death?
   Suicide—or have they attempted suicide?

Any young person who has four or more symptoms of depression for longer than a few weeks, or who is doing poorly in school, seems socially withdrawn, uncaring, overly impulsive, and no longer interested in activities once enjoyed, should be checked for a possible depressive illness. A trained therapist or counselor can help depressed young people learn more positive ways to think about themselves, change behavior, cope with problems, or handle relationships. A physician can prescribe the medications to help relieve the symptoms of depression. (See also ADOLESCENT DEPRESSION.)

young people's suicide Dr. Neal D. Ryan, assistant professor of psychiatry at the

University of Pittsburgh, has found that depressed teenagers intent on killing themselves show chemical abnormalities in their brain that appear to predispose them to suicide. Earlier studies have found similar abnormalities in the brain of suicidal adults, although experts are divided as to what conclusions can be drawn. Ryan's research is believed to be the first that demonstrates neurochemical abnormalities in suicidal adolescents. From 1980 to 1987 Dr. Ryan and his coworkers monitored the growth hormone secretion of 140 boys and girls ranging in age from 12 to just under 18. The tests were conducted while the subjects slept. According to Ryan, most growth hormone secretion occurs during sleep, especially during the first several hours.

APPENDIXES

1. WHO COLLABORATIVE STUDY ON STANDARDIZED ASSESSMENT OF DEPRESSIVE DISORDERS

Source: World Health Organization, *Depressive Disorders in Different Cultures* (Geneva: WHO, 1983).

Comparisons between selected characteristics of the five catchment areas (data provided by the field research centers)

Selected characteristics	Basel	Montreal	Nagasaki	Teheran	Tokyo
(A) *Geographical and demographic characteristics*					
(1) Area (km²)	37	2,673	4,069	25,434	17,164
(2) Population	224,630	2,802,480	1,570,000	3,492,500	25,647,067
(3) Population density per km²	6,071	1,027	383	111	1,494
(4) Percentage rural population	0	0	41	12.5	18
(5) Percentage population aged 0–14	16.3	27.4	28	46	24.3
(6) Percentage population aged 60+	22.1	11.0	12	6	12.3
(7) Birth rate per 1,000	10.1	12.3	not available	36.8	20.1
(8) Infant mortality per 1,000 live births	15.4	17.0	15.2	120	10.6
(9) Deaths in age group 60+ as percentage of all deaths	83.8	69.9	71.5	not available	71.8
(10) Deaths due to cancer, cardiovascular, and cerebrovascular diseases as percentage of all deaths	68.2	71.9	52.8	22	57.2
(11) Suicide rates per 100,000	31	12.1	15.4	2.1	15.3
(12) Percentage households with five or more members	7.7	41.7 (4+ members)	33	39	27.2
(13) Percentage of one-person households	29.3	14.9	9	5.5	18.3
(14) Minorities exceeding 5% of population	Italians	Greeks and Italians	none	none	none
(15) Percentage of population age 7+ with no schooling	data not available	data not available	1.6	73.1	0.38

Comparisons between selected characteristics of the five catchment areas (data provided by the field research centers)

Selected characteristics	Basel	Montreal	Nagasaki	Teheran	Tokyo
(B) *Health services*					
(1) Hospital beds per 1,000	15.8	8.1	12.2	data not available	8.49
(2) Psychiatric beds per 1,000	2.8	3.3	3.9	0.6	1.74
(3) Number of physicians per 1,000	1.46	1.1	1.33	0.2	1.51
(4) Number of psychiatrists	94	335	104	96	2,170
(5) Year when first psychiatric facility established	1842	1875	1913	1920	1879
(6) Year when first psychiatrist started work in area	1861	1875	1907	1937	1879
(7) Annual number of admissions (including readmissions) to psychiatric facilities in area	2,154	9,056	data not available	18,000	60,250
(8) Average length of stay in facilities of center (days)	data not available	25[a]	150	30	60
(9) Percentage of all admitted patients:					
(a) All psychoses	47.9	43.3	69	84.4	84
(b) Schizophrenia	21	20.3	46	52.3	20.8
(c) Affective psychoses	16.9	11.8	2	23.5	21.2
(d) All neuroses	9.1	20.6	2	7.6	14.3
(e) Alcohol dependence	13.6	18.2	6	0.1	4
(f) Drug dependence	6.8	1.7	less than 1	0.9	1
(g) Other diagnoses	21.1	16.2	22	6.8	38.7

[a]Average length for the hospital's facilities not calculated.

Percentage distribution of the patients by age and sex in the different centers

Years of age	Basel M (N = 44)	F (N = 92)	All (N = 136)	Montreal M (N = 36)	F (N = 72)	All (N = 108)	Nagasaki M (N = 50)	F (N = 58)	All (N = 108)
Under 15	–	–	–	–	–	–	–	–	–
15–24	6.8	10.9	9.6	13.9	19.4	17.6	16.0	17.2	16.7
25–34	27.3	16.3	19.8	22.2	16.7	18.5	18.0	6.9	12.0
35–44	11.4	22.8	19.1	30.6	19.4	23.1	38.0	25.9	31.5
45–54	27.3	26.1	26.5	13.9	25.0	21.3	20.0	27.6	24.1
55–64	20.4	16.3	17.6	16.7	15.3	15.7	4.0	17.2	11.1
≥65	6.8	7.6	7.3	2.8	4.2	3.7	4.0	5.2	4.6
Totals (%)	100.0	100.0	100.0	100.0	100.0	100.0	100.0	100.0	100.0

Years of age	Teheran M (N = 43)	F (N = 64)	All (N = 107)	Tokyo M (N = 63)	F (N = 51)	All (N = 114)	All centers M (N = 236)	F (N = 337)	All (N = 573)
Under 15	–	1.6	0.9	–	–	–	–	0.3	0.2
15–24	18.6	29.7	25.2	11.1	21.6	15.8	13.1	19.0	16.6
25–34	46.5	23.4	32.7	20.6	13.7	17.5	26.3	15.7	20.1
35–44	16.3	17.2	16.8	30.2	25.5	28.1	25.8	22.0	23.6
45–54	11.6	20.3	16.8	23.8	15.7	20.2	19.9	23.4	22.0
55–64	7.0	6.2	6.6	7.9	19.6	13.1	10.6	14.8	13.1
≥65	–	1.6	0.9	6.3	3.9	5.3	4.2	4.7	4.5
Totals (%)	100.0	100.0	100.0	100.0	100.0	100.0	100.0	100.0	100.0

Marital status of patients (%) by center

Center	Single never married	Married including common-law marriage	Divorced	Separated	Widowed	Total
Basel (N = 136)	26.5	53.7	11.0	4.4	4.4	100
Montreal (N = 108)	31.5	50.9	2.8	6.5	8.3	100
Nagasaki (N = 108)	21.2	65.8	5.6	0.9	6.5	100
Teheran (N = 107)	28.0	59.9	2.8	0.9	8.4	100
Tokyo (N = 114)	21.0	72.9	1.7	—	4.4	100
All centers (N = 573)	25.6	60.4	5.1	2.7	6.2	100

Economic status of patients (%) by center

Center	High	Medium	Low	Impossible to estimate	Total
Basel (N = 136)	6.6	63.2	26.5	3.7	100
Montreal (N = 108)	16.7	32.4	35.2	15.7	100
Nagasaki (N = 108)	11.1	80.6	6.5	1.8	100
Teheran (N = 107)	3.7	41.2	55.1	—	100
Tokyo (N = 114)	19.3	75.4	5.3	—	100
All centers (N = 573)	11.3	59.0	25.5	4.2	100

Distribution (%) of study population by occupation and by center

Occupational group	Basel $N = 136$	Montreal $N = 108$	Nagasaki $N = 108$	Teheran $N = 107$	Tokyo $N = 114$	All centers $N = 573$
Professionals, executives, civil servants and freelance occupations	8.8	8.3	11.1	—	14.9	8.7
Skilled technical occupations (e.g., technicians, secretaries, nurses)	10.3	2.8	2.8	4.7	13.2	7.0
Skilled industrial workers	0.7	2.8	—	3.7	2.6	1.9
Unskilled and semiskilled workers and employees	20.6	22.1	18.5	23.4	17.6	20.4
Self-employed persons (e.g., trade, craftsmanship)	19.9	7.4	6.5	6.5	7.9	10.1
Agricultural workers	—	1.9	9.2	1.9	—	2.4
Students	2.9	3.7	5.6	4.7	4.4	4.2
Housewives	25.8	36.1	26.8	43.0	21.9	30.4
Retired persons and invalids	3.7	1.9	—	—	2.6	1.8
Unemployed	0.7	11.1	13.9	9.3	8.8	8.4
Other or not known	6.6	1.9	5.6	2.8	6.1	7.7
Total (%)	100	100	100	100	100	100

Highest level of education reached (%) by center

Center	Illiterate, no school	Less than 5 years of school	5–12 years of school	More than 12 years of school, including completed or uncompleted university education	Postgraduate education completed	Unknown	Total
Basel ($N = 136$)	0.7	2.2	83.9	12.5	0.7	—	100
Montreal ($N = 108$)	0.9	3.7	67.6	23.1	2.8	1.9	100
Nagasaki ($N = 108$)	—	0.9	82.4	16.7	—	—	100
Teheran ($N = 107$)	43.0	12.2	41.1	0.9	1.9	0.9	100
Tokyo ($N = 114$)	—	2.6	45.6	50.0	0.9	0.9	100
All centers ($N = 573$)	8.4	4.2	64.9	20.6	1.2	0.7	100

Distribution of patients according to the classification system proposed by the Basel center

Center	Periodic depression[a]			Involutional Depression (late depression)			Cyclic (manic-depression) depression			Schizo-affective disorder			Exhaustion depression			Neurotic depression			Reactive depression			Other or not classified			Total		
	%(a)	N	%(b)	%(a)	N	%(b)	%(a)	N	%(b)	%(a)	N	%(b)	%(a)	N	%(b)	%(a)	N	%(b)	%(a)	N	%(b)	%(a)	N	%(b)	%(a)	N	%(b)
Basel	10.4	20	14.7	33.3	29	21.3	28.3	13	9.6	50.0	4	2.9	67.6	25	18.4	20.3	24	17.6	27.6	16	11.8	18.5	5	3.7	23.7	136	100
Montreal	12.5	24	22.2	10.3	9	8.3	23.9	11	10.2	25.0	2	1.9	5.4	2	1.9	34.7	41	38.0	27.6	16	14.8	18.5	5	4.6	18.8	108	100
Nagasaki	27.6	53	49.1	28.7	25	23.1	23.9	11	10.2							3.4	4	3.7	12.1	7	6.5	22.2	6	5.6	18.8	108	100
Teheran	21.3	41	38.3	8.1	7	6.5	6.5	3	2.8	12.5	1	0.9	24.3	9	8.4	18.6	22	20.6	24.1	14	13.1	37.0	10	9.3	18.7	107	100
Tokyo	28.1	54	47.4	19.5	17	14.9	17.4	8	7.0	12.5	1	0.9	2.7	1	0.8	22.9	27	23.7	8.6	5	4.4	3.7	1	0.9	19.9	114	100
All centers	100	192	33.5	100	87	15.2	100	46	8.0	100	8	1.4	100	37	6.5	100	118	20.6	100	58	10.1	100	27	4.7	100	573	100

a % (a) = vertical percentages, i.e., by centers; % (b) = horizontal percentages, i.e., by diagnosis.

Distribution of patients according to broader diagnostic groups

Center	Endogenous[a]			Psychogenic			Other			Total		
	% (a)	N	% (b)	% (a)	N	% (b)	% (a)	N	% (b)	% (a)	N	% (b)
Basel	19.1	62	45.6	30.5	65	47.8	25.7	9	6.6	23.7	136	100
Montreal	13.5	44	40.7	27.7	59	54.6	14.3	5	4.6	18.8	108	100
Nagasaki	27.4	89	82.4	5.2	11	10.2	22.9	8	7.4	18.8	108	100
Teheran	15.7	51	47.7	21.1	45	42.0	31.4	11	10.3	18.7	107	100
Tokyo	24.3	79	69.3	15.5	33	28.9	5.7	2	1.8	19.8	114	100
All centers	100	325	56.7	100	213	37.2	100	35	6.1	100	573	100

a% (a) = vertical percentages, i.e., by center; % (b) = horizontal percentages, i.e., by diagnosis.

2. NIMH EPIDEMIOLOGIC CATCHMENT AREA (ECA) PROGRAM

Source: Robins, L. et al., "Lifetime Prevalence of Specific Psychiatric Disorders in Three Sites," *Archives of General Psychiatry,* 41(October 1984).

Urbanization of Area of Residence and *DSM-III* Lifetime Diagnosis (St. Louis Only)*

	Central City, % N = 983	Inner Suburb, % N = 1,267	Small Town/Rural, % N = 740
Cognitive impairment[†]	2.6 (0.5)	0.7 (0.2)	0.6 (0.3)
Drug abuse/dependence[‡]	8.1 (1.6)	5.6 (0.8)	4.3 (0.8)
Alcohol abuse/dependence[‡]	19.4 (2.1)	15.9 (1.1)	14.0 (1.7)
Antisocial personality[‡]	5.7 (1.5)	3.1 (0.7)	2.4 (0.6)
Schizophrenia[§]	1.9 (0.5)	0.8 (0.3)	0.8 (0.4)
Panic[‖]	1.7 (0.5)	0.8 (0.2)	2.1 (0.6)
Dysthymia	4.9 (1.2)	4.5 (0.7)	2.7 (0.6)
Agoraphobia	4.6 (0.9)	4.3 (0.6)	3.7 (0.9)

*Numbers in parentheses are SEs.
[†]$P < .001$, central city v others.
[‡]$P < .05$, central city v small town/rural.
[§]$P < .05$, central city v suburbs.
[‖]$P < .05$, suburb v small town.

Urbanization of Area of Residence and *DSM-III* Lifetime Diagnosis (St. Louis Only)*

	Central City, % N = 983	Inner Suburb, % N = 1,267	Small Town/Rural, % N = 740
Somatization	0.4 (0.2)	0.2 (0.1)	0.0 (0.0)
Manic episode	1.7 (0.7)	0.7 (0.3)	1.1 (0.5)
Major depressive episode	6.4 (1.0)	5.1 (0.9)	5.5 (1.0)
Anorexia nervosa	0.2 (0.2)	0.0 (0.0)	0.1 (0.1)
Simple phobia	6.6 (1.1)	7.6 (0.9)	6.3 (1.1)
Obsessive-compulsive	1.5 (0.3)	2.4 (0.5)	1.7 (0.6)
Schizophreniform disorder	0.0 (0.0)	0.3 (0.2)	0.0 (0.0)
Any of the covered diagnoses[‡]	33.7 (2.2)	32.2 (1.6)	27.5 (2.0)

*Numbers in parentheses are SEs.
[†]*P*<.001, central city *v* others.
[‡]*P*<.05, central city *v* small town/rural.
[§]*P*<.05, central city *v* suburbs.
[ǁ]*P*<.05, suburb *v* small town.

Lifetime Prevalence of DSM-III Diagnoses by Race*

	New Haven, Conn, %		Baltimore, %		St Louis, %	
	Black N = 334	Nonblack N = 2,708	Black N = 1,182	Nonblack N = 2,299	Black N = 1,158	Nonblack N = 1,846
Simple phobia	5.1 (1.6)	6.4 (0.5)	27.6 (1.4)	17.4 (1.1)†	11.1 (1.2)	5.9 (0.7)†
Agoraphobia	4.4 (1.0)	3.4 (0.3)	13.4 (1.2)	7.2 (0.7)†	4.4 (0.7)	4.1 (0.6)
Drug abuse/dependence	6.4 (1.3)	5.7 (0.5)	7.3 (0.9)	4.9 (0.5)‡	6.4 (1.0)	5.3 (0.7)
Cognitive impairment	1.9 (0.6)	1.3 (0.2)	1.8 (0.3)	1.1 (0.2)	2.2 (0.3)	0.7 (0.2)†
Schizophrenia	2.1 (0.7)	1.9 (0.3)	2.4 (0.5)	1.2 (0.2)‡	1.0 (0.3)	1.0 (0.3)
Manic episode	1.0 (0.5)	1.2 (0.2)	0.5 (0.2)	0.7 (0.2)	2.5 (0.8)	0.7 (0.2)‡
Somatization	0.7 (0.4)	0.1 (0.0)	0.1 (0.1)	0.1 (0.1)	0.4 (0.2)	0.1 (0.1)
Major depressive episode	5.7 (1.5)	6.8 (0.5)	3.7 (0.7)	3.8 (0.4)	4.9 (0.8)	5.7 (0.7)
Anorexia nervosa	0.0 (0.0)	0.1 (0.0)	0.0 (0.0)	0.1 (0.1)	0.0 (0.0)	0.1 (0.1)
Schizophreniform disorder	0.0 (0.0)	0.1 (0.1)	0.4 (0.2)	0.3 (0.1)	0.0 (0.0)	0.1 (0.1)
Dysthymia	3.3 (1.1)	3.2 (0.4)	1.8 (0.5)	2.3 (0.3)	3.6 (0.7)	3.9 (0.5)
Panic	1.3 (0.6)	1.5 (0.2)	1.6 (0.4)	1.3 (0.2)	1.1 (0.3)	1.6 (0.4)
Obsessive-compulsive	2.7 (0.8)	2.6 (0.3)	2.7 (0.5)	3.1 (0.4)	1.5 (0.4)	2.0 (0.4)
Alcohol abuse/dependence	14.3 (2.4)	11.1 (0.6)	14.6 (1.1)	13.2 (0.8)	14.7 (1.6)	16.0 (1.1)
Antisocial personality	1.7 (0.6)	2.1 (0.3)	2.3 (0.5)	2.7 (0.4)	3.9 (0.9)	3.1 (0.5)
Any of the covered diagnoses	30.5 (3.1)	28.6 (1.0)	45.1 (1.8)	34.7 (1.1)†	34.9 (1.9)	30.1 (1.4)‡

*Numbers in parentheses are SEs.
†P<.001.
‡P<.05.

Lifetime Prevalence of *DSM-III* Diagnoses by Education*

	New Haven, Conn, %		Baltimore, %		St Louis, %	
	College Graduate N = 839	Other N = 2,218	College Graduate N = 303	Other N = 3,174	College Graduate N = 416	Other N = 2,498
Cognitive impairment	0.3 (0.2)	1.7 (0.3)†	0.2 (0.2)	1.4 (0.2)†	0.0 (0.0)	0.8 (0.1)†
Simple phobia	3.8 (0.8)	7.2 (0.5)†	12.8 (2.3)	21.4 (0.9)‡	5.1 (1.5)	7.2 (0.7)
Agoraphobia	2.2 (0.5)	4.1 (0.4)§	4.4 (1.1)	9.6 (0.6)†	2.1 (0.8)	4.5 (0.5)§
Schizophrenia	0.5 (0.3)	2.5 (0.3)†	0.6 (0.4)	1.7 (0.3)	0.6 (0.3)	1.1 (0.3)
Schizophreniform disorder	0.0 (0.0)	0.1 (0.1)	0.0 (0.0)	0.3 (0.1)†	0.0 (0.0)	0.1 (0.1)
Alcohol abuse/dependence	9.5 (1.0)	12.2 (0.8)§	12.1 (2.4)	13.8 (0.7)	15.3 (2.3)	15.9 (1.0)
Somatization	0.0 (0.0)	0.2 (0.1)§	0.0 (0.0)	0.1 (0.1)	0.1 (0.1)	0.2 (0.1)
Panic	1.6 (0.4)	1.4 (0.3)	1.1 (0.6)	1.5 (0.2)	0.5 (0.3)	1.7 (0.4)§
Manic episode	0.7 (0.3)	1.3 (0.3)	0.3 (0.3)	0.7 (0.2)	0.6 (0.4)	1.1 (0.3)
Antisocial personality	0.9 (0.4)	2.5 (0.4)	1.5 (0.8)	2.7 (0.3)	2.3 (1.0)	3.4 (0.5)
Major depressive episode	7.1 (1.1)	6.6 (0.5)	5.5 (1.2)	3.6 (0.3)	4.6 (0.9)	5.7 (0.6)
Dysthymia	2.2 (0.6)	3.5 (0.4)	2.5 (1.0)	2.1 (0.2)	3.7 (0.9)	3.9 (0.5)
Obsessive-compulsive	2.7 (0.5)	2.6 (0.3)	1.9 (0.7)	3.1 (0.4)	2.1 (0.8)	1.9 (0.4)
Drug abuse/dependence	5.2 (0.8)	6.0 (0.6)	8.2 (1.4)	5.4 (0.5)	4.5 (1.3)	5.8 (0.6)
Anorexia nervosa	0.0 (0.0)	0.1 (0.0)	0.0 (0.0)	0.1 (0.1)	0.2 (0.2)	0.1 (0.1)
Any of the covered diagnoses	25.1 (1.8)	30.2 (1.1)†	30.9 (3.1)	38.7 (1.0)†	25.6 (2.7)	31.9 (1.2)§

*Numbers in parentheses are SEs.
†P<.01.
‡P<.001.
§P<.05.

Lifetime Prevalence Rates of DIS/*DSM-III* Disorders, Three ECA Sites*

Disorders	New Haven, Conn, % 1980–1981 (N = 3,058)	Baltimore, % 1981–1982 (N = 3,481)	St Louis, % 1981–1982 (N = 3,004)
Any DIS disorder covered	28.8 (0.9)	38.0 (0.9)	31.0 (1.2)
Any DIS disorder except phobia	24.9 (0.9)	23.9 (0.8)	26.2 (1.1)
Any DIS disorder except substance use disorders	19.3 (0.8)	29.5 (0.9)	18.6 (1.0)
Substance use disorders	15.0 (0.7)	17.0 (0.7)	18.1 (0.9)
Alcohol abuse/dependence	11.5 (0.6)	13.7 (0.7)	15.7 (0.9)
Drug abuse/dependence	5.8 (0.4)	5.6 (0.5)	5.5 (0.6)
Schizophrenic/schizophreniform disorders	2.0 (0.3)	1.9 (0.3)	1.1 (0.2)
Schizophrenia	1.9 (0.3)	1.6 (0.2)	1.0 (0.2)
Schizophreniform disorder	0.1 (0.1)	0.3 (0.1)	0.1 (0.1)
Affective disorders	9.5 (0.6)	6.1 (0.4)	8.0 (0.7)
Manic episode	1.1 (0.2)	0.6 (0.2)	1.1 (0.3)
Major depressive episode	6.7 (0.5)	3.7 (0.3)	5.5 (0.6)
Dysthymia	3.2 (0.4)	2.1 (0.2)	3.8 (0.4)
Anxiety/somatoform disorders	10.4 (0.6)	25.1 (0.8)	11.1 (0.7)
Phobia	7.8 (0.4)	23.3 (0.8)	9.4 (0.6)
Panic	1.4 (0.2)	1.4 (0.2)	1.5 (0.3)
Obsessive-compulsive	2.6 (0.3)	3.0 (0.3)	1.9 (0.3)
Somatization	0.1 (0.1)	0.1 (0.1)	0.1 (0.1)
Eating disorders			
Anorexia	0.0 (0.0)	0.1 (0.0)	0.1 (0.1)
Personality disorders			
Antisocial personality	2.1 (0.3)	2.6 (0.3)	3.3 (0.5)
Cognitive impairment (severe)	1.3 (0.2)	1.3 (0.2)	1.0 (0.2)

*DIS indicates Diagnostic Interview Schedule; ECA, Epidemiologic Catchment Area; numbers in parentheses are SEs.

3. CENTRAL MONOAMINE SYSTEMS

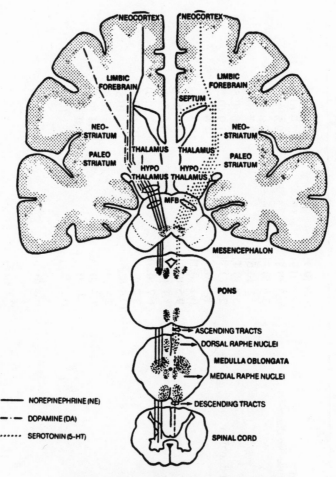

The monoamine neurotransmitter system. These neurotransmitters are widely distributed throughout the central nervous system, lending support to hypotheses implicating them in the etiology of the affective illnesses and accounting for their influence over a range of varied symptoms.

Source: Corfman, Eunice, *Depression, Manic-Depressive Illness and Biological Rhythms,* National Institute of Mental Health Science Reports #1 (Rockville, Maryland: NIMH, 1982; DHHS #(ADM)82-899).

4. DISTRIBUTION OF PSYCHIATRIC ADMISSIONS

Source: Department of Health and Human Services, Survey and Reports Branch, Division of Biometry and Applied Sciences, National Institute of Mental Health, Rockville, Maryland 20857.

Number and percent distribution of admissions under age 18 to selected inpatient psychiatric services of mental health organizations, by selected primary psychiatric diagnoses: United States, 1986.

Selected primary psychiatric diagnoses	Total	State and county mental hospitals	Private psychiatric hospitals	Inpatient psychiatric service				
					Non-federal general hospitals			Multi-service
				Total	Public	Nonpublic	
				Number				
Total, all diagnoses	112,215	15,953	42,502	45,587	11,856	33,731	8,173
Schizophrenia and related disorders	6,384	*	1,877	3,460	811	*	*
Alcohol/drug disorders	7,960	1,677	3,054	2,516	764	*	713
Affective disorders	35,728	1,607	18,559	13,215	2,366	10,849	2,347
				Percent Distribution				
Total, all diagnoses	100.0%	100.0%	100.0%	100.0%	100.0%	100.0%	100.0%
Schizophrenia and related disorders	5.7	*	4.4	7.6	6.8	*	*
Alcohol/drug disorders	7.1	10.5	7.2	5.5	6.4	*	8.7
Affective disorders	31.8	10.1	43.7	29.0	20.0	32.2	28.7

*Based on five or fewer sample cases; estimate not shown because it does not meet standards of reliability.

Number and percent of admissions age 17 and under with bipolar affective disorder and with any affective disorder, by type of psychiatric inpatient service, United States, 1986

Type of psychiatric inpatient service	Bipolar affective disorder*		Any affective disorder		Total admissions age 17 and under
	N	%	N	%	N
State and county mental hospitals	76	0.5	1,607	10.1	15,953
Private psychiatric hospitals	1,135	2.7	18,559	43.7	42,502
Non-federal general hospitals with separate psychiatric inpatient services	2,098	4.6	13,215	29.0	45,587
Multiservice mental health organizations	462	5.7	2,347	28.7	8,173
Total	3,771	3.4	35,728	31.8	112,215

Unpublished survey data from the Patient Survey Programs, Survey and Reports Branch, Division of Biometry and Applied Sciences, National Institute of Mental Health.
*Of the 3,771 cases of bipolar affective disorder, 3,601 were between the ages of 14 and 17. Only 170 cases in private psychiatric hospitals were less than age 14.

Number and percent of admissions with bipolar affective disorder and with major depression, by type of psychiatric inpatient service and age, United States, 1986

Type of psychiatric inpatient service and age	Bipolar affective disorder		Major depression		Total admissions
	N	%	N	%	N
Total	134,846	9.5	276,553	19.5	1,416,901
State and county mental hospitals					
Age 17 and under	76*	0.5*	484*	3.0*	15,953
18–24	1,850	3.2	4,078	7.0	58,111
25–34	13,264	10.7	6,776	5.5	123,575
35–64	15,468	13.7	4,050	3.6	113,310
65+	1,415*	9.5*	893*	6.0*	14,853
Private psychiatric hospitals					
Age 17 and under	1,135*	2.7*	10,657	25.1	42,502
18–24	1,232	5.6	5,569	25.4	21,931
25–34	5,533	11.4	12,902	26.6	48,487
35–64	10,775	14.1	26,644	34.8	76,472
65+	1,811	10.0	7,699	42.7	18,047

Non-federal general hospitals with separate psychiatric inpatient services				
Age 17 and under	2,098	4.6	8,064	17.7	45,587
18–24	5,595	4.7	20,958	17.5	119,667
25–34	24,589	10.6	39,590	17.0	232,794
35–64	35,785	11.4	81,562	26.0	313,906
65+	7,094	8.6	38,817	47.3	82,106
Multiservice mental health organizations					
Age 17 and under	462*	5.7*	1,216	14.9	8,173
18–24	604	5.0	365	3.0	11,995
25–34	1,435	5.0	1,732	6.0	28,740
35–64	4,447	12.1	3,518	9.5	36,858
65+	178*	4.6*	979	25.5	3,834

Unpublished survey data from the Patient Survey Program, Survey and Reports Branch, Division of Biometry and Applied Sciences, National Institute of Mental Health.

*Based on five or fewer sample cases.

5. CHEMICAL AND TRADE NAMES OF PSYCHIATRIC DRUGS

For easy reference the following listing provides chemical and trade names at a glance for many of the commonly used medications for depression and related disorders. Throughout this volume there are separate entries for the major medications. Each is described under the entry for the chemical (generic) name with the trade name in parentheses. Trade names are cross-referenced. For more detailed information check the separate entries.

CHEMICAL NAME	TRADE NAME	CHEMICAL NAME	TRADE NAME
alprazolam	Xanax	hexafluorodiethyl ether	Indoklon
amitriptyline hydrochloride	Elavil, Endep, SK-Amitriptyline	imipramine hydrochloride	Imavate, Janimine, SK-Pramine, Tofranil
amoxapine	Asendin		
amphetamine sulfate	Benzedrine	iproniazid	Marsilid
barbital	Veronal	isocarboxazid	Marplan
benzphetamine hydrochloride	Didrex	lithium carbonate	Eskalith, Lithane, Lithonate
buspirone hydrochloride	BuSpar	lorazepam	Ativan
bupropion hydrochloride	Wellbutrin	maprotiline hydrochloride	Ludiomil
carbamazepine	Tegretol		
carbidopa-Levodopa	Sinemet	mazindol	Sanorex
chlordiazepoxide hydrochloride	Librium	meprobamate	Miltown
		methylphenidate hydrochloride	Ritalin
clonazepam	Klonopin		
clonidine	Catapres	nortriptyline hydrochloride	Aventyl, Pamelor
clorazepate dipotassium	Tranxene, Azene		
chlorpromazine	Thorazine	oxazepam	Serax
clozapine	Clozaril	Phenobarbital	Luminal
dextroamphetamine sulfate	Dexedrine	phenelzine sulfate	Nardil
		prazepam	Verstram, Centrax
desipramine hydrochloride	Norpramin	protriptyline hydrochloride	Vivactil
diazepam	Valium	reserpine	Serpasil, Serpate
doxepin hydrochloride	Adapin, Sinequan	selegiline hydrochloride	Deprenyl, Eldepryl
flurazepam hydrochloride	Dalmane	temazepam	Restoril
		tranylcypromine sulfate	Parnate
fluoxetine hydrochloride	Prozac	trazodone hydrochloride	Desyrel
haloperidol	Haldol	triazolam	Halcion
halazepam	Paxipam	trimipramine maleate	Surmontil

210

6. SOURCES OF INFORMATION

This section contains selected major sources of information on depression, including some organizations that provide treatment. Further information on treatment programs is usually available from national or local government agencies.

UNITED STATES

National Associations, Institutes,
   Organizations and Government Agencies
Community Mental Health Centers
State-by-State Mental Health Centers
D/ART Community Partnerships
Self Help/Support Organizations and Hot
   Lines

CANADA

Provincial and Territorial Agencies

SPECIALIZED AGENCIES OF THE UNITED NATIONS

OTHER FOREIGN ORGANIZATIONS

MAJOR ENGLISH-LANGUAGE JOURNALS, NEWSPAPERS AND PERIODICALS

UNITED STATES NATIONAL ASSOCIATIONS, INSTITUTES, ORGANIZATIONS AND GOVERNMENT AGENCIES

Acupuncture Research Institute
313 W. Andrix St.
Monterey Park, CA 91754

Alcoholic and Drug Problem Association of
   North America
1101 Fifteenth St., NW, #204
Washington, DC 20005

Alcohol, Drug Abuse, and Mental Health
   Administration
Department of Health and Human Services
5600 Fishers Lane
Rockville, MD 20857
301-443-3738

Alcoholics Anonymous
General Service Staff
468 Park Ave. S.
New York, NY 10016
212-686-1100

Alternative Medical Association
7909 S.E. Stark St.
Portland, OR 97215
503-253-4031

Alzheimer's Disease and Related Disorders
   Association, Inc.
70 E. Lake Street, Suite 600
Chicago, IL 60601
312-853-3060

American Academy of Clinical
   Psychiatrists
P.O. Box 3212
San Diego, CA 92103
619-460-2675

American Academy of Family Physicians
1740 West 92nd St.
Kansas City, MO 64114
800-821-2512

American Acupuncture Association
4262 Kissena Blvd.
Flushing, NY 11355

American Association Against Addiction
1668 Bush Street
San Francisco, CA 94109

American Association for Acupuncture and
   Oriental Medicine
5473 66th St. N.
St. Petersburg, FL 33709

American Association for Advancement of
    Health Education
1900 Association Drive
Reston, VA 22091
703-476-3440

American Association for Marriage and
    Family Therapy
924 West Ninth Street
Upland, CA 91786
714-981-0888

American Association of Professional
    Hypnotherapists
P.O. Box 731
McLean, VA 22101
703-448-9623

American Association of Psychiatric
    Services for Children
1133 Fifteenth Street, NW, Suite 1000
Washington, DC 20005
202-429-9440

American Association of Suicidology
    (AAS)
2459 S. Ash St.
Denver, CO 80222
303-692-0985

American Holistic Medical Association,
2002 Eastlake Ave. E.
Seattle, WA 98102
206-322-6842

American Institute of Family Relations
5287 Sunset Boulevard
Los Angeles, CA 90027

American Medical Association
535 No. Dearborn St.
Chicago, IL 60610
312-645-5000

American Mental Health Counselors
    Association
5999 Stevenson Ave.
Alexandria, VA 22304
703-823-9800

American Mental Health Foundation
2 E. 86th St.
New York, NY 10028
212-737-9027

American Psychiatric Association
1400 K Street, NW
Washington, DC 20005
202-682-6000

American Psychological Association
1200 17th St., NW
Washington, DC 20036
202-955-7600

American Sociological Association
1722 North Street, NW
Washington, DC 20036

Association for Advancement of Behavior
    Therapy
15 W. 36th St.
New York, NY 10170
212-279-7970

Barr-Harris Center for the Study of
    Separation and Loss During Childhood
Institute for Psychonalysis
180 North Michigan Ave.
Chicago, IL 60601
312-726-6300

BASH Treatment and Research Center for
    Eating and Mood Disorders
6125 Clayton Ave., Suite 215
St. Louis, MO 63139
314-567-4080

Bereavement and Loss Center of New York
170 E. 83rd St.
New York, NY 10028
212-879-5655

Big Brother, Big Sister of America
117 E. 17th St.
Suite 1200
Philadelphia, PA 19103
215-567-2748

Biofeedback Society of America
11200 W. 44th Ave., #304
Wheat Ridge, CO 80033
303-422-8436

Center for Attitudinal Healing
19 Main St.
Tiburon, CA 94920
415-435-5022

Center for Cognitive Therapy
Room 602
133 South 36th St.
Philadelphia, PA 19104
215-898-4100

Center for Suicide Research and Prevention
Rush-Presbyterian-St. Luke's Medical
  Center
1753 West Congress Parkway
Chicago, IL 60612

Center on Parent Education (COPE)
Barnert Memorial Hospital Center
660 Broadway
Paterson, NJ 07514
201-977-6661

Centers for Disease Control
Department of Health and Human Services
1600 Clifton Road, NE, 3-SSB33
Atlanta, GA 30329

Committee on Problems of Drug
  Dependence
4105 Dunnel Lane
Kensington, MD 20795

Dept. of Health, Education, and Welfare
26 Federal Plaza
New York, NY 10017
212-264-5285

Dept. of Health and Human Services
Freedom of Information Office
Office of Communication
Public Health Service
Room 9-46, Parklawn
5600 Fishers Lane
Rockville, MD 20857
301-443-5252

Depression Awareness Recognition and
  Treatment Project
National Institute of Mental Health
  DART/Program
5600 Fishers Lane
Rockville, MD 20857

Division of Biometry and Applied Sciences
National Institute of Mental Health
5600 Fishers Lane
Rockville, MD 20857

Division of Vital Statistics
U.S. Public Health Service
5600 Fishers Lane
Rockville, MD 20857

Dr. Edward Bach Healing Society
463 Rockaway Ave.
Valley Stream, NY 11580
516-825-1677

Fair Oaks Hospital
19 Prospect St.
Summit, NJ 07901

Family Service Association of America
44 East 23rd St.
New York, NY 10010
212-674-6100

Food and Drug Administration (FDA)
Consumer Inquiries, HFI-10
5600 Fishers Lane
Rockville, MD 20857

Foundation for Better Living
Box 183
201 E. 87th St.
New York, NY 10128
212-860-2339

Foundation for Depression and Manic
  Depression
7 E. 67th St.
New York, NY 10021

Grief Education Institute
2422 South Downing St.
Denver, CO 80210
303-777-8234

Grief Recovery Institute
8306 Wilshire Blvd., #21-A
Los Angeles, CA 90211

Health Insurance Association of America
1025 Connecticut Ave., NW
Washington, DC 20036

Indian Health Service
5600 Fishers Lane, Room 5A-55
Rockville, MD 20857
301-443-1083

Institute for the Advancement of Human
   Behavior
P.O. Box 7226
Stanford, CA 94305
415-851-8411

Institute for Research in Behavioral
   Neuroscience
360 E. 72nd St.
New York, NY 10021
212-517-9070

Institute for Research in Hypnosis and
   Psychotherapy
133 W. 72nd Street
New York, NY 10023
212-874-5290

Institute for Scientific Information
3501 Market St.
Philadelphia, PA 19104

Institute for Social Research
University of Michigan
Rm. 2213
Box 1249
Ann Arbor, MI 48108

Institute for Studies of Destructive
   Behavior/Suicide Prevention Center
1041 South Menlo Ave.
Los Angeles, CA 90006
213-386-5111

International Phototherapy Association,
   Inc.
3260 Euclid Hts. Blvd.
Cleveland Heights, OH 44118
216-929-8301, ext. 381

Karen Horney Psychoanalytic Center
329 E. 62nd St.
New York, NY 10021

Lithium Information Center
Public Affairs Department
Center for Health Sciences

University of Wisconsin-Madison
Madison, WI 53705

Mental Health Clinic Research Center for
   Affective Disorders
Western Psychiatric Institute and Clinic
University of Pittsburgh
School of Medicine
Pittsburgh, PA 15260

Mental Health Material Center
20 E. 29th St.
New York, NY 10016

Mood, Anxiety and Personality Disorder
   Research Branch
National Institute of Mental Health
5600 Fishers Lane, Room 10C-24
Rockville, MD 20587

Mothertime
140 Christie St.
Leonia, NJ 07605
201-585-0845

Narcotics Education
6830 Laurel Ave., NW
Washington, DC 20012
202-723-4774

Narcotics Educational Foundation of
   America
5055 Sunset Boulevard
Los Angeles, CA 90027
213-663-5171

Nathan S. Kline Institute for Psychiatric
   Research
Orangeburg, NY 10962
914-365-2000

National Academy of Science
Institute of Medicine
Committee for Division of Mental Health
   and Behavior Medicine
2101 Constitution Ave., NW
Washington, DC 20418

National Alliance for the Mentally Ill
1901 North Fort Myer Drive
Suite 500
Arlington, VA 22209

National Alliance for Research on
   Schizophrenia and Depression
208 S. LaSalle St.
Suite 1438
Chicago, IL 60604

National Alliance of Mental Patients
P.O. Box 618
Sioux Falls, SD 57101
605-334-4067

National Anorexic Aid Society, Inc.
5796 Karl Road
Columbus, OH 43229
614-436-1112

National Association of Anorexia Nervosa
   and Associated Disorders
Box 7
Highland Park, IL 60035
312-831-3438

National Association of Social Workers
7981 Eastern Avenue
Silver Spring, MD 20910
301-565-0333

National Association of State Mental
   Health Program Directors
1101 King St.
Suite 160
Alexandria, VA 22314
703-739-9333

National Association on Drug Abuse
   Problems
355 Lexington Ave.
New York, NY 10017
212-986-1170

National Center for Health Statistics
U.S. Department of Health & Human
   Services
3700 East-West Highway, Room I-57
Hyattsville, MD 20782

National Clearing House for Alcohol and
   Drug Information
P.O. Box 2345
Rockville, MD 20852

National Clearing House for Mental Health
5600 Fishers Lane
Rockville, MD 20857
301-443-4513

National Committee for the Prevention of
   Alcoholism and Drug Dependency
6830 Laurel Street, NW
Washington, DC 20012

National Committee on Youth Suicide
   Prevention
67 Irving Place South
New York, NY 10003

National Council on Alcoholism
12 West 21st St.
New York, NY 10010

National Depressive and Manic Depressive
   Association
Merchandise Mart
Box 3395
Chicago, IL 60654

National Federation of Parents for Drug
   Free Youth
8730 George Avenue, Suite 200
Silver Spring, MD 20901

National Foundation for Depressive Illness,
   Inc.
P.O. Box 2257
New York, NY 10116
212-620-7637

National Institute of Alcohol Abuse and
   Alcoholism (NIAA)
P.O. Box 2345
Rockville, MD 20852

National Institute of Mental Health (NIMH)
Public Inquiries
Parklawn Building, Room 15C-05
5600 Fishers Lane
Rockville, MD 20857

National Institute on Drug Abuse
5600 Fishers Lane
Rockville, MD 20857

National Medical Association
1012 10th St., NW
Washington, DC 20001

National Mental Health Association
1021 Prince St.
Alexandria, VA 22314
703-684-7722

National Mental Health Consumers'
   Association
311 South Juniper St.
Room 902
Philadelphia, PA 19107
215-735-2465

National Organization for Seasonal
   Affective Disorder
P.O. Box 40133
Washington, DC 20016

National Sudden Infant Death Syndrome
   (SIDS) Foundation
8200 Professional Place
Suite 104
Landover, MD 20785
800-221-SIDS

OCD Foundation, Inc.
P.O. Box 9573
New Haven, CT 06535
203-772-0565, 0575

Parents Without Partners
7910 Woodmont Ave.
Washington, DC 20014
301-654-8850

Parkinson's Educational Program
1800 Park Newport, #302
Newport Beach, CA 92660
714-640-0218

Phobia Society of America
133 Rollins Ave.
Suite 4B
Rockville, MD 20852
301-231-9350

Pill Addicts Anonymous
P.O. Box 278
Reading, PA 19603
215-372-1128

Recovery, Inc.
802 North Dearborn St.
Chicago, IL 60610

Runaway Suicide Prevention Network
Human Services Development Institute
University of Southern Maine
246 Deering Avenue
Portland, ME 04102
207-780-4430

Scientific and Technical Information
   Branch
Division of Data Services
National Center for Health Statistics
3700 East-West Highway
Hyattsville, MD 20782

Seasons: Suicide Bereavement
1358 Sunset Dr.
Salt Lake City, UT 84116
803-596-2341

Social Psychiatry Research Institute
150 E. 69th St.
New York, NY 10021
212-628-4800

Society of Behavioral Medicine
P.O. Box 8530 University Station
Knoxville, TN 37996
615-974-5164

Survivors
P.O. Box 134
993 "C" S. Santa Fe Ave.
Vista, CA 92083
619-727-5682

Tardive Dyskinesia/Tardive Dystonia
   National Association
600 East Pine St.
Seattle, WA 98122
206-522-3166

Texas Tech Alzheimer's Disease Center
Texas Tech University Health Sciences
   Center
Lubbock, TX 79430

U.S. Department of Health & Human
   Services
Public Health Service
Rockville, MD 20857

Wellness Associates
Box 5433

Mill Valley, CA 94942
415-383-3806

Women For Sobriety
Box 618
Quakertown, PA 18951
215-536-8026

COMMUNITY MENTAL HEALTH CENTERS IN THE UNITED STATES

Superintendent of Documents
U.S. Government Printing Office
Washington, DC 20402
202-783-3238

A *Mental Health Directory* (stock number 017-024-01230) published by the National Institute of Mental Health is available through the Government Printing Office. The directory includes inpatient, outpatient, partial care and supportive care organizations for emotionally ill adults and children. The cost is $9.00. Please note that prices of publication's are subject to change.

National Council of Community Mental
  Health Centers
12300 Twinbrook Parkway
Suite 320
Rockville, MD 20852
301-984-6200

Publishes a directory of member community mental health centers. For further information and cost contact the council directly.

STATE-BY-STATE MENTAL HEALTH CENTERS AND REGIONAL REFERRALS FOR THE TREATMENT OF DEPRESSION*

ALABAMA

Birmingham

University of Alabama
School of Medicine
University Station

*Mental Health Clinic Research Center for Affective Disorders, Western Psychiatric Institute and Clinic, University of Pittsburgh, School of Medicine, Pittsburgh, Pennsylvania.

Birmingham, AL 35294
(205) 934-2011

Mobile

University of Southern Alabama
College of Medicine
307 University Boulevard
Mobile, AL 36688
(205) 471-7476

ARIZONA

Tucson

Southern Arizona Mental Health Center
1930 E. 6th Street
Tucson, AZ 85719
(602) 628-5221

ARKANSAS

Little Rock

University of Arkansas for Medical
  Sciences
4301 West Markham
Little Rock, AR 72205
(501) 661-5266

CALIFORNIA

Los Angeles

University of California at Los Angeles
Affective Disorders Clinic
10966 LeConte
Los Angeles, CA 90024
(213) 825-0764, 0271 or 0491

University of Southern California
School of Medicine
Department of Psychiatry
Tower Hall
1711 N. Griffen Avenue
Los Angeles, CA 90033
(213) 226-5731

Harbor-UCLA Medical Center
Building F-5
Torrance, CA 90509
(213) 533-3775, 3776

Northern: San Francisco

Langley Porter Neuropsychiatric Inst.
401 Parnassus Avenue
San Francisco, CA 94143
(415) 681-8080, x 478

Orange County

University of California at Irvine
Medical Center
Department of Psychiatry and Human
  Behavior
101 City Drive South
Orange, CA 92668
(714) 634-5886

San Diego

La Jolla V.A. Hospital
3350 La Jolla Village Drive
San Diego, CA 92161
(714) 453-7500, x 3471

UCSD Gifford Mental Health Clinic
3427 4th Avenue
San Diego, CA 92103
(714) 299-3510

Stanford (Palo Alto)

Stanford University
Department of Psychiatry and Behavioral
  Science
V.A. Hospital
Stanford, CA 94305
(415) 493-5000, x 5461

COLORADO

Denver

University of Colorado Medical Center
4200 East 9th Avenue
Denver, CO 80220
(303) 394-8403

CONNECTICUT

New Haven

Connecticut Mental Health Center
34 Park Street
New Haven, CT 06519
(203) 789-7300

Yale New Haven Hospital
Dana Psychiatric Clinic
789 Howard Avenue
New Haven, CT 06504
(203) 436-1650

DELAWARE

No medical school in the state; refer to
  Philadelphia, Pennsylvania.

FLORIDA

Miami

Mount Sinai Medical Center
4300 Alton Road
Miami Beach, FL 33140
(305) 674-2194

University of Miami Medical Center
Box 520875
Biscayne Annex
Miami, FL 33152
(305) 325-6862

Tampa

University of Southern Florida
Department of Psychiatry
12901 North 30th Street
Tampa, FL 33612
(813) 974-4355

Tarpon Springs

Anclote Manor Hospital
P.O. Box 1224
Tarpon Springs, FL 33589
(813) 937-4211

GEORGIA

Atlanta

Emory University School of Medicine
Emory Outpatient Clinic
1440 Clifton Road, NE
Atlanta, GA 30322
(404) 321-0111

HAWAII

Honolulu

University of Hawaii
Department of Psychiatry
1356 Lusapana Street
Honolulu, HI 96813
(808) 548-3420

St. Francis Hospital
Honolulu, HI 96813
(808) 595-6387

IDAHO

No medical school; refer to Oregon or
Nevada.

ILLINOIS

Chicago

Illinois State Psychiatric Institute
1601 W. Taylor Street
Chicago, IL 60612
(312) 996-1065

Rush Medical College
1720 W. Polk Street
Chicago, IL 60612
(312) 942-5372

University of Chicago
Pritzker School of Medicine
Department of Psychiatry
Chicago, IL 60637
(312) 947-6477

INDIANA

Indianapolis

LaRue D. Carter Memorial Hospital
1315 West Tenth Street
Indianapolis, IN 46202
(317) 634-8401

IOWA

Iowa City

University of Iowa
Department of Psychiatry
500 Newton Road

Iowa City, IA 52242
(319) 353-3719

KANSAS

Kansas City

University of Kansas
School of Medicine
Department of Psychiatry
Kansas City, KS 66103
(913) 588-6464

Topeka

Menninger Clinic
P.O. Box 829
Topeka, KS 66601
(913) 234-9566

KENTUCKY

Lexington

University of Kentucky
Department of Psychiatry
Lexington, KY 40506
(606) 233-5492

LOUISIANA

New Orleans

Tulane Medical Center
Department of Psychiatry
1415 Tulane Avenue
New Orleans, LA 70112
(504) 588-5236

Shreveport

Louisiana State University
School of Medicine
Department of Psychiatry
P.O. Box 33932
Shreveport, LA 71130
(318) 674-6040

MAINE

No medical school in Maine; refer to
Boston.

MARYLAND AND WASHINGTON, D.C.

Bethesda

National Institute of Mental Health
9000 Rockville Pike
Building 10, Room 45-239
Bethesda, MD 20014
(301) 496-5755, 2141

National Institute of Mental Health
9000 Rockville Pike
Building 10
Bethesda, MD 20014
(301) 496-3465

MASSACHUSETTS

Belmont

McLean Hospital
115 Mill Street
Belmont, MA 02178
(617) 855-2255, ×3342

Boston

Massachusetts General Hospital
Department of Psychiatry
Boston, MA 02114
(617) 726-5568

Massachusetts Mental Health Center
74 Fenwood Road
Boston, MA 02115
(617) 731-2921

MICHIGAN

Ann Arbor

University of Michigan Hospital
Clinical Studies Unit
ATH-6
Ann Arbor, MI 48109
(313) 763-4382

Detroit

Lafayette Clinic
951 Lafayette
Detroit, MI 48206
(313) 256-9418

Lansing

Michigan State University
Psychiatry Clinics
Affective Disorders Clinic
E. Lansing, MI 48824
(517) 353-3070

MINNESOTA

Minneapolis

University of Minnesota
Medical School
Minneapolis, MN 55455
(612) 373-8868

MISSISSIPPI

Jackson

University of Mississippi
School of Medicine
Department of Psychiatry and Human
    Behavior
2500 North State Street
Jackson, MS 39216
(601) 987-6565

MISSOURI

St. Louis

Washington University
School of Medicine
4940 Audubon Avenue
St. Louis, MO 63110
(314) 454-3348

MONTANA

No medical school in the state; refer to
    Colorado or North Dakota.

NEBRASKA

Omaha

University of Nebraska
College of Medicine
Department of Psychiatry
42nd and Dewey Avenue
Omaha, NE 68105
(402) 559-5100

University of Nebraska
Nebraska Psychiatric Institute
602 S. 45th Street
Omaha, NE 68106
(402) 559-5019

NEVADA

Reno

University of Nevada Medical School
Department of Psychiatry and Behavioral
  Science
Reno, NV 89557
(702) 784-4917

NEW HAMPSHIRE

Hanover

Dartmouth-Hitchcock Medical Center
Community Mental Health Center
Hanover, NH 03755
(603) 643-4000, 3694

NEW JERSEY

Summit

Fair Oaks Hospital
19 Prospect Street
Summit, NJ 07901
(201) 277-2300

NEW MEXICO

Albuquerque

University of New Mexico
School of Medicine
Albuquerque, NM 87131
(505) 277-2223

NEW YORK

New York City

Mt. Sinai Medical Center
1 Gustave Levy Place
New York, NY 10029
(212) 650-7191

New York University Medical Center
560 First Avenue
New York, NY 10016
(212) 340-5707

Psychiatric Institute
722 West 168th Street
New York, NY 10032
(212) 960-2200

Psychiatric Institute Annex
722 West 168th Street
New York, NY 10032
(212) 960-2307

Rochester

University of Rochester
Department of Psychiatry
Affective Disorders Clinic
300 Crittenden Boulevard
Rochester, NY 14642
(716) 275-3071

NORTH CAROLINA

Chapel Hill

University of North Carolina
School of Medicine
Division of Health Affairs
Chapel Hill, NC 27514
(919) 966-1480

NORTH DAKOTA

Fargo

University of North Dakota
Medical Education Center
1919 North Elm
Fargo, ND 58102
(701) 293-4113

OHIO

Cincinnati

University of Cincinnati
College of Medicine
Central Outpatient Clinic
Intake Department
231 Bethesda Avenue
Cincinnati, OH 45267
(513) 872-5856

Cleveland

University Hospital
2040 Abington Road
Cleveland, OH 44106
(216) 444-3450

OKLAHOMA

Oklahoma City

University of Oklahoma
Health Sciences Center
Department of Psychiatry
P.O. Box 26901
Oklahoma City, OK 73190
(405) 271-5251

OREGON

Portland

Portland Division V.A.
3710 South West U.S.
Veterans Hospital Road
P.O. Box 1034
Portland, OR 97207
(503) 222-9221

PENNSYLVANIA

Philadelphia

Center for Cognitive Therapy
133 S. 36th Street
Philadelphia, PA 19104
(215) 243-4102

Girard Bank Building
Suite 309
133 S. 36th Street
Philadelphia, PA 19102
(215) 387-4814

University of Pennsylvania Hospital
Biological Psychiatry
Philadelphia, PA 19104
(215) 662-3462, 2844

University Hospital
Depression Clinic
203 Piersol Building-G1
3400 Spruce Street
Philadelphia, PA 19104
(215) 662-2844, 3560

V.A. Ambulatory Care Center
Mental Hygiene Clinic (16A)
1421 Cherry Street
Philadelphia, PA 19102
(215) 597-7168, 7169

Pittsburgh

Western Psychiatric Institute and Clinic
Mood Disorders Clinic
3811 O'Hara Street
Pittsburgh, PA 15213
(412) 624-2000

RHODE ISLAND

Providence

V.A. Hospital of Providence
Providence, RI 02908
(401) 273-7100

SOUTH CAROLINA

Charleston

Medical University of South Carolina
Outpatient Department
171 Ashlet Avenue
Charleston, SC 29403
(803) 792-3051

SOUTH DAKOTA

Refer to Nebraska.

TENNESSEE

Memphis

University of Tennessee
Department of Psychiatry
66 North Pauline, Suite 633
Memphis, TN 38105
(901) 528-6628

Nashville

Vanderbilt University
Department of Psychiatry
Nashville, TN 37232
(615) 322-4927

TEXAS

Dallas

University of Texas
Health Science Center
Department of Psychiatry
5323 Harry Hines
Dallas, TX 75235
(214) 688-3300

Galveston

University of Texas Medical Branch
Department of Psychiatry
Behavorial Science
1200 Graves Building
Galveston, TX 77550
(713) 765-3901

Houston

Baylor College of Medicine
Texas Medical Center
Department of Psychiatry
1200 Moursund Avenue, Room 115 D
Houston, TX 77030
(713) 790-4889

San Antonio

University of Texas
Health Science Center at San Antonio
Medical School
Department of Psychiatry
7703 Floyd Curl Drive
San Antonio, TX 78284
(512) 691-7315

UTAH

Salt Lake City

University of Utah
College of Medicine
Department of Psychiatry
50 North Medical Drive
Salt Lake City, UT 84132
(801) 581-7955

VERMONT

Burlington

University of Vermont
Department of Psychiatry
Medical Alumni Building
Burlington, VT 05401
(802) 656-4560

VIRGINIA

Norfolk

Eastern Virginia Medical School
Department of Psychiatry and Behavioral
   Science
P.O. Box 1980
Norfolk, VA 23501
(804) 446-5888

Richmond

Medical College of Virginia
Department of Psychiatry
Box 710
Richmond, VA 23298
(804) 786-9157

WASHINGTON

Harbor View Medical Center
Psychiatry Department
2H Harbor View Hall
325 9th Avenue
Seattle, WA 98104
(206) 223-3404

WEST VIRGINIA

Recommend WPIC in Pittsburgh.

WISCONSIN

Madison

Clinical Sciences Center
Department of Psychiatry
600 Highland Avenue
Madison, WI 53792
(608) 263-6075

WYOMING

No medical school in Wyoming; refer to
   Colorado or Utah.

D/ART COMMUNITY PARTNERSHIPS*
STATE PROGRAMS

Indiana

Carrie Giannakos
Director of Education and Media
Mental Health Association in Indiana
1443 North Meridian
Indianapolis, IN 46202
(317) 638-3501

Michigan

Tom Sovine, Executive Director
Mental Health Association in Michigan
15920 W. 12 Mile Road
Southfield, MI 48076
(313) 557-6777

Minnesota

George D. Carr, Executive Director
Mental Health Association of Minnesota
328 E. Hennepin
Minneapolis, MN 55414
(612) 331-6840

New York

Leila Salmon, Executive Director
Mental Health Association in
   New York State
75 New Scotland Avenue
Albany, NY 12208
(518) 434-0439

North Dakota

Allen Koss, Ph.D.
Coordinator of Planning and Prevention
Division of Mental Health
Department of Human Services
State Capitol Building
Bismarck, ND 58505
(701) 224-3268

Myrt Armstrong, Executive Director
Mental Health Association in
   North Dakota
Box 160
Bismarck, ND 58502
(701) 255-3692

Pennsylvania

Marta Peck, Director
Advocacy Services
Mental Health Association of
   Pennsylvania
900 Market Street
Harrisburg, PA 17101
(717) 236-9363

Lisa Rossi, Chairperson
Southwest Pennsylvania Regional
   D/ART Campaign
c/o Division of Public Relations
DeSoto at O'Hara Streets
Pittsburgh, PA 15213
(412) 647-7182

Utah

Tia Davis, D/ART Chairperson
Mental Health Association of Utah
3760 Highland Drive, Suite 200
Salt Lake City, UT 48106
(801) 273-3944

TARGETED AREAS

Central Florida

Pamela Davis, Executive Director
Mental Health Association of Central
   Florida
608 Mariposa Street
Orlando, FL 32801
(407) 843-1564

Houston, Texas

Diane Long
Coordinator of Professional and
   Education Services
Mental Health Association of Houston
   and Harris County
2211 Norfolk, Suite 810

*This material on state mental health programs was provided by the National Institute of Mental Health's D/ART Depression Campaign.

Houston, TX 77098
(713) 523-8963

Huntsville, Alabama

Molly Pitts-Jones
Executive Director
Mental Health Association in
   Madison County
701 Andrew Jackson Way
Huntsville, AL 35801-3504
(205) 536-9441

Kansas City, Kansas

Fenna Swenson, Associate Director
Mental Health Association of Johnson
   County
9728 Rosehill Road
Lenexa, KS 66215
(913) 888-5663

Metropolitan Washington, D.C.
   Metro Consortium

Harriet Guttenberg, Chair
Executive Director
Mental Health Association of
   Montgomery County
1000 Twinbrook Parkway
Rockville, MD 20851
(301) 424-0656

Robert Simon, Executive Director
Mental Health Association of Alexandria
3112 Mt.Vernon Avenue
Alexandria, VA 22305
(703) 548-0010

Anita Bellamy-Shelton
Executive Director
Mental Health Association-D.C.
1628 16th Street, NW
Washington, DC 20001
(202) 265-6363

Mary Lynne Reynolds,
   Executive Director
Mental Health Association of
   Prince Georges County
6607 Riverdale Road

Riverdale, MD 20737
(301) 577-3140

Elizabeth McManus, Executive Director
Mental Health Association of
   Northern Virginia
Suite 232
100 North Washington Street
Falls Church, VA 22046
(703) 536-4100

Michigan

Tom Sovine, Executive Director
Mental Health Association in Michigan
15920 W. 12 Mile Road
Southfield, MI 48076
(313) 557-6777

Napa, California

Maryellen Vander Sluis
D/ART Chair
Mental Health Association of
   Napa County
1627A Lincoln Avenue
Napa, CA 94558
(707) 224-9033

Redding, California

Richard Baxter, Director
Family Service Agency of Shasta County
225 Locust Street, Suite 200
Redding, CA 96001
(916) 243-2024

Roanoke, Virginia

Diane Kelly, Executive Director
Mental Health Association of
   Roanoke Valley
920 S. Jefferson Street, Suite 201
Roanoke, VA 24016
(703) 344-0931

Sacramento, California

Joan Reiss, Executive Director
Mental Health Association—
   Sacramento/Placer Counties
5370 Elvas Avenue, Suite B
Sacramento, CA 95819
(916) 456-2070

San Bernardino, California

Deborah Reff
Mental Health Education Coordinator
Department of Mental Health
San Bernardino County
700 East Gilbert St., Bldg. 5
San Bernardino, CA 92415-0920
(714) 387-7049

Seattle, Washington

Eleanor Owen, Executive Director
Washington Advocates for the
   Mentally Ill
225 N. 70th Street
Seattle, WA 98103
(206) 789-7722

Southwestern New Jersey

Wenllian J. Stallings, Executive Director
Mental Health Association in
   Southwestern New Jersey
505 Cooper Street
Camden, NJ 08102
(609) 966-6767

Springfield, Missouri

Pat Kloberdanz, President
Mental Health Association of the Ozarks
1675 E. Seminole, Suite 6200
Springfield, MO 65804
(417) 882-4677/4691

Tulsa, Oklahoma

Judy Leaver, Executive Director
Mental Health Association in Tulsa
1502 S. Denver
Tulsa, OK 74119
(918) 585-1213

Washington (Eastern)

Vicki Johnson, President
Alliance for the Mentally Ill of
   Washington State
East 11115 -23rd Avenue
Spokane, WA 99206
(509) 928-1536

SELF HELP/SUPPORT
ORGANIZATIONS AND HOT LINES*

Many of the following groups maintain a hot
line so that those in need will have constant
access to information and an understanding
listener.

ARIZONA

CoDependents Anonymous
P.O. Box 33577
Phoenix, AZ 85067

The Rainy Day People
P.O. Box 422
Scottsdale, AZ 85252
(602) 840-1029

CALIFORNIA

California Self-Help Center
2349 Franz Hall, UCLA
405 Hilgard Avenue
Los Angeles, CA 90024
(213) 825-1799; in CA: (800) 222-LINK

San Francisco Self-Help Clearinghouse
2398 Pine Street
San Francisco, CA 94115
(415) 921-4401

For information about other clearinghouses in California, contact the California
Self-Help Center.

Families Anonymous
P.O. Box 528
Van Nuys, CA 91408
(818) 989-7841

Narcotics Anonymous
P.O. Box 9999
Van Nuys, CA 91409
(818) 780-3951

*Source: Self-Help Clearinghouse, Saint Clares-River-
side Medical Center, Pocono Road, Denville, NJ 07834;
(201) 625-7101. The Self-Help Clearinghouse also publishes *The Self-Help Sourcebook,* which lists other self
help/support organizations and hot lines throughout the
country. It is available from the foregoing address. Cost:
$8.00 (book rate postage) or $9.00 (first class postage).

Parents Anonymous
6733 South Sepulveda Blvd.
Suite 270
Los Angeles, CA 90045
(213) 410-9732

Parents United
P.O. Box 952
San Jose, CA 95108
(408) 280-5055

CONNECTICUT

Self-Help Mutual Support Network
19 Howe Street
New Haven, CT 06115
(203) 789-7645

FLORIDA

Hotline Information and Referral
P.O. Box 13087
St. Petersburg, FL 33733
(813) 531-4664

ILLINOIS

Compassionate Friends, Inc.
P.O. Box 3696
Oak Brook, IL 60522
(312) 990-0010

Self-Help Center
1600 Dodge Center, Suite S122
Evanston, IL 60201
(312) 328-0470

Self-Help Center
405 State Street
Champaign, IL 61820
(217) 352-0099

INDIANA

Indianapolis Hotline
(317) 926-HELP

KANSAS

Self-Help Network
Wichita State University, Box 34
Wichita, KS 67208
(316) 689-3170

MASSACHUSETTS

Cooperative Extension Service
University of Massachusetts
113 Skinner Hall
Amherst, MA 01003
(413) 545-2313

MICHIGAN

Berrien County Self-Help Clearinghouse
Riverwood Community Mental Health
  Center
1485 Highway M-139
Benton Harbor, MI 49022
(616) 925-0585

Michigan Self-Help Clearinghouse
109 W. Michigan Avenue, Suite 900
Lansing, MI 48933
(517) 484-7373; in MI: (800) 752-5858

MINNESOTA

Emotions Anonymous
P.O. Box 4245
St. Paul, MN 55104

Mutual Help Resource Center
Wilder Foundation, Community Care
  Unit
919 Lafond Avenue
St. Paul, MN 55104
(612) 642-4060

MISSOURI

Kansas City Mental Health Association
706 West 42nd Street
Kansas City, MO 64111
(816) 561-1800

NEBRASKA

Self-Help Information Services
1601 Euclid Avenue
Lincoln, NE 68502
(402) 476-9668

NEW JERSEY

New Jersey Self-Help Clearinghouse
St. Clare's Hospital-Riverside Medical
   Ctr.
Pocono Road
Denville, NJ 07834
(201) 625-9565; in NJ: (800) 367-6274

NEW YORK

Depressives Anonymous
329 E. 62nd St.
New York, NY 10021
(212) 689-2600

Long Island Self-Help Clearinghouse
New York Institute of Technology
Carleton Avenue
Central Islip, NY 11722
(516) 348-3030

National Self-Help Clearinghouse
Graduate School and University Center
   of the City University of New York
Room 620
25 West 43rd St.
New York, NY 10036
(212) 642-2944

New York City Self-Help Clearinghouse
P.O. Box 022812
Brooklyn, NY 11201
(718) 596-6000

New York State Self-Help Clearinghouse
Council on Children and Families
Empire State Plaza
Erastus Corning Tower 2, 28th Floor
Albany, NY 12223
(518) 473-4329

Westchester Self-Help Clearinghouse
Westchester Community College
Academic/Arts Building
75 Grasslands Road
Valhalla, NY 10595
(914) 347-3620

For information about other clearinghouses in New York state, contact the New
York State Self-Help Clearinghouse.

OHIO

Ohio Self-Help Clearinghouse
Family Service Association
184 Salem Avenue
Dayton, OH 45406
(513) 222-9481

OREGON

Northwest Regional Self-Help
   Clearinghouse
718 West Burnside
Portland, OR 97209
(503) 226-9360

PENNSYLVANIA

Depression After Delivery
P.O. Box 1282
Morrisville, PA 19067
(215) 295-3994

Self-Help Group Network
710 1/2 South Avenue
Pittsburgh, PA 15221
(412) 247-5400

Self-Help Information Network
   Exchange
SHINE Voluntary Action Center
225 N. Washington Avenue
Scranton, PA 18503
(717) 961-1234

Theos
Suite 410
Office Building
Penn Hills Mall
Pittsburgh, PA 15235
(412) 243-4299

UNITE, INC
c/o Jeanes Hospital
7600 Central Ave.
Philadelphia, PA 19111
(215) 728-2082

RHODE ISLAND

Support Group Helpline
Rhode Island Dept. of Health
Cannon Building

Davis Street
Providence, RI 02908
(401) 277-2223

SOUTH CAROLINA

Support Group Network
Lexington Medical Center
2720 Sunset Blvd.
West Columbia, SC 29169
(803) 791-9227

TENNESSEE

Support Group Clearinghouse
Mental Health Center of Knox County
6712 Kingston Pike, Suite 203
Knoxville, TN 37196
(615) 588-9747

TEXAS

Dallas Self-Help Clearinghouse
Dallas County Mental Health Association
2500 Maple Avenue
Dallas, TX 75201
(214) 871-2420

Greater San Antonio Self-Help
  Clearinghouse
Mental Health in Greater San Antonio
1407 North Main
San Antonio, TX 78212
(512) 222-1571

Houston Self-Help Clearinghouse
Mental Health Assn. in Houston &
  Harris County
2211 Norfolk, Suite 810
Houston, TX 77098
(713) 523-8963

Tarrant County Self-Help Clearinghouse
Tarrant County Mental Health
  Association
3136 West 4th Street
Fort Worth, TX 76102
(817) 335-5405

Texas Self-Help Clearinghouse
Mental Health Association in Texas
1111 W. 24th Street

Austin, TX 78705
(512) 476-0611

WASHINGTON, D.C.

Family Stress Services of D.C.
2001 O Street, NW, Suite 6
Washington, DC 20036
(202) 628-FACT

Greater Washington Self-Help Coalition
100 N. Washington Street, Suite 232
Falls Church, VA 22046
(703) 536-4100

Parents Without Partners
7910 Woodmont Ave.
Washington, DC 20014
(301) 654-8850

WISCONSIN

Health and Human Services Outreach
University of Wisconsin-Madison
414 Lowell Hall, 610 Langdon Street
Madison, WI 53706
(608) 263-4432

Mutual Aid Self-Help Association
P.O. Box 09304
Milwaukee, WI 53209
(414) 461-1466

SELF-HELP CLEARINGHOUSE
TELEPHONE NUMBERS

California*   1-800-222-LINK (in CA only)
Connecticut   (203) 789-7645
Illinois   1-800-322-M.A.S.H. (in IL)
Kansas   (316) 686-1205
Massachusetts   (413) 545-2313
Michigan*   1-800-752-5858 (in MI)
Minnesota   (612) 642-4060
Missouri-Kansas City   (816) 361-5007
Nebraska   (402) 476-9668
New Jersey   1-800-FOR-M.A.S.H. (in NJ)
New York State*   (518) 474-6293
N.Y.-Long Island   (516) 348-3030
N.Y.-New York City   (718) 596-6000

---

*Maintains listings of additional local clearinghouses
operating within that state

N.Y.-Westchester   (914) 347-3620
Oregon-Portland   (503) 222-5555
PA-Pittsburgh   (412) 247-5400
PA-Scranton   (717) 961-1234
South Carolina   (803) 791-2426
Texas-Dallas   (214) 871-2420
Vermont   1-800-442-5356
Greater Washington, DC   (703) 536-4100

For national U.S. listings and directories:
Self-Help Clearinghouse, NJ
   (201) 625-7101
Self-Help Center, Illinois   (312) 328-0470
National Self-Help Clearinghouse,
   N.Y. City   (212) 840-1259

OTHER HELPFUL ORGANIZATIONS

O.D.P.H.P. National Health Information
   Clearinghouse (U.S.)   1-800-336-4797
National Organization for Rare Disorders
   (U.S.)   1-800-447-6673

CANADA
PROVINCIAL AND TERRITORIAL
AGENCIES

ALBERTA—Branch Contacts—
CANADIAN MENTAL HEALTH
ASSOCIATION

Canadian Mental Health Association
Barrhead Branch
c/o F.C.S.S.
Box 488
5115 - 45 Street
Barrhead, Alberta TOG OEO
Telephone: 403-674-3341

Canadian Mental Health Association
Brooks Branch
General Delivery
Scandia, Alberta TOJ 2Z0

Canadian Mental Health Association
#328, 9707-110 Street
Edmonton, Alberta T5K 2L9
Telephone: 403-482-6576

Canadian Mental Health Association
Camrose Branch

R.R. 2
New Norway, Alberta TOB 3L0
Telephone: 403-855-2493

Canadian Mental Health Association
Claresholm Branch
Box 1354
Claresholm, Alberta TOL 0T0
Telephone: 403-625-4404

Canadian Mental Health Association
Fort McMurray Branch
c/o Peter Pond Community School
Room 22B, 9601 Franklin Avenue
Fort McMurray, Alberta T9H 2J8
Telephone: 403-743-1053

Canadian Mental Health Association
Pincher Creek Branch
Box 1544
Pincher Creek, Alberta TOK 1W0
Telephone: 403-627-3513

ALBERTA—Regional Contacts—
CANADIAN MENTAL HEALTH
ASSOCIATION

North Region
#201, 10118-101 Avenue
Grande Prairie, Alberta
T8V 0Y2
Telephone: 403-539-6660

North Central Region
9th Floor
One Twelve Professional Building
10050-112 Street
Edmonton, Alberta
T5K 2J1
Telephone: 403-482-6091

Central Region
#2, 5015-48 Street
Red Deer, Alberta
T4N 1S9
Telephone: 403-342-2266

South Central Region
#201, 723-14 Street, N.W.
Calgary, Alberta
T2N 2A4

Telephone: 403-283-7491
FAX: 403-270-3066

South Region
505-7th Street South
Lethbridge, Alberta
T1J 2G8
Telephone: 403-329-4775

Southeast Region
379 Aberdeen Street, S.E.
Medicine Hat, Alberta
T1A 0R3
Telephone: 403-529-6011

Suicide Information and Education
   Centre/Suicide Prevention Training
   Program
#201, 1615-10 Avenue, S.W.
Calgary, Alberta
T3C 0J7
Telephone: 403-245-3900

Psychologists Assoc. of Alberta
Dr. Stan Whitsett (President & Delegate)
Alberta Children's Hospital
1820 Richmond Road South West
Calgary, Alberta
T2T 5C7
Telephone: 403-229-7959 (B)
403-246-4570 (H)

BRITISH COLUMBIA

British Columbia Psychological Assoc.
Dr. Greg Banwell (President & Delegate)
Suite 1610, Marine Building
355 Burrard Street
Vancouver, B.C.
V6C 2G8
Telephone: 604-689-1717

Canadian Mental Health Association
#207, 96 East Broadway
Vancouver, B.C. V5T 4N9
Telephone: 604-873-1633

MANITOBA

Canadian Mental Health Association
2-836 Ellice Avenue

Winnipeg, Manitoba R3G 0C2
Telephone: 204-775-8888

Psychological Association of Manitoba
Dr. Jim Newton (President & Delegate)
Manitoba Adolescent Treatment Centre
120 Tecumseh Avenue
Winnipeg, Manitoba
R3E 2A9
Telephone: 204-477-6391 (B)
204-255-6655 (H)

NEW BRUNSWICK

Campbellton Regional Hospital
Psychiatric Unit
35 Arran Street
Campbellton, N.B.
E3N 1L1

Canadian Mental Health Association
65 Brunswick Street
Fredericton, N.B. E3B 1G5
Telephone: 506-455-5231
506-362-2970

Centracare Saint John Inc.
P.O. Box 3220, Station B
Saint John, N.B.
E2M 4H7

Chaleur Regional Hospital
Psychiatric Unit
P.O. Drawer S
Bathurst, N.B.
E2A 4A4

Dr. Everett Chalmers Hospital
Psychiatric Unit
P.O. Box 9000
Fredericton, N.B.
E3B 5N5

College of Psychologists of
   New Brunswick
Juanita Mureika (President & Delegate)
University of New Brunswick
Learning Centre
Division of Educational Foundations
Faculty of Education
Fredericton, N.B.
E3B 6E3

Department of Health
P.O. Box 6000
348 King Street
Fredericton, New Brunswick
   E3B 4H1

Department of Psychiatry
Georges Dumont Hospital
330 Archibald Street
Moncton, N.B.
E1C 2Z3

Edmundston Regional Hospital
Psychiatric Unit
54, 21st Avenue
Edmundston, N.B.
E3V 2C1

Moncton City Hospital
Psychiatric Unit
135 MacBeath Avenue
Moncton, N.B.
E1C 6Z8

Restigouche Hospital Center
P.O. Drawer 10
Campbellton, N.B.
E3N 3G2

Saint John Regional Hospital
Psychiatric Unit
P.O. Box 2100
Saint John, N.B.
E2L 4L2

NEW BRUNSWICK—Mental Health
Commission

Region I
Mental Health Clinic/Clinique de Santé
   Mentale
Hôpital Stella-Maris de Kent
Ste-Anne-de Kent
New Brunswick
E0A 2N0
Telephone: 902-743-2436

Region II
Mental Health Clinic/Clinique de Santé
   Mentale
Professional Arts Building

100 Arden Street, 2nd Fl.
Moncton, N.B.
E1C 4B7
Telephone: 902-856-2444

Region III
Mental Health Clinic
116 Coburg Street
Saint John, N.B.
E2L 3K1
Telephone: 902-632-8090

Mental Health Clinic
Sussex Health Center
Sussex, N.B.
E0E 1P0
Telephone: 902-433-3100, x334

Region IV
Mental Health Clinic/Clinique de Santé
   Mentale
P.O. Box 280
Prince William Street
St. Stephen, N.B.
E3L 2X2
Telephone: 902-466-1140, 5020

Region V
Mental Health Clinic/Clinique de Santé
   Mentale
Victoria Health Center
P.O. Box 5001
Fredericton, N.B.
E3B 5G1
Telephone: 902-453-2132

Region VI
Mental Health Clinic/Clinique de Santé
   Mentale
P.O. Box 5001
200 King Street
Woodstock, N.B.
E0J 2B0
Telephone: 902-328-9979

Region VII
Clinique de Santé Mentale
Carrefour Assomption
Edmundston, N.B.
E3V 2C1
Telephone: 902-735-2070

Clinique de Santé Mentale
C.P. 5001
Grand Falls, N.B.
E0J 1M0
Telephone: 902-473-4686

Region VIII
Mental Health Clinic/Clinique de Santé
   Mentale
Hotel-Dieu St. Joseph
6 rue Arran
Campbellton, N.B.
E3N 3G2
Telephone: 902-753-7753

Region IX
Mental Health Clinic/Clinique de Santé
   Mentale
C.P. 5001
Bathurst, N.B.
E2A 4H4
Telephone: 902-547-2020

Region X
Mental Health Clinic/Clinique de Santé
   Mentale
C.P. 5001
Caraquet, N.B.
E0B 1K0
Telephone: 902-727-6574

Region XI
Mental Health Clinic/Clinique de Santé
   Mentale
Hotel-Dieu Hospital
Chatham, N.B.
E1N 2W9
Telephone: 902-773-4464

NEWFOUNDLAND

Assoc. of Newfoundland Psychologists
Madonna Tracey (Past President &
   Delegate)
5 Exeter Avenue
St. John's, Newfoundland
A1B 1R1
Telephone: 709-722-9765

Canadian Mental Health Association
P.O. Box 5788

St. John's, Newfoundland
A1C 5X3
Telephone: 709-753-8550

Department of Health
Confederation Building
St. John's, Newfoundland
A1C 5T7
Telephone: 709-737-2300

NOVA SCOTIA

Assoc. of Psychologists of Nova Scotia
Dr. Joe Byrne (President & Delegate)
APNS, P.O. Box 594, Station M
Halifax, N.S.
B3J 2R7
Telephone: 902-428-8454 (B)
902-429-3568 (H)

Canadian Mental Health Association
5739 Inglis Street
Halifax, Nova Scotia
B3H 1K5
Telephone: 902-422-5800

ONTARIO

Canadian Medical Association
Box 8650
Ottawa, Ontario
K1G 0G8
Telephone: 613-731-9331

Canadian Mental Health Association
56 Wellesley St. W. (4th flr.)
Toronto, Ontario
M4S 2S3
Telephone: 416-964-9611

Canadian Psychiatric Association
222 Lisgar St., Suite 103
Ottawa, Ontario
K2P0C6

Canada Psychiatric Research Foundation
220 Yonge St. Suite 206
P.O. Box 607
Toronto, Ontario
M5B 2H1

Clark Institute of Psychiatry
250 College St.
Toronto, Ontario
M5T 1R8
Telephone: 416-979-2221

Ontario Association of Distress Centres
811A Queen St., East
Toronto, Ontario
M4M 1HB
Telephone: 416-463-6606

Ontario Psychological Association
730 Yonge St., Suite 221
Toronto, Ontario
M4Y 2B7
Telephone: 416-961-5552

Royal Ottawa Hospital
1145 Carling Avenue
Ottawa, Ontario
K12 7K4
Telephone: 613-722-6521, x574

PRINCE EDWARD ISLAND

Canadian Mental Health Association
96 Sydney St., P.O. Box 785
Charlottetown, P.E.I.
C1A 7L9
Telephone: 902-566-3034

Psychological Association of
   Prince Edward Island
Dr. Philip Smith (President & Delegate)
University of Prince Edward Island
Department of Psychology
Charlottetown, P.E.I.
C1A 4P3
Telephone: 902-566-0563 (B)
902-838-2042 (H)

QUEBEC

Canadian Mental Health Association
550 Sherbrooke St. W., #310
Montreal, Quebec
H3A 1B9
Telephone: 514-849-3291

Canadian Psychological Association
Chemin Vincent Rd.
Old Chelsea, Quebec
J0X 2N0
Telephone: 819-827-3927

SASKATCHEWAN

Canadian Mental Health Asssociation
1810 Albert Street
Regina, Saskatchewan
S4P 2S8
Telephone: 306-525-5601

Saskatchewan Psychological Association
Dr. Carl von Baeyer (Delegate)
Psychology Division
University Hospital
Saskatoon, Saskatchewan
S7N 0X0
Telephone: 306-966-2344 (B)
306-652-6546 (H)

NORTHWEST TERRITORIES

Assoc. of Psychologists of the Northwest
   Territories
Andrew Langford (President & Delegate)
Department of Social Services
Government of Northwest Territories
Yellowknife, Northwest Territories
X1A 2L9
Telephone: 403-873-7429 (B)
403-873-8814 (H)

Canadian Mental Health Association
P.O. Box 2580
Yellowknife, N.W.T. X1A 2P9
Telephone: 403-873-3190

YUKON

Canadian Mental Health Association
8 Green Street
Whitehorse, Yukon
Y1A 4R9
Telephone: 403-667-5413 (B)
403-667-4358 (H)

Self-Help Clearinghouses in Canada
Calgary: (403) 262-1117
Montreal: (514) 484-7406
Saskatchewan: (306) 652-7817
Toronto: (416) 487-4512
Winnipeg: (204) 589-5500 or 633-5955
National newsletter, *Initiative*:
   (613) 728-1865 (C.C.S.D. in Ottawa)

SPECIALIZED AGENCIES OF THE UNITED NATIONS

Association Medica Pan Americana
222 Kent Terrace
West Palm Beach, FL 33407

Pan American Health Organization (WHO)
Regional Office of the WHO
525 Twenty-third Street, NW
Washington, DC 20037

United Nations
Division of Narcotic Drugs (DND)
P.O. Box 500
A-1400 Vienna, Austria

United Nations Education, Scientific and
   Cultural Organization (UNESCO)
7, Place de Fontenoy
F-7500 Paris, France

World Health Organization (WHO)
1211 Geneva 27
Switzerland

World Health Organization (WHO)
Regional Office for Europe
Scherfigsvej, 8
DK-2100 Copenhagen, Denmark

World Health Organization (WHO)
Regional Office for Western Pacific
P.O. Box 2932
2115 Manila, Philippines

OTHER FOREIGN ORGANIZATIONS

Australian Psychological Society
National Science Center
191 Royal Parada
Parkville, Victoria 3052
Australia

AWARE
Depression Research Unit
St. Patrick's Hospital
Fenian Chambers
37-38 Fenian Street
Dublin, Ireland

Bundeskanzleramt
Sektion VI
Dr. Lambrecht Wissgott
Abteilung 7
Ballhausplatz 2
A-1014 Wien
Austria
Telephone: (01143) 1/ 53 11 50

Byran for psykiatrisk vard
Informationssekretariatet
Social styrelsen
S-106 30 Stockholm
Sweden

Department of Health
Box 5013
Wellington, New Zealand

Director of Information
Institute of Psychiatry
P.O. Box 1
Rozelle NSW 2039
Australia

The Health Research Board
73 Lr. Baggot Street
Dublin 2, Ireland

Helsedirektoratet [Directorate of Health]
P.O. Box 8128 Dep.
0032 Oslo 1
Norway

Institute of Psychiatry
de Grespigny Park
Denmark Hill, London SE56AF
England

Instituto Mexicano Del Seguro Social
Paseo De La Reforma 476
Mexico, 06698 D.F.
Mexico
Telephone: (1-905) 211-0018

Instituto Mexicano De Psiquiatria
Ant. Camino A Xochimilco 101
Mexico, 14370 D.F.
Apartado Postal 20-587
Mexico
Telephone: (1-905) 655-2811

Ministry of Social Affairs and Health
Dept. of International Relations
Snellmaninkatu 4-6
00170 Helsinki, Finland

National Health and Medical Research
  Council
GPO Box 9848
Cambra ACT 2601
Australia

The Netherlands Institute of Mental Health
P.O. Box 5103
3502 JC Utrecht
The Netherlands
Telephone: 011-31-30-935141

Oesterreichische Aerztekammer
Weihburggasse 10-12
A-1010 Wien
Austria
Telephone: (01142) 1/ 52 69 44

Psychological Association of Finland
Snellmaninkatu 9.11
00170 Helsinki, Finland

Secretaria De Salud [Ministry of Health]
Lieja 7- 1ER Piso
06696 Mexico, D.F.
Mexico
Telephone: (1-905) 553-0758
            553-1353

Sundhedsministeriet
Christiansborg Slotsplads 1
DK-1218 Copenhagen K.
Denmark
Telephone: (33) 92.33.60.

Suomen Mielenterveysseura [Mental Health
  Association of Finland]
Lauttasaarentie 28-30
00200 Helsinki, Finland

MAJOR ENGLISH LANGUAGE JOURNALS, NEWSPAPERS AND PERIODICALS

Alcohol Health and Research World
P.O. Box 2345
Rockville, MD 20852

Alcoholism: The National Magazine
P.O. Box C19051
Queen Anne Station
Seattle, WA 98109

The Alcoholism Report
744 National Press Building
Washington, DC 20045

American Journal of Drug and Alcohol
  Abuse
Marcel Dekker Journals, Inc.
270 Madison Avenue
New York, NY 10016

American Journal of Epidemiology
Johns Hopkins University
School of Hygiene and Health
615 N. Wolfe Street
Baltimore, MD 21205

American Journal of Pharmacy and the
  Sciences Supporting Public Health
Philadelphia College of Pharmacy and
  Science
43rd Street and King Sessing Hall
Philadelphia, PA 19104

American Journal of Psychiatry
American Psychiatric Association
1700 18th Street, NW
Washington, DC 20009

American Journal of Psychoanalysis
Agathon Press, Inc.
111 Eighth Avenue
New York, NY 10011

American Journal of Psychology
University of Illinois Press
Urbana, IL 61801

American Journal of Psychotherapy
Association for Advancement of

Psychotherapy
114 E. 78th St.
New York, NY 10021

American Journal of Public Health
American Public Health Association
1015 18th Street, NW
Washington, DC 20036

American Journal of Sociology
University of Chicago Press
5801 South Ellis Avenue
Chicago, IL 60637

Annals of Internal Medicine
American College of Physicians
4200 Pine Street
Philadelphia, PA 19104

Annals of the New York Academy of
    Science
The New York Academy of Sciences
2 East 63rd Street
New York, NY 10021

Archives of General Psychiatry
American Medical Association
535 N. Dearborn Street
Chicago, IL 60610

British Journal of Addiction
Longman Group, Ltd.
Journals Division
43-45 Annandale Street
Edinburgh EH7 4AT, Scotland
United Kingdom

British Journal of Psychiatry
Headley Bros., Ltd.
Ashford
Kent TN 24 8HH, England
United Kingdom

British Journal on
    Alcohol and Alcoholism
Grosvenor Crescent
London SWIX 7EE, England
United Kingdom

British Medical Journal
British Medical Association

B.M.A. House, Tavistock Square
London WCI, England
United Kingdom

Canadian Journal of Psychiatry
294 Albert Street-Suite 204
Ottawa, Ontario
K1P 6E6
Canada

Canadian Medical Association Journal
Canadian Medical Association
Box 8650
Ottawa, Ontario
K1G 068
Canada

Clinical Pharmacology and Therapeutics
C.V. Mosby Co.
11830 Westline Industrial Drive
St. Louis, MO 63141

Clinical Toxicology
Marcel Dekker Journals
270 Madison Avenue
New York, NY 10016

Contempory Drug Problems
Federal Legal Publications, Inc.
95 Morton Street
New York, NY 10014

Crime and Delinquency
National Council on Crime and
    Delinquency
411 Continental Plaza
Hackensack, NJ 07601

Criminology
Sage Publications, Inc.
275 S. Beverly Drive
Beverly Hills, CA 90212

Crisis: International Journal of Suicide and
    Crisis Studies
C.J. Hogrefe, Inc.
525 Eglinton Avenue East
Toronto, Ontario
M4P IN5
Canada

Culture, Medicine and Psychiatry
Reidel Publishing Co.
Box 17, 3300 AA Dordrecht
Netherlands

Current Comments
Institute for Scientific Information
3501 Market St.
Philadelphia, PA 19104

Digest of Alcoholism Theory and
    Application (DATA)
10700 Olson Memorial Highway
Minneapolis, MN 55441

Diseases of the Nervous System
Physicians Post Graduate Press
Box 38293
Memphis, TN 38138

Drug Abuse and Alcoholism Newsletter
Vista Hill Foundation
3420 Camino del Rio North, Suite 100
San Diego, CA 92108

Drug Forum
Baywood Publishing Co., Inc.
120 Marine Street
Farmingdale, NY 11735

Drugs and Alcohol Dependence
Elsevier Sequoia S.A.
Box 851
CH-1001 Lausanne 1, Switzerland

Essence: Issues in the Study of Aging,
    Dying and Death
Atkinson College Press
4700 Keele Street
Downview, Ontario M3J 2R7
Canada

European Journal of Clinical Pharmacology
Springer-Verlag
175 Fifth Avenue
New York, NY 10010

The Grapevine
The Alcoholics Anonymous Grapevine,
    Inc.
468 Park Avenue South
New York, NY 10016

Human Pathology
Saunders Co.
West Washington Square
Philadelphia, PA 19105

International Journal of the Addictions
Marcel Dekker Journals
270 Madison Avenue
New York, NY 10016

International Journal of Psychoanalysis
Institute of Psychoanalysis
Bailliere Tindall
24-28 Oval Road
London, N.W. 17DX
England

The Journal
Addiction Research Foundation
33 Russell Street
Toronto, Ontario
M5S 2S1
Canada

Journal of Abnormal Psychology
American Psychological Association
1200 17th Street, NW
Washington, DC 20036

Journal of Affective Disorders
Elsevier Science Publishing Company
Box 211, 1000 A.E.
Amsterdam, Netherlands

Journal of Altered States of Consciousness
Baywood Publishing Co., Inc.
43 Central Drive
Farmingdale, NY 11735

Journal of the American Medical
    Association (JAMA)
535 North Dearborn Street
Chicago, IL 60610

Journal of the American Psychoanalytic
    Assoc.
Theodore Shapiro International Universities
    Press Inc.
Journal Dept. 59
Boston Road
P.O. Box 1524
Madison, CT 06443

Journal of Clinical Psychology
Clinical Psychology Publishing Co., Inc.
4 Conant Square
Brandon, Vermont 05733

Journal of Consulting and Clinical
 Psychology
American Psychological Association
1200 17th Street, NW
Washington, DC 20036

Journal of Drug Education
Baywood Publishing Co., Inc.
120 Marine Street
Farmingdale, NY 11735

Journal of Drug Issues
Box 4021
Tallahassee, FL 32303

Journal of General Psychology
Journal Press
2 Commercial Street
Provincetown, MA 02657

Journal of Health and Social Behavior
American Sociological Association
1722 North Street, NW
Washington, DC 20036

Journal of Nervous and Mental Diseases
Williams and Wilkins Co.
428 East Preston Street
Baltimore, MD 21202

Journal of Personality
Duke University Press
6697 College Station
Durham, NC 27708

Journal of Personality and Social
 Psychology
American Psychological Association
1200 17th Street, NW
Washington, DC 20036

Journal of Pharmacology and Experimental
 Therapeutics
Williams and Wilkins Co.
428 East Preston Street
Baltimore, MD 21202

Journal of Pharmacy and Pharmacology
Pharmaceutical Society of Great Britain
One Lambeth High Street
London SE1 7JN, England
United Kingdom

Journal of Psychoactive Drugs
Transaction Periodicals Consortium,
 Department 2000
Rutgers, The State University
New Brunswick, NJ 08903

Journal of Studies on Alcohol
Rutgers Center of Alcohol Studies
Publication Division
New Brunswick, NJ 08903

Journal of Youth and Adolescents
Plenum Press
233 Spring Street
New York, NY 10013

Journal on Alcohol and Drug Education
1120 East Oakland
P.O. Box 10212
Lansing, MI 48901

Lancet
Lancet Ltd.
7 Adam Street
London WC2N6AD
England

New England Journal of Medicine
Massachusetts Medical Society
10 Shattuck Street
Boston, MA 02115

Newslink
American Association of Suicidology
2459 South Ash Street
Denver, CO 80222

New York State Journal of Medicine
Medical Society of the State of New York
420 Lakeville Road
Lake Success, NY 11040

Omega: Journal of Death and Dying
Baywood Publishing Co., Inc.
120 Marine Street
P.O. Box D
Farmingdale, NY 11735

Personality and Social Psychology Bulletin
Sage Publications, Inc.
2111 W. Hillcrest Drive
Newbury Park, CA 91320

Psychiatry
William Alanson White Psychiatric
   Foundation, Inc.
1610 New Hampshire Avenue, NW
Washington, DC 20009

Psychoanalytic Quarterly
Psychoanalytic Quarterly, Inc.
175-5th Avenue
Room 210
New York, NY 10010

Psychological Medicine
Cambridge University Press
Edinburgh Bldg.
Shaftesbury Rd.
Cambridge CB22RU
England

Psychological Reports
Box 9229
Missoula, MT 59801

Psychology
Box 6495, Station C
Savannah, GA 31405

Psychology Today
80 Fifth Ave.
New York, NY 10011

Psychopharmacology
Springer-Verlag

174 Fifth Avenue
New York, NY 10010

Psychosomatics
American Psychiatric Press
1400 K Street, NW
Suite 1101
Washington, DC 20005

Science News
Science Service, Inc.
1719 N Street, NW
Washington, DC 20036

Social Problems
Society for the Study of Social Problems
114 Rockwell Hall
State University College
Buffalo, NY 14222

Sociology Quarterly
Midwest Sociological Society
Department of Sociology
Southern Illinois University
Carbondale, IL 62901

Suicide and Life-Threatening Behavior
Guilford Publications, Inc.
200 Park Avenue South
New York, NY 10003

U.S. Journal of Drug and Alcohol
   Dependence
2119-A Hollywood Boulevard
Hollywood, FL 33020

BIBLIOGRAPHY

Abramson, L.Y., Alloy, L.B. and Metalsky, G.I., "Learned Helplessness in Humans: Critique and Reformulation," *Journal of Abnormal Psychology*, 87(1978), 49–59.

Agee, James, *A Death in the Family*. New York: Avon Books, 1957.

Ahmed, S. Haroon, "Treatment Response and the Clinical Continuum of Illness," in *Mental Disorders, Alcohol-and-Drug-Related Problems* (Amsterdam: Excerpta Medica, 1985).

Ahmed, S. Haroon and Arif, M., "Culture and Symptomatology in Depression," *Pakistan Journal of Medical Research*, 21(April-June 1982).

Akhund, F., Khan, M., Mohsin, A. and Ahmed, S.H., "Psychiatric Disorders in General Practice," *Journal of the Pakistan Medical Association*, 37(January 1987).

Alcohol, Drug Abuse and Mental Health Administration, *A Consumer's Guide to Mental Health Services*. Rockville, Maryland: DHHS, 1987.

———, *Depressive Disorders: Treatments Bring New Hope*. Rockville, Maryland: DHHS, 1986.

———, *Helpful Facts About Depressive Disorders*. Rockville, Maryland: DHHS, 1987.

———, *You Are Not Alone*. Rockville, Maryland: DHHS, 1985.

Alsop, Stewart, *Stay of Execution: A Sort of Memoir*. Philadelphia: J.B. Lippincott, 1973.

Altschul, Sol (ed.), *Childhood Bereavement and Its Aftermath*. Madison, Connecticut: International Universities Press, 1988.

Alvarez, A., *The Savage God*. New York: Random House, 1970.

American Psychiatric Association, *Diagnostic and Statistical Manual of Mental Disorders*, (DSM-III-R), 3rd edition, revised. Washington, D.C.: American Psychiatric Association, 1987.

Amoroso, Mary, "When A Hope and a Dream Are Stillborn," *The* [Hackensack, N.J.] *Record*, July 21, 1987.

———, "When A Young Sibling Dies," *The* [Hackensack, N.J.] *Record*, March 19, 1989.

Andreasen, N.C., "Ariel's Flight: The Death of Sylvia Plath," *Journal of the American Medical Association*, 228:5(April 29, 1974).

———, *Broken Brain*. New York: Harper, 1985.

———, "Creativity and Mental Illness: Prevalence Rates in Writers and Their First-Degree Relatives," *American Journal of Psychiatry*, 144:10(October 1987).

Andreasen, N.C. and Canter, A., "The Creative Writer: Psychiatric Symptoms and Family History," *Comprehensive Psychiatry*, 15:2(March/April 1974).

Andreasen, N.C. and Glick I., "Bipolar Affective Disorder and Creativity: Implications and Clinical Management," *Comprehensive Psychiatry*, 29:3(May/June 1988).

Associated Press, "Computer Helps Cure Depression," *New Haven Register*, January 30, 1990.

———, "Stronger Cases Made for Link Between Genetics, Depression," *The* [Hackensack, N.J.] *Record*, October 8, 1987.

———, "Study Casts Doubt on Idea Grief Can Kill," *The* [Hackensack, N.J.] *Record*, August 12, 1988.

Baier, Marjorie, "The 'Holiday Blues' as a Stress Reaction," *Perspectives in Psychiatric Care*, 24:2(1987/1988).

Baldessarini, R.J., "Current Status of Antidepressants: Clinical Pharmacology and Therapy," *Journal of Clincal Psychiatry*, 50:4(April 1989).

Baron, Miron, "Defective Genes Linked to Manic Depressive Illness," *The Psychiatric Times*, December 1987.

Bebbington, P., Katz, R. et al., "The Risk of Minor Depression Before Age 65: Results from a Community Survey," *Psychological Medicine*, 19(1989).

Beck, Aaron, T., *Depression: Causes and Treatment*. Philadelphia: University of Pennsylvania Press, 1967.

———, *Love Is Never Enough*. New York: Harper & Row, 1988.

Beck, Aaron T. et al., *Cognitive Therapy of Depression*. New York: Guilford Press, 1979.

———, "An Inventory for Measuring Depression," *Archives of General Psychiatry*, 4(1961).

Beck, Melinda et al., "Miscarriages," *Newsweek*, August 15, 1988.

Becker, Ernest, *The Denial of Death*. New York: Macmillan, 1973.

Becker, R., "Depression in Schizophrenia," *Hospital Community Psychiatry*, 39:12(December 1988).

Becker, Robert and Heimberg, Richard, "Treatment of Dysthymic Disorder," to be published in a professional journal.

Becker, R., Heimberg, R. and Bellack, A.S., *Social Skills Training Treatment for Depression*. New York: Pergamon, 1988.

Begley, Sharon, "The Stuff That Dreams Are Made Of," *Newsweek*, August 14, 1989.

Behar, David et al., "Familial Subtypes of Depression: A Clinical View," *Journal of Clinical Psychiatry*, 42:2(February 1980).

Bell, Carl C. and Mehta, Harshad, "The Misdiagnosis of Black Patients With Manic Depressive Illness," *Journal of the National Medical Association*, 72:2(1980).

———, "Misdiagnosis of Black Patients With Manic Depressive Illness: Second in a Series," *Journal of the National Medical Association*, 73:2(1981).

Bell, Glennys, "A New Light on the Blues," *The Bulletin*, July 25, 1989.

Belmaker, R.H. and VanPraag, H.M., *Mania, An Evolving Concept*. New York: Spectrum, 1980.

Benson, George, *What to Do When You're Depressed*. Minneapolis: Augsburg Publishing House, 1975.

Benson, Herbert, *The Mind-Body Effect*. New York: Berkley, 1980.

Berchtold, Nancy and Goldberger, Peter, "When a Woman Is Driven to Kill Her Baby," *The New York Times* (Letters), May 23, 1988.

Berger, Milton M., (ed.), *Videotape Techniques in Psychiatric Training and Treatment*. New York: Brunner/Mazel, 1978.

Berlin, Irving, N. "Effects of Changing Native American Cultures on Child Development," *Journal of Community Psychology*, 15(July 1987).

———, "Prevention of Adolescent Suicide Among Some Native American Tribes," *Adolescent Psychiatry*, 12(1985).

———, "Psychopathology and Its Antecedents Among American Indian Adolescents," in Benjamin B. Lahey and Alan E. Kazdin (eds.), *Advances in Clinical Child Psychology*, vol. 9. New York: Plenum, 1986.

———, "Suicide Among American Indian Adolescents: An Overview," *Suicide and Life Threatening Behavior*, 17(Fall 1987).

Besedovsky, H.O., Sorkin, E., Felix, D. et al., "Hypothalamic Changes During The Immune Response," *European Journal of Immunology*, 7(1977), 323–325.

Black, Donald W. et al., "Treatment and Outcome in Secondary Depression: A Naturalistic Study of 1087 Patients," *Journal of Clinical Psychiatry*, 48:11(1987).

Blair, Gwenda, *Almost Golden*. New York: Simon & Schuster, 1988.

Blakeslee, Sandra, "New Methods Help Researchers Explore the Dark World of Dreams," *The New York Times*, August 11, 1988.

———, "New Research Links Depression With Asthma Deaths in Children," *The New York Times*, May 30, 1989.

Blalock, J.E., "The Immune System As a Sensory Organ," *Journal of Immunology*, 132(1984), 1067–1070.

Blazer, D., "Psychiatric Disorders: A Rural Urban Comparison," *Archives of General Psychiatry*, 42(1985).

Bower, B., "Bereavement: Reeling in the Years," *Science News*, 131(February 7, 1987).

Bowlby, J., *Loss: Sadness and Depression* (Attachment and Loss, Vol. 3). New York: Basic Books, 1980.

Braiker, Harriet, *Getting Up When You're Feeling Low: A Woman's Guide to Overcoming and Preventing Depression*. New York: Putnam, 1988.

Bristol-Myers Company, *Bristol-Myers Company Annual Report for 1984*. New York: Bristol-Myers, 1985.

———, "Desyrel: A New Generation of Antidepressants," *Bristol-Myers Third Quarter Report*. New York: Bristol-Myers, 1982.

Brody, Jane, "Personal Health," *The New York Times*, April 20, 1989.

Brown, R., "U.S. Experience with Valproate in Manic Depressive Illness: A Multicenter Trial," *Journal of Clinical Psychiatry*, 50(March 1989).

Brown, R.S., "Jogging: Its Uses and Abuses," *Virginia Medical*, July 1979.

Brown, R.S., Ramirez, D.E. and Taub, J.M., "The Prescription of Exercise for Depression," in *The Physician and Sportsmedicine*, 6:12(December 1978).

Burns, David B., *The Feeling Good Handbook*. New York: William Morrow, 1989.

_____, *Feeling Good: The New Mood Therapy*. New York: New American Library, 1980.

_____, *The Feeing Good Workbook*. New York: New American Library, 1988.

Caine, Lynne, *Widow*. New York: Bantam Books, 1974.

Calabrese, Joseph R. et al., *Alterations in Immunocompetence During Stress, Bereavement, and Depression: Focus on the Interplay Between the Immunologic Apparatus and Neuroendocrine Regulation*. Cleveland: Cleveland Clinic Foundation, n.d.

California-Berkeley, University of, "A Special Kind of Grief," *University of California-Berkeley Wellness Letter*, August 1988.

Cammer, Leonard, *Up from Depression*. New York: Pocket Books, 1969.

Caputo, Philip, "Styron's Choice," *Esquire*, December 1986.

Centers for Disease Control, *Chronic Fatigue Syndrome*. Atlanta: DHHS, 1989.

Clark, Patrick and Marques, Stuart, "Birth Blues Clear Baby-Killer Mom," *New York Daily News*, October 1, 1988.

Clayton, P.J., "Mortality and Morbidity in the First Year of Widowhood," *Archives of General Psychiatry*, 30(1974), 747–750.

Cohen, Daniel, *The Body Snatchers*. Philadelphia: J. B. Lippincott, 1975.

Cohen, Sherry Suib, "The Amazing Power of Touch," *Ladies' Home Journal*, June 1982.

Colby, C.A. and Gotlib, I.H., "Memory Deficits in Depression," *Cognitive Therapy and Research*, 12:6(1988).

Colp, Ralph, Jr., *To Be an Invalid: The Illness of Charles Darwin*. Chicago: University of Chicago Press, 1977.

Consensus Development Conference on Mood Disorders, *Mood Disorders: Pharmacologic Prevention of Recurrences*, consensus statement (5:4). National Institutes of Health in conjunction with the National Institute of Mental Health. April 24–26, 1984.

Cook, B.L. and Winokur, G., "Nosology of Affective Disorders," in John G. Howells (ed.), *Perspectives in the Psychiatry of the Affective Disorders*. New York: Brunner Mazel, 1989.

Cool, Lisa Collier, "Fatigue: Are You Fighting an Internal Clock?" *McCall's*, December 1987.

Corfman, Eunice, *Depression, Manic-Depressive Illness, and Biological Rhythms*. Rockville, Maryland: Alcohol, Drug Abuse, and Mental Health Administration, 1982; DHHS 82–889.

Coryell W.H. and Zimmerman M., "Personality Disorder in the Families of Depressed, Schizophrenic, and Never-Ill Probands," *American Journal of Psychiatry*, 146:4(April 1989).

Cousins, Norman, *Anatomy of an Illness As Perceived By the Patient*. New York: Bantam, 1981.

_____, *Head First: The Biology of Hope*. New York: E.P. Dutton, 1989.

Currents in Affective Illness, "Carbamazepine and Affective Disorders," *Currents in Affective Illness*, 5:2(1986).

DeRosis, Helen, *The Book of Hope*. New York: Macmillan, 1976.

_____, *Women and Anxiety*. New York: Delacorte Press, 1979.

Diamond, John, "Winter Blues Officially an Illness," *The* [Hackensack, N.J.] *Record* (Associated Press), November 30, 1987.

Dietz, Jean, "Study: Sorrow May Weaken Body," *Boston Globe*, February 1, 1984.

Dobson, K.S., "A Meta-Analysis of the Efficacy of Cognitive Therapy for Depression," *Journal of Consulting and Clinical Psychiatry*, in press.

Dobson, K.S. and Shaw, B.F., "Cognitive Assessment with Major Depressive Disorders," *Cognitive Therapy and Research*, 10:1(1988).

Doherty, Matthew J., "L-tryptophan Is Still Around Despite Recall," *The* [Hackensack, N.J.] *Record*, December 1, 1989.

Donnelly, Katherine Fair, *Recovering from the Loss of a Parent*. New York: Dodd, Mead, 1987.

Dowrick, P.W. and Biggs, S.J.(eds.), *Using Video: Psychological and Social Applications*. New York: John Wiley, 1983.

Duke, Patty, *Call Me Anna*. New York: Bantam, 1987.

Eaton, W.W. et al., "The Design of the Epidemiologic Catchment Area Surveys," *Archives of General Psychiatry*, 41(October 1984).

Egeland, J.A. and Hostetter, A.M., "Amish Study I: Affective Disorders Among the Amish, 1976–1980," *American Journal of Psychiatry*, 140(1983), 56–61.

Egeland, J.A., Hostetter, A.M. and Eshleman, S.K., "Amish Study III: The Impact of Cultural Factors on Diagnosis of Bipolar Illness," *American Journal of Psychiatry*, 140(1983), 67–71.

Egeland, J.A. et al., "Bipolar Affective Disorders Linked to DNA Markers on Chromosome 11," *Nature*, 325(February 1987).

Elkin, Irene et al., "NIMH Treatment of Depression Collaborative Research Program," *Archives of General Psychiatry*, 42(1985), 305–316.

Ellis, Albert, *Reason and Emotion in Psychotherapy*. New York: Lyle Stuart, 1962.

Ellis, Albert and Harper, R.A., *A New Guide to Rational Living*. North Hollywood, California: Wilshire Book Co., 1975.

Emery, G., *A New Beginning*. New York: Simon and Schuster, 1981.

Encyclopedia Americana, "Funerals," *Encyclopedia Americana*. New York: Grolier, 1985.

Encyclopedia Brittanica, "Funerals," *Encyclopedia Brittanica*, 15th ed. Chicago: University of Chicago, 1986.

Endler, Norman S., *Holiday of Darkness*. New York: John Wiley, 1982.

Essex, Marilyn J., "Depression Associated with Lack of Intimacy in Older Women," *Geriatric Medicine Today*, 6:3(March 1987).

Evans, Glen and Farberow, Norman L., *The Encyclopedia of Suicide*. New York: Facts On File, 1988.

Evans, Jocelyn, *Living With a Man Who Is Dying: A Personal Memoir*. New York: Taplinger, 1971.

Faraday, A., *Dream Power*. New York: Berkley, 1973.

Faulkner, William, *As I Lay Dying*. New York: Random House, 1964.

Feifel, Herman, *New Meanings of Death*. New York: McGraw-Hill, 1977.

Feifel, Herman (ed.), *The Meaning of Death*. New York: McGraw-HIll, 1959.

Fieve, Ronald, *Moodswing: The Third Revolution in Psychiatry*. New York: William Morrow, 1975.

Folkenberg, Judy, "Multi-Site Study of Therapies for Depression," *ADAMHA News*, August 1986.

———, *Using Drugs to Lift That Dark Veil of Depression*. Rockville, Maryland: DHHS, 1985; DHHS (FDA) 84–3140.

Foster, Valerie, "Foods That Set the Mood," *The* [Hackensack N.J.] *Record*, May 24, 1989.

Freedman, Daniel X., "Psychiatric Epidemiology Counts," *Archives of General Psychiatry*, 41(October 1984).

Freedman, Russell, *Lincoln: A Photobiography*. New York: Clarion Books, 1987.

Freud, Sigmund, *Beyond the Pleasure Principle*. London: Hogarth Press, 1950.

———, "Mourning and Melancholia," in *Collected Papers*, vol. 4. London: Hogarth Press, 1949.

Frosch, William A., "Moods, Madness, and Music," *Outlook*, Fall 1988.

Fryrear, J.L. and Fleshman, B. (eds.), *Videotherapy in Mental Health*. Springfield, Illinois: Charles C. Thomas, 1981.

Furman, Erna, *A Child's Parent Dies: Studies in Childhood Bereavement*. New Haven, Connecticut: Yale University Press, 1974.

Gaffney, Donna A., *The Seasons of Grief*. New York: New American Library, 1988.

Gallagher, Dolores E. and Thompson, Larry W., "Treatment of Major Depressive Disorder in Older Adult Outpatients with Brief Psychotherapies," *Psychotherapy Theory, Research and Practice*, 19:4(Winter 1982).

Gallagher, Winifred, "The Dark Affliction of Mind and Body," *Discover*, May 1986.

Garfield, Patricia, *Creative Dreaming*. New York: Ballentine, 1976.

Gershon, S. And Shopsin, B. (eds.), *Lithium: Its Role in Psychiatric Research and Treatment*. New York: Plenum Press, 1973.

Giannini, A.J. et al., "Clonidine in Mania," *Drug Development Research*, 3(1983), 101–103.

Gilman, A.G., Goodman, L.S., Rall, T.W. and Murad, F. (eds.), *Goodman and Gilman's: The Pharmacological Basis of Therapeutics*. New York: Macmillan, 1985.

Glick, I.O., Weiss, R.S. and Parkes, C.M., *The First Year of Bereavement*. New York: John Wiley, 1974.

Gold, Mark S., *Good News About Depression*. New York: Villard Books, 1987.

———, "Hypothyroidism and Depression," *Journal of the American Medical Association*, 295:19(May 15, 1981).

———, "Hypothyroidism—Or Is It Depression?" *Psychosomatics*, 24:7(July 1983).

Gold, Mark S. and Kronig, Michael H., "Comprehensive Thyroid Evaluation in Psychiatric Patients," in *Handbook of Psychiatric Diagnostic Procedures*, Hall, R. and Bresford, T. (eds.), New York: Spectrum Publications, n.d.

Gold, Mark S., with Morris, Lois B., *The Good News About Depression*. (New York: Bantam, 1988).

Gold, Mark S. et al., "Diagnosis of Depression in the 1980s," *Journal of the American Medical Association*, 245:15(April 17, 1981).

Goleman, Daniel, "Clues to Suicide: A Brain Chemical Is Implicated," *The New York Times*, October 8, 1985.

——, "Depressed Parents Put Children At a Greater Risk of Depression," *The New York Times*, March 30, 1989.

——, "Obsessive Disorder: Secret Toll Is Found," *The New York Times*, December 13, 1988.

——, "New Studies Find Many Myths About Mourning," *The New York Times*, August 8, 1989.

——, "Study of Normal Mourning Process Illuminates Grief Gone Awry," *The New York Times*, March 29, 1988.

Gordon, Audrey K. and Klass, Dennis, *They Need to Know: How to Teach Children About Death*. Englewood Cliffs, New Jersey: Prentice-Hall, 1979.

Gotham, A.M. et al., "Depression in Parkinson's Disease: A Quantitative and Qualitative Analysis," *Journal of Neurological Neurosurgical Psychiatry*, 49(1986), 381–9.

Gotlib, Ian H. and Colby, C.A., *Treatment of Depression: An Interpersonal Systems Approach*. Elmsford, New York: Pergamon Press, 1987.

Gotlib, Ian H. and Hooley, Jill M., "Depression and Marital Distress: Current Status and Future Directions," in S.W. Duck (ed.), *Handbook of Personal Relationships*. New York: John Wiley, 1988.

Graedon, Joe, *The People's Pharmacy*. New York: St. Martin's Press, 1985.

Green, E. and Green A., *Beyond Biofeedback*. New York: Delacorte Press, 1977.

Greist, J.H. and Jefferson, J.W., *Depression and Its Treatment*. New York: Warner Books, 1984.

Greist, J.H., Jefferson, J.W. and Marks, I.M., *Anxiety and Its Treatment: Help Is Available*. Washington, D.C.: American Psychiatric Press, 1986.

Greist, J.H., Jefferson, J.W. and Spitzer, R.L., *Treatment of Mental Disorders*. New York: Oxford University Press, 1982.

Grollman, Earl A., *Explaining Death to Children*. Boston: Beacon Press, 1968.

Gunther, John, *Death Be Not Proud*. New York: Harper and Row, 1949.

Gurin, Carol Duchow (with Joel Gurin), "Depression: Is There a Quick Fix for This Dangerous Disease?" *Ms*, December 1987.

Haberman, Clyde, "Florence's Art Makes Some Go to Pieces," *The New York Times*, May 15, 1989.

Handke, Peter, *A Sorrow Beyond Dreams: A Life Story*. London: Souvenir Press, 1976.

Handkoff, L.D. and Einsidler, B., *Suicide Theory and Clinical Aspects*. Littleton, Massachusetts: PSG Publishing, 1979.

Harrison, W.M. et al., "Treatment of Premenstrual Depression With Nortriptyline: A Pilot Study," *Journal of Clinical Psychology*, 50:4(April 1989).

Harvard Medical School Health Letter, "Chronic Fatigue—What Does It Mean?" *Harvard Medical School Health Letter*, 14:5(March 1989).

Hazleton, Lesley, *The Right to Feel Bad*. New York: Dial Press, 1984.

Heilveil, Ira, *Video in Mental Health Practice: An Activities Handbook*. New York: Springer, 1983.

Hendin, David, *Death As a Fact of Life*. New York: Warner Books, 1974.

Henig, Robin M., "Beyond the Beat: Doctors Take New Look At Hypertension," *AARP BULLETIN*, July-August 1989.

Hirschfeld, R.M., *Depression, What We Know*. Rockville, Maryland: National Institute of Mental Health, n.d.

Hirschfeld, R.M. et al., "Premorbid Personality Assessments of First Onset of Major Depression," *Archives of General Psychiatry*, 46:4(April 1989).

HMSO, *On the State of the Public Health, 1987*. London: HMSO, October 1988.

Horowitz, M.J., *Introduction to Psychodynamics*. New York: Basic Books, 1988.

——, "A Model of Mourning: Change in Schemas of Self and Other," *The Journal of Psychoanalytic Association*, In press.

Horowitz, M.J., Wilner, N., Marmar, C. and Krupnick, J., "Pathological Grief and the Activation of Latent Self Images," *American Journal of Psychiatry*, 137:1157–1162.

Hughes, Donna Yount, "Alzheimer's Disease and Psychiatric Nursing: Treating the Depression," *Perspectives in Psychiatric Care*, 24:1(1987).

Hughes, Langston and Bontemps, Anna (eds.), *The Book of Negro Folklore*, New York: Dodd, Mead, 1959.

Hutton, J.T., "Alzheimer's Disease: Evolving Clinical Concepts and Management Strategies," *Comprehensive Therapy*, 13:9(September 1987).

Hutton, J.T. and Morris, J.L., "Long-Acting Levodopa Preparations," *Neurology Supplement*, October 1989.

Jackson, Edgar N., *Understanding Grief*. Nashville, Tennessee: Abington Press, 1957.

———, *You and Your Grief*. New York: Hawthorne Books, 1961.

Jackson, Stanley W., *Melcancholia and Depression—From Hippocratic Times to Modern Times*. New Haven, Connecticut: Yale University Press, 1986.

Jacobson, M.S. et al., "Marital Therapy and Spouse Involvement in the Treatment of Depression, Agoraphobia, and Alcoholism," *Journal of Consulting Cinical Psychology*. 57:1(February 1989).

James, John W. and Cherry, Frank, *The Grief Recovery Handbook*. New York: Harper & Row, 1988.

Jamison, Kay Redfield, "Mood Disorders and Patterns of Creativity in British Writers and Artists," *Psychiatry*, 52(May 1980).

Jefferson, J.W., "Lithium: A Therapeutic Magic Wand," *Journal of Clinical Psychiatry*, 50:3(March 1989).

Jefferson, J.W. and Greist, J.H., *Primer of Lithium Therapy*. Baltimore, Maryland: Williams & Wilkins, 1977.

Jefferson, J.W., Greist, J.H. et al., *Lithum Encyclopedia for Clinical Practice*, Washington, D.C.: American Psychiatric Press, 2nd ed., 1987.

Johnson, F. Neil, *The History of Lithium Therapy*. London and Basingstoke: Macmillan Press Ltd., 1984.

Johnson, F. Neil (ed.), *Handbook of Lithium Therapy*. Baltimore, Maryland: University Park Press, 1980.

Johnson, F. Neil (ed.), *Lithium Research and Therapy*. New York: Academic Press, 1975.

Jones, Billy E. et al., "Major Affective Disorders in Blacks: A Preliminary Report," *Integr. Psychiatry*, 6(1988).

Judd, L.I. et al., "The Effect of Lithium Carbonate on the Cognitive Functions of Normal Subjects," *Archives of General Psychiatry*, 34(1977), 355–57.

Kaplan, Harold J. and Sadock, Benjamin J. (eds.), *Comprehensive Textbook of Psychiatry*, 2 vols., 4th ed. Baltimore: Williams & Wilkins, 1985.

Kaslof, Leslie J., *The Bach Remedies: A Self-Help Guide*. New Canaan, Connecticut: Keats Publishing, 1988.

Katz, Lillian G., "More Than Just the Blues," *Parents Magazine*, June 1988.

Kerr, Norine J., "Signs and Symptoms of Depression and Principles of Nursing Intervention," *Perspectives in Psychiatric Care*. 24:2(1987/88).

Kiev, Ari, *Recovery from Depression*. New York: Dutton, 1982.

Kinney, J. and Leaton G., *Loosening the Grip: A Handbook of Alcohol Information*. St. Louis: C.V. Moseby, 1986.

Klein, D.F. and Wender, P.H., *Do You Have a Depressive Illness?* New York: New American Library, 1988.

Kleiner, Art, "How Not to Commit Suicide," *CoEvolution Quarterly*, 30(Summer 1981).

Kleinman, A. "Neurasthenia and Depression: A Study of Somatization and Culture in China," *Cultural and Medical Psychiatry*, 6(1982).

Klerman, Gerald, "The Age of Melancholy," *Psychology Today*, 1979.

———, "The Current Age of Youthful Melancholia," *British Journal of Psychiatry*, 152(1988), 4–14.

Klerman, G., Lavori, P., Rice, J. et al., "Birth Cohort Trends in Rates of Major Depressive Disorder Among Relatives of Patients With Affective Disorder," *Archives of General Psychiatry*, 42(1985).

Klerman G.L. and Weissman M.M., "Increasing Rates of Depression," *Journal of American Medical Association*, 261:15(April 21, 1989).

Klerman, Gerald and Weissman, Myrna, *Inte,personal Psychotherapy of Depression*. New York: Basic Books, 1984.

Kline, Nathan S., *From Sad to Glad*. New York: Putnam, 1974.

Knauth, P., *A Season in Hell*. New York: Harper and Row, 1975.

Kochakian, Mary Jo, "A Therapist's Guide to Explaining Death to Children," *The* [Hackensack, N.J.] *Record* (special from *The Hartford Courant*), July 8, 1988.

Kolata, Gina, "Experts Say Treatments Affect Recall," *The New York Times*, October 19, 1988.

———, "Manic-Depression Gene Tied to Chromosome 11," *Science*, March 6, 1987.

_____, "Researcher Gains Support for Tests of Novel Theory of Drugs and the Brain," *The New York Times*, June 21, 1988.

_____, "Researchers Find New Drug Slows Parkinson's Pace," *The New York Times*, August 4, 1989.

_____, "Study Finds 31% Rate of Miscarriage," *The New York Times*, July 27, 1988.

Kong, Dolores, "No Higher Cancer Risk for Depressed," *The* [Hackensack, N.J.] *Record* (special from *The Boston Globe*), September 1, 1989.

Krauss, D.A. and Fryrear, J.L. (eds.), *Phototherapy in Mental Health*. Springfield, Illinois: Charles C. Thomas, 1983.

Kronfol, Z., Nasrallah, H.A., Chapman, S. and House, J.D. "Depression, Cortisol Metabolism, and Lymphocytopenia," *Journal of Affective Disorders*, 9(1985), 169–173.

Kronfol, Z., Silva, J., Greden, J. et al., "Impaired Lymphocyte Function in Depressive Illness," *Life Science*, 33(1983), 241–247.

Kubler-Ross, Elisabeth, *Death: The Final Stage of Growth*. Englewood Cliffs, New Jersey: Prentice-Hall, 1975.

_____, *On Death and Dying*. New York: Macmillan, 1969.

_____, *Questions and Answers on Death and Dying*. New York: Macmillan, 1974.

_____, *To Live Until We Say Goodbye*. Englewood Cliffs, New Jersey: Prentice-Hall, 1978.

Kushner, Harold, *When All You Ever Wanted Isn't Enough*. New York: Summit Books, 1986.

Laitner, Bill, "Laugh Until It Stops Hurting," *The* [Hackensack, N.J.] *Record* (Knight-Ridder News Service), September 17, 1989.

Lang, L.H., "A New Prescription: The Family," *American Health* (World Wide Medical Press), Fall 1980.

Lee, C.M. and Gotlib, I.H., "Clinical Status and Emotional Adjustment of Children of Depressed Mothers," *American Journal of Psychiatry*, 146:4(April 1989).

Leerhsen, Charles et al., "Depression." *Newsweek*, May 4, 1987.

LeShan, Eda, *Learning to Say Goodbye: When A Parent Dies*. New York: Macmillan, 1978.

Lesse, Stanley, "The Masked Depression Syndrome—Results of a Seventeen-Year Clinical Study," *American Journal of Psychotherapy*, 37:4(October, 1983).

Levinson, Daniel J. et al., *The Seasons of a Man's Life*. New York: Alfred A. Knopf, 1978.

Lewis, C.S., *A Grief Observed*. New York: Seabury Press, 1961.

Lewis, David A. and Winokur, George, "Depression," *Medical Grand Rounds*, 3:4(1984).

Lewis, Howard and Martha E., *Psychosomatics: How Your Emotions Can Damage Your Health*. New York: Viking, 1972.

Lindemann, Eric, "Symptomology and Management of Acute Grief," *American Journal of Psychiatry*, 101(1944), 7–21.

Liston, E., Jarvik, L. and Gerson, S., "Depression in Alzheimer's Disease: An Overview of Adrenergic and Cholinergic Mechanisms," *Psychiatry*, 28:5(September-October 1987).

Lithium Information Center, *Lithium and Manic Depression: A Guide*. Madison, Wisconsin: Lithium Information Center, 1984.

Lynch, James J., *The Broken Heart*. New York: Basic Books, 1977.

Maltz, Maxwell, *Creative Living for Today*. New York: Trident Press, 1967.

Marshall, E., "Psychotherapy Works, but for Whom?" *Science*, 207(February 1, 1980).

Matarazzo, J.D. et al. (eds.), *Behavioral Health*. New York: John Wiley, 1984.

Matteson, Stefanie, "Death From a So-called Broken Heart," *The* [Hackensack, N.J.] *Record*. Hackensack, N.J. March 16, 1980.

Mayeux, Richard et al., "Altered Serotonin Metabolism in Depression Patients with Parkinson's Disease," *Neurology*, 34(1984), 642–6.

_____, "The Relationship of Serotonin to Depression in Parkinson's Disease," *Movement Disorders*, 3:3(1988).

_____, "Clinical and Biochemical Features of Depression in Parkinson's Disease." *American Journal of Psychiatry*, 143(1986), 756–9.

McCormick, W.O., "Epidemiology of Depression," *Psychiatric Journal-University of Ottawa*, 14:2(1989).

McGuffin, P. and Katz, R., "The Genetics of Depression and Manic-Depressive Disorder," *The British Journal of Psychiatry* (in press, 1989).

McHargue, Georgess, *Mummies*. (Philadelphia: J.B. Lippincott), 1972.

248 Bibliography

McKnew, Donald H., Cytryn, Leon, and Yahraes, Herbert, *Why Isn't Johnny Crying?* New York: W.W. Norton, 1983.

Medical Research Council, *MRC Handbook 1987*. London: Medical Research Council, 1987.

Medenwald, J.R., Greist, J.H., and Jefferson, J.W., *Carbamazepine and Manic Depression: A Guide*. Madison: Lithium Information Center, University of Wisconsin, 1987.

Mendara, Edward J. and Meese, Abigail (eds.), *The Self-Help Sourcebook*. Denville, New Jersey: Self-Help Clearinghouse, St. Clares-Riverside Medical Center, 1988.

Michels, Robert, Cavenar, Jesse O. et al., *Psychiatry*, 6 vols. New York: Basic Books and J.B. Lippincott, 1986.

Miller, Bruce D. and Strunk Robert C., "Circumstances Surrounding the Deaths of Children Due to Asthma," *American Journal of Diseases of Children*, November 1989.

Mitford, Jessica, *The American Way of Death*. New York: Simon and Schuster, 1963.

Morris, Sarah, *Grief and How to Live With It*. New York: Grosset and Dunlap, 1972.

Morrison, J.R., *Your Brother's Keeper*. Chicago: Nelson-Hall, 1981.

Mosko S. et al., "Self-Reported Depressive Symptomatology, Mood Ratings, and Treatment Outcome in Sleep Disorders Patients," *Journal of Clinical Psychology*, 45:1(January 1989).

Murphy, J., Sobol, A., Neff, R., Olivier, D. and Leighton, A., "Stability of Prevalence: Depression and Anxiety Disorders," *Archives of General Psychiatry*, 41(1984).

Myers, Edward, *When Parents Die*. New York: Viking, 1986.

Myers, J., Weissman, M., Tischler, G. et al., "Six-month Prevalance of Psychiatric Disorders in Three Communities," *Archives of General Psychiatry*, 41(1984).

National Depressive and Manic-Depressive Association, *Q & A: The Amish Study Findings*. Chicago: National Depressive and Manic-Depressive Association, March 1987.

National Institute of Mental Health, *Depression—What We Know*. Rockville, Maryland: DHHS, 1985.

———, *Depressive Disorders: Causes and Treatment*. Rockville, Maryland: DHHS, 1983.

Neeld, Elizabeth Harper, *Unfinished Grieving*. New York: Clarkson N. Potter, 1989.

New York Times, "Joshua Logan, Stage and Screen Director, Dies at 79," *New York Times*, July 13, 1988.

O'Brien, Robert and Cohen, Sidney, *The Encyclopedia of Drug Abuse*. New York: Facts On File, 1984.

O'Brien, Robert, Evans, Glen and Chafetz, Morris, *The Encyclopedia of Alcoholism*. New York: Facts On File, 1982, 1991.

O'Connor, A. and Walsh, D., *Activities of Irish Psychiatric Hospitals and Units 1986*. Dublin: The Health Research Board, 1989.

O'Connor, Joan, "Probing the Biology of Affective Disorder," *Psychiatric News*, November 6, 1987.

Osterweiss, M., Solomon, F. and Green, M., *Bereavement Reactions, Consequences and Care*. Washington, D.C.: National Academy of Sciences Press, 1984.

Ostrow, David G., "Models for Understanding the Psychiatric Consequences of AIDS" in T. Peter Bridge et al. (eds.), *Psychological, Neuropsychiatric, and Substance Abuse Aspects of AIDS*. New York: Raven Press, 1988.

Ostrow, David G. et al., "Assessment and Management of the AIDS Patient with Neuropsychiatric Disturbances," *The Journal of Clinical Psychiatry*, 49(May 1988).

Parkes, Colin Murray, *Bereavement: Studies of Grief in Adult Life*. New York: International Universities Press, 1972.

———, "The First Year of Bereavement: A Longitudinal Study of the Reaction of London Widows to the Death of Their Husbands," *Psychiatry*, 33(November 1970).

———, "Recent Bereavement as a Cause of Mental Illness," *British Journal of Psychiatry*, 110(1964).

Patient Care, "Insomnia," *Patient Care*, August 15, 1980.

Peterson, C. and Seligman, M.E.P., "Causal Explanations As a Risk Factor for Depression: Theory and Evidence," *Psychological Review*, 91(1984).

Peterson, C., Seligman, M.E.P. and Vaillant, G., "Pessimistic Explanatory Style As a Risk Factor for Physical Illness: A Thirty-Five Year Longitudinal Study," *Journal of Personality and Social Psychology*, 1988.

Post, Robert M. et al., "Antidepressant Effects of Carbamazepine," *American Journal of Psychiatry*, 143:1(January 1986).

———, "Correlates of Antimanic Response to Carbamazepine," *Psychiatry Research*, 21(1986), 71–83.

Pottash, A. et al., "The Use of the Clinical Laboratory," in *Inpatient Psychiatry—Diagnosis and Treatment*, Lloyd I. Sederer (ed.) Baltimore: Williams & Wilkins, n.d.

Prien, Robert A., *Information on Lithium*. Rockville, Maryland: National Institute of Mental Health, 1981: DHHS (ADM) 81–1078.

Princeton Religious Research Center, "Prayer, Bible Reading Cited Often As Ways to Beat Depression," *Emerging Trends*, 9:7(September 1987).

Rainèy, J.M., Aleem A. et al., "A Laboratory Procedure for the Induction of Flashbacks," *American Journal of Psychiatry* (in press).

Record, The, "Boomers Sing The Blues," *The* [Hackensack, N.J.] *Record*, October 9, 1988.

———, Quicker Cures for Depressed Women," *The* [Hackensack, N.J.] *Record*, (L.A. Times News Service), August 13, 1989.

———, "Young Adults Have Epidemic of 'The Blues'," *The* [Hackensack, N.J.] *Record*, October 10, 1988.

Reeves, Robert B., "The Hospital Chaplain Looks At Grief," a paper reprinted by *Horizons*, 490 Riverside Drive, New York, New York; no date is given.

Regier, D.A. et al., "The NIMH Epidemiologic Catchment Area Program," *Archives of General Psychiatry*, 41(October 1984).

Richards, R.L. et al., "Creativity in Manic-Depressives, Cyclothymes, and Their Normal First-Degree Relatives: A Preliminary Report," *Journal of Abnormal Psychology*, 97(1988).

Richardson, M.A. et al., "Tardive Dyskinesia and Depressive Symptoms in Schizophrenics," *Psychopharmacology Bulletin*, 21(1985).

Robins, L., Helzer, J., Weissman, M. et al., "Lifetime Prevalence of Specific Psychiatric Disorders in Three Sites," *Archives of General Psychiatry*, 41(1984), 949–58.

Robinson, Miranda, "Molecular Genetics of the Mind," *Nature*, February 1987.

Roesch, Roberta, "How Dreams Work For You," *The American Legion*, October 1983.

Rohter, Larry, "In Mexico, This Is Not the Day to Bury Mirth," *The New York Times*, November 2, 1988.

Romney, Elizabeth, "Breaking Through," *NARSAD Research Newsletter*, 1(Spring 1988).

Rosellini, Gayle and Worden, Mark, *Here Comes the Sun: Finding Your Way Out of Depression*. New York: Harper & Row, 1988.

Rosenthal, Norman E. and Wehr, Thomas A., "Seasonal Affective Disorders," *Psychiatric Annals*, 17:10 (October 1987).

Rovner, Sandy, "Down But Not Out," *The Washington Post* (Health: A Weekly Journal), February 12, 1986.

Rubenstein, J.L. et al., "Suicidal Behavior in 'Normal' Adolescents: Risk and Protective Factors," *American Journal of Orthopsychiatry*, 59:1(January 1989).

Rubin, E.H. et al., "Overlapping Symptoms of Geriatric Depression and Alzheimer-type Dementia," *Hospital Community Psychiatry*, 39:10(October 1988).

Sargent, Marilyn, *Depressive Disorders: Treatments Bring New Hope*. Rockville, Maryland: DHHS, 1986; (ADM) 86-1491.

Sartorius, N., "Cross-Cultural Research on Depression," *Psychopathology*, 19:Suppl. 2 (1986).

Sartorius, N. et al., *Depressive Disorders in Different Cultures*. Geneva: World Health Organization, 1983.

Schatzberg, A.F. and Cole, J.O., *Manual of Clinical Psychopharmacology*. Washington, D.C.: American Psychiatric Press, 1986.

Scheiffelin, E., "The Cultural Analysis of Depressive Affect: An Example from New Guinea," unpublished manuscript. (University of Pennsylvania).

Schiff, Harriet S., *The Bereaved Parent*. New York: Crown, 1977.

Schleifer, S.J., Keller, S.E., Meyerson, A.T. et al., "Lymphocyte Function in Major Depressive Disorder," *Archives of General Psychiatry*, 41(1984), 484–486.

Schleifer, S.J., Keller, S.E., Siris, S.G. et al., "Depression and Immunity," *Archives of General Psychiatry*, 42(1985), 129–133.

Schmeck, Harold M., Jr., "Depression and Anxiety Seen as Cause of Much Addiction," *The New York Times*, November 15, 1988.

———, "Depression Studies Bring New Drugs and Insights," *The New York Times*, February 16, 1988.

Schoenberg, Bernard, et al. (eds.), *Anticipatory Grief*. New York: Columbia University Press, 1974.
———, *Bereavement: Its Psychosocial Aspects*. New York: Columbia University Press, 1975.
———, *Loss and Grief: Psychological Movement in Medical Practice*. New York: Columbia University Press, 1970.
Seiden, Henry and Lukas, Christopher, *Silent Grief: Living in the Wake of Suicide*. New York: Scribner's, 1988.
Seligman, M.E.P., *Helplessness: On Depression, Development, and Death*. San Francisco: Freeman, 1975.
———, "Why Is There So Much Depression Today?" G. Stanley Hall Lecture Series; Washington, D.C., 1988.
Selmi, P., Klein, M., Greist, J. et al., "Computer-Administered Cognitive-Behavioral Therapy for Depression," *American Journal of Psychiatry*, January 1990.
Selye, Hans, *The Stress of Life*, 2nd ed. New York: McGraw-Hill, 1978.
Shaw, E.D. et al., "Effects of Lithium Carbonate on Association Productivity and Idiosyncrasy in Bipolar Outpatients," *American Journal of Psychiatry*, 143(1986), 1166–69.
Sheehy, Gail, *Passages: Predictable Crises of Adult Life*. New York: Bantam Books, 1976.
Shopsin, B., *Manic Illness*. New York: Raven Press, 1966.
Showater, Elaine, *The Female Malady: Women, Madness, and English Culture, 1830–1980*. New York: Pantheon Books, 1985.
Siegel, Bernie S., *Love, Medicine & Miracles*. New York: Harper & Row/Perennial Library, 1988.
Silfverskiold, P. and Risberg, J., "Regional Cerebral Blood Flow in Depression and Mania," *Archives of General Psychiatry*, 46:3(March 1989).
Silver, F.W. and Ruckle J.L., "Depression: Management Techniques in Primary Care," *Postgraduate Medicine*, 85:4(March 1989).
Spiegel, Yorick, *The Grief Process: Analysis and Counseling*. Nashville: Abingdon Press, 1973.
Squires, Sally, "How to Help Yourself," *Parade Magazine*, March 26, 1989.
Stack, Jack M., "Grief Reactions and Depression in Family Practice: Differential Diagnosis and Treatment," *The Journal Of Family Practice*, 14:2(1982).
Stamm, Karen, "Images for Research, *The Mission*, 16:3(Summer 1989). Published by the University of Texas Health Science Center at San Antonio.
Steiner, M., "The Neurochemistry of Mood," *Psychiatric Journal of the Univerity of Ottawa*, 14:2(1989).
Steinfels, Peter and Veatch, Robert M. (eds.), *Death Inside Out*. New York: Harper and Row, 1975.
Sternbach, Harvey A. et al., "Thyroid Failure and Protirelin (Thyrotropin-Releasing Hormone) Test Abnormalities in Depressed Outpatients," *Journal of American Medical Association*, 249:12(March 25, 1983).
Stewart, Walter A. and Freeman, Lucy, *The Secrets of Dreams*. New York: Macmillan, 1972.
Stoneman Z. et al., "Marital Quality, Depression, and Inconsistent Parenting: Relationship With Observed Mother-Child Conflict," *American Journal of Orthopsychiatry*, 59:1(January 1989).
Strunk, Robert C. et al., "Physiologic and Psychological Characteristics Associated With Deaths Due to Asthma in Childhood," *Journal of the American Medical Association*, September 6, 1985.
Sturgeon, Wina, *Depression: How to Recognize It, How to Treat It, and How to Grow From It*. Englewood Cliffs, New Jersey: Prentice-Hall, 1979.
Styron, William, "Why Primo Levi Need Not Have Died," *The New York Times*, December 19, 1988.
Temes, Roberta, *Living With an Empty Chair*. Amherst, Maine: Mandala Press, 1977.
Thompson, L., Gallagher, D. and Breckenridge, J.S., "Comparative Effectiveness of Psychotherapies for Depressed Elders," *Journal of Consulting and Clinical Psychology*, 55:3(1987).
Tiger, Lionel, *Optimism: The Biology of Hope*. New York: Simon & Schuster, 1979.
Travis, John and Ryan, Regina, *Wellness Workbook*. Berkeley, California: Ten Speed Press, 1981.
Tsuang, Ming T. and Vandermey, R., *Genes and the Mind, Inheritance of Mental Illness*. New York: Oxford University Press, 1980.
Toufexis, A. et al., "Why Mothers Kill Their Babies," *Time*, June 20, 1988.
Ubell, Earl, "You Can Fight Depression," *Parade*, May 6, 1988.
United Press International, "Seek Help, Victims of Depression Are Urged," *The* [Hackensack, N.J.] *Record*, November 29, 1988.
University of Texas Health Science Center at San Antonio. "Images for Research," *The Mission*, 16:3(Summer 1989).

U.S. Department of Health and Human Services, *Sixth Special Report to the U.S. Congress on Alcohol and Health*. (Washington, D.C.: Government Printing Office, 1987; DHHS No. (ADM) 87-1519.

VanValkenburg, Charles et al., "Depressed Women: With Panic Attacks," *Journal of Clinical Psychiatry*, 45:9(September 1984).

Vlamis, Gregory, *Flowers to the Rescue*. Wellingborough, New York: Thorsons Publishing Group, 1986.

Wasserman, Harry and Danforth, Holly E., *The Human Bond: Support Groups and Mutual Aid*. New York: Springer Publishing, 1988.

Weeks, Nora, *The Medical Discoveries of Edward Bach, Physician*. New Canaan, Connecticut: Keats Publishing, 1979.

Weissman, Myrna et al., "Affective Disorders in Five United States Communities," *Psychological Medicine*, 18(1988).

Wells, Kenneth B. et al., "The Functioning and Well-being of Depressed Patients," *Journal of the American Medical Association*, 262:7(August 18, 1989).

Wender, Paul H. and Klein, Donald F., *Mind, Mood and Medicine*. New York: Farrar, Straus & Giroux, 1981.

Wenzloff, Richard and Grozier, Sherilyn, "Depression and the Magnification of Failure," *Journal of Abnormal Psychology*, 9:1(1988).

Wesner, Robert B. and Winokur, George, "An Archival Study of Depression Before and After Age 55," *Journal of Geriatric Psychiatry and Neurology*, 1(October-December 1988).

Westburg, Granger E., *Good Grief*. New York: Fortress Press, 1962.

Winokur, George, *Depression: The Facts*. New York: Oxford University Press, 1981.

_____, "The Schizoaffective Continuum: Euclid's Second Axiom," *Annals of Clinical Psychiatry*, 1(1989), 19–24.

Winokur, George et al., "Depressions Secondary to Other Psychiatric Disorders and Medical Illnesses," *American Journal of Psychiatry*, 145:2(February 1988).

_____, "The Iowa 500: Affective Disorder in Relatives of Manic and Depressed Patients," *American Journal of Psychiatry*, 139:2(February 1982).

_____, "Neurotic Depression: A Diagnosis Based on Preexisting Characteristics," *European Archives of Psychiatry and Neurological Sciences*, 236(1987), 343–348.

Wolfenstein, M., "How Is Mourning Possible?" *Psychoanalytic Study of the Child*, 21(1966), 93–123.

Woods, Ralph L. and Greenhouse, Herbert B., *The New World of Dreams*. New York: Macmillan, 1974.

World Book, "Funeral Customs," *World Book Encyclopedia*. Chicago: World Book, 1988.

Wurtman, Judith, *Managing Your Mind and Mood Through Food*. New York: Harper & Row, 1989.

Wurtman, Richard J. and Judith J., "Carbohydrates and Depression," *Scientific American*, January 1989.

Yates, William R. and Sieleni, Bruce, "Anorexia and Bulimia," *Primary Care*, 14:4(December 1987).

Yglesias, Helen, *How She Died*. Boston: Houghton Mifflin, 1972.

Zimmerman, M. and Coryell, W., "The Validity of a Self-Report Questionnaire for Diagnosing Major Depressive Disorder," *Archives of General Psychiatry*, 45(August 1988).

Zimmerman, M. et al., "Diagnostic Criteria for Melancholia: The Comparative Validity of DSM-III and DSM-III-R," *Archives of General Psychiatry*, 46:4(April 1989).

Zisook, Sidney and Schuckit, Marc, "Male Primary Alcoholics With and Without Family Histories of Affective Disorder," *Journal of Studies on Alcohol*, 48:4(1987).

Zisook, Sidney et al., "The Dexamethasone Suppression Test and Unipolar/Bipolar Distinctions," *Journal of Clinical Psychiatry*, 46:11(November 1985).

_____, "Efficacy and Safety of Fezolamine in Depressed Patients," *Neuropsychobiology*, 17(1987),133–138.

Zonderman, Jon, "Schizophrenia: The Postneuroleptic Era," *NARSAD Research Newsletter*, 2(Summer 1989).

INDEX

Bold face numbers indicate main heading.